Emergency Anesthesia Procedures

T0177807

ANESTHESIA ILLUSTRATED

Keith J. Ruskin, MD, and Barbara K. Burian, PhD
Series Editors

Published and Forthcoming Titles:

Pediatric Anesthesia Procedures, edited by Anna Clebone and Barbara Burian

Ultrasound Guided Procedures and Radiologic Imaging for Pediatric Anesthesiologists, edited by Anna Clebone, Joshua Finkle, and Barbara Burian

Emergency Anesthesia Procedures, edited by Lauren C. Berkow

Cancer Pain Procedures, edited by Amit Gulati

Radiologic Imaging for the Anesthesiologist, edited by Keith Ruskin and Abraham Dachman

Emergency Anesthesia Procedures

EDITED BY

Lauren C. Berkow, MD, FASA
Professor of Neuroanesthesia
Department of Anesthesiology
University of Florida College of Medicine
Gainesville, FL, USA

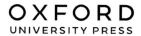

OXFORD
UNIVERSITY PRESS

Oxford University Press is a department of the University of Oxford. It furthers
the University's objective of excellence in research, scholarship, and education
by publishing worldwide. Oxford is a registered trade mark of Oxford University
Press in the UK and certain other countries.

Published in the United States of America by Oxford University Press
198 Madison Avenue, New York, NY 10016, United States of America.

Library of Congress Cataloging-in-Publication Data
Names: Berkow, Lauren C., 1968– editor.
Title: Emergency anesthesia procedures / edited by Lauren C. Berkow.
Other titles: Anesthesia illustrated.
Description: New York, NY : Oxford University Press, 2023. |
Series: Anesthesia illustrated |
Includes bibliographical references and index.
Identifiers: LCCN 2022040759 (print) | LCCN 2022040760 (ebook) |
ISBN 9780190902247 (paperback) | ISBN 9780190902261 (epub) |
ISBN 9780190902278 (online)
Subjects: MESH: Anesthesia | Emergencies
Classification: LCC RD82 (print) | LCC RD82 (ebook) |
NLM WO 200 | DDC 617.9/6042—dc23/eng/20221109
LC record available at https://lccn.loc.gov/2022040759
LC ebook record available at https://lccn.loc.gov/2022040760

DOI: 10.1093/med/9780190902247.001.0001

Printed by Integrated Books International, United States of America

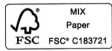

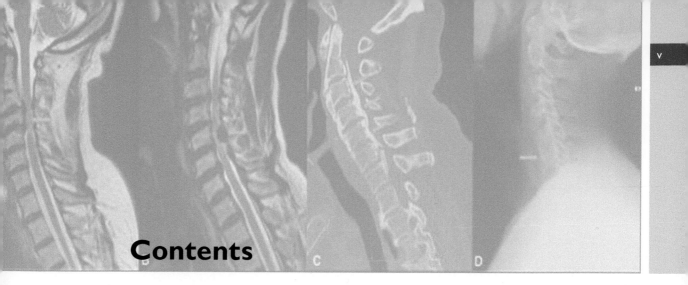

Contents

Contributors ix

PART 1   AIRWAY, BREATHING, LUNGS

1. Airway Fire 3
   Pavel Balduyeu and Robert G. Loeb

2. Bronchospasm 9
   Joseph LaGrew II, Adam Chadwick, Sandra Gonzalez, and Sonia Mehta

3. Foreign Bodies in the Airway and Esophagus 15
   Lauren Moore, Tracy Wester, and Alison Ellis

4. Laryngospasm 25
   Joseph LaGrew II, Adam Chadwick, Sandra Gonzalez, and Sonia Mehta

5. One-Lung Ventilation 33
   Patricia Nwajuaku, Dustin L. Hegland, and Joseph C. Goldstein

6. Unanticipated Difficult Airway 43
   Lauren C. Berkow

7. Tracheostomy Complications 55
   Matthew Hernandez and Arturo Torres

PART 2   CARDIAC

8. Arrhythmias 71
   Loren R. Francis and Eric W. Nelson

9. Cardiac Tamponade 85
   Matthew M. Andoniadis

10. Myocardial Ischemia 95
    Alberto Bursian and Basma Mohamed

11. Pulseless Electrical Activity (PEA) and Asystole 103
    Claudia Sotillo and Basma Mohamed

12. Management of Ventricular Tachycardia and Ventricular Fibrillation 113
    Amanda Redding, Marc Hassid, and Ryan Smith

13. Tension Pneumothorax 123
    Matthew Desmond and Yury Zasimovich

Contents

14. Vascular Access: Peripheral Venous, Central Venous, and Intraosseous Access 133
Linda Le-Wendling, Jayme N. Looper, and Lisa Gu

15. Venous Air Embolism 147
Sindhu Reddy Nimma and Christoph Nikolaus Seubert

PART 3   BLEEDING, BLOOD, TRANSFUSIONS

16. Hemorrhage and Massive Transfusion Protocols 157
Christopher Heine and Tod Brown

17. Intraoperative Management of the Bleeding Patient 167
Renuka M. George and Loren R. Francis

18. Post-Tonsillectomy Bleeding 177
Rhae Battles, Adrian Ching, Sandra Gonzalez, and Sonia Mehta

19. Transfusion Reactions 185
Geoffrey D. Panjeton, Alex Coons, Jayme N. Looper, and Jeffrey D. F. White

PART 4   NEUROLOGIC

20. Management of the Unstable Cervical Spine 195
Peggy White and Christopher W. Maxwell Jr.

21. Emergent Craniotomy 207
Nelson N. Algarra and Taylor Johnson

22. Perioperative Complications of Neuraxial Anesthesia 217
Richa Wardhan and Adejuyigbe Olusegun Adaralegbe

PART 5   ALLERGIC REACTION, TOXICITY

23. Anaphylaxis 227
Richa Sutaria and Cosmin Guta

24. Angioedema 235
Alberto Bursian and Yury Zasimovich

25. Local Anesthetic Systemic Toxicity (LAST) 243
Timothy V. Feldheim and Rene Przkora

PART 6   METABOLIC

26. Malignant Hyperthermia 253
Cameron R. Smith

PART 7   OB, NEONATAL

27. Amniotic Fluid Embolism 263
Adam Wendling and Brandon Lopez

28. Anesthetic Management of Emergency Cesarean Delivery 273
M. Anthony Cometa and Adam L. Wendling

29. Anesthetic Management of Morbidly Adherent Placenta
(Accreta/Increta/Percreta) 283
Brandon M. Lopez and M. Anthony Cometa

PART 8 EQUIPMENT, FACILITIES, CRM

30. Anesthesia Machine Failures 293
    Isaac Luria and Robert G. Loeb

31. Operating Room Fires 307
    Jennifer R. Matos and David Gutman

32. Crisis Resource Management 315
    Lauren C. Berkow and Keith Ruskin

Index 323

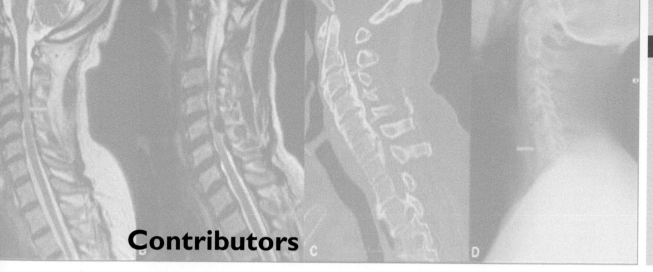

Contributors

Adejuyigbe Olusegun Adaralegbe, MD

Department of Anesthesiology, Rutgers University New Jersey Medical School, Newark, NJ, USA

Nelson N. Algarra, MS, MD

Department of Anesthesiology, University of Central Florida, Ocala, FL, USA

Matthew M. Andoniadis, MD

Department of Anesthesiology, University of Florida College of Medicine, Gainesville, FL, USA

Pavel Balduyeu, MD

Department of Anesthesiology, University of Florida College of Medicine, Gainesville, FL, USA

Rhae Battles, MD

Department of Pediatric Anesthesiology, University of Texas Southwestern, Dallas, TX, USA

Lauren C. Berkow, MD, FASA

Department of Anesthesiology, University of Florida College of Medicine, Gainesville, FL, USA

Taylor Johnson, MD

Department of Anesthesiology, Northside Anesthesiology Clinicians LLC, Northside Hospital, Atlanta, GA, USA

Tod Brown, MD

Department of Anesthesia and Perioperative Medicine, Medical University of South Carolina, Charleston, SC, USA

Alberto Bursian, MD

Department of Interventional Pain Management, Wright Patterson Air Force Base, Dayton, OH, USA

Adam Chadwick, MD

Department of Anesthesiology, Northwestern University, Chicago, IL, USA

Adrian Ching, MD

Department of Anesthesiology, University of Florida College of Medicine, Gainesville, FL, USA

M. Anthony Cometa, MD

Department of Anesthesiology, University of Florida College of Medicine, Gainesville, FL, USA

Alex Coons, MD

Department of Anesthesiology, Anesthesia Associates of Pinellas County, Clearwater, FL, USA

Matthew Desmond, MD

Department of Anesthesiology and Perioperative Medicine, University of California, Los Angeles, Los Angeles, CA, USA

Alison M Ellis, MD, MBA

Department of Anesthesiology and Perioperative Medicine, UPMC Children's Hospital of Pittsburgh, Pittsburgh, PA,USA

Timothy V. Feldheim, MD, MA

Department of Anesthesiology, Divisions of Chronic Pain, Multi-specialty Anesthesia, and Vascular Anesthesia, University of Florida College of Medicine, Gainesville, FL, USA

Loren R. Francis, MD

Department of Anesthesia and Perioperative Medicine, Medical University of South Carolina, Charleston, SC, USA

Renuka M. George, MD

Regional Anesthesia and Acute Pain Management, Department of Anesthesia and Perioperative Medicine, Medical University of South Carolina, Charleston, SC, USA

Joseph C. Goldstein, MD

Department of Anesthesiology, Malcom Randall VA Medical Center, Gainesville, FL, USA

Sandra Gonzalez, MD

Department of Anesthesiology, University of Florida College of Medicine, Gainesville, FL, USA

Lisa Gu, MD

Department of Anesthesiology, University of Texas Southwestern Dallas, TX, USA

Cosmin Guta, MD, MBA

Department of Anesthesiology, University of Miami, Miami, FL, USA

David Gutman

Department of Anesthesia and Perioperative Medicine, Medical University of South Carolina, Charleston, SC, USA

Marc Hassid, MD
Department of Anesthesia and
Perioperative Medicine, Medical
University of South Carolina,
Charleston, SC, USA

Dustin L. Hegland, MD
Department of Anesthesiology,
Malcom Randall VA Medical
Center, Gainesville, FL, USA

Christopher Heine, MD
Department of Anesthesia and
Perioperative Medicine, Medical
University of South Carolina,
Charleston, SC, USA

Matthew Hernandez, DO
Department of Anesthesia,
Division of Critical Care,
University of Kentucky
College of Medicine,
Lexington, KY, USA

Joseph LaGrew II, MD
Department of Anesthesiology,
Pediatric Anesthesiologist and
Department Chief Ft. Myers
Division US Anesthesia Partners
Ft. Myers, FL, USA

Linda Le-Wendling, MD
Department of Anesthesiology,
University of Florida College of
Medicine, Gainesville, FL, USA

Robert G. Loeb, MD
Department of Anesthesiology,
University of Florida College of
Medicine, Gainesville, FL, USA

Jayme N. Looper, MD
Department of Anesthesiology,
University of Florida College of
Medicine, Gainesville, FL, USA

Brandon M. Lopez, MD
Department of Anesthesiology,
University of Florida College of
Medicine, Gainesville, FL, USA

Isaac Luria, MD
Department of Anesthesiology,
University of Florida College of
Medicine, Gainesville, FL, USA

Jennifer R. Matos, MD
Department of Anesthesia and
Perioperative Medicine, Medical
University of South Carolina,
Charleston, SC, USA

Christopher W. Maxwell Jr.
Department of Anesthesiology
Langley AFB, United States Air
Force, Hampton, VA, USA

Sonia Mehta, MD
Department of Anesthesiology,
University of Florida College
of Medicine, Gainesville, FL, USA

Basma Mohamed, MBChB
Department of Anesthesiology,
University of Florida College
of Medicine, Gainesville, FL, USA

Lauren Moore, MD
Department of Anesthesiology,
Medical University of South
Carolina, Charleston, SC, USA

Eric W. Nelson, DO, FASA
Medical Director, Cardiothoracic
Anesthesia, Adjunct Associate
Professor Anesthesia Practice
Consultants, Michigan State
University, Grand Rapids, MI, USA

Sindhu R. Nimma, MD
Department of Anesthesiology
and Perioperative Medicine
Mayo Clinic, Jacksonville, FL, USA

Patricia Nwajuaku, MD
Department of Anesthesiology
David Geffen School of Medicine
at UCLA, Los Angeles, CA, USA

Geoffrey D. Panjeton, MD
Department of Anesthesiology
and Critical Care, Saint Louis
University, St. Louis, MO, USA

Rene Przkora, MD, PhD
Department of Anesthesiology,
University of Florida College of
Medicine, Gainesville, FL, USA

Amanda Redding, MD
Department of Anesthesia and
Perioperative Medicine, Medical
University of South Carolina,
Charleston, SC, USA

Keith Ruskin, MD
Department of Anesthesia and
Critical Care, University of
Chicago, Chicago, IL, USA

**Christoph N. Seubert, MD,
PhD, DABNM**
Department of Anesthesiology,
University of Florida College of
Medicine, Gainsville, FL, USA

Cameron R. Smith, MD, PhD
Department of Anesthesiology,
University of Florida College of
Medicine, Gainesville FL, USA

Ryan Smith, MD
Department of Anesthesia and
Perioperative Medicine, Medical
University of South Carolina,
Charleston, SC, USA

Claudia Sotillo, MD
Department of Anesthesiology,
Tufts Medical Center
Boston, MA, USA

Richa Sutaria, MD
Department of Pain Management,
Neuspine Institute, Tampa, FL, USA

Arturo Torres, MD
Department of Anesthesiology,
Division of Critical Care,
Anes & CCM Services
Atlanta, GA, USA

Richa Wardhan, MD
Department of Anesthesiology,
University of Florida College of
Medicine, Gainesville, FL, USA

Adam Wendling, MD
Department of Anesthesiology,
University of Florida College of
Medicine, Gainesville, FL, USA

Tracy Wester, MD
Department of Anesthesiology,
Medical University of South
Carolina, Charleston, SC, USA

Jeffrey D. F. White, MD
Department of Anesthesiology,
University of Florida College of
Medicine, Gainesville, FL, USA

Peggy White, MD
Department of Anesthesiology;
Director, Multidisciplinary
Adult Critical Care Medicine
Fellowship, MD-ANEST Critical
Care Med, University of Florida
College of Medicine, Gainesville,
FL, USA

Yury Zasimovich, MD
Department of Anesthesiology,
University of Florida College of
Medicine, Gainesville, FL, USA

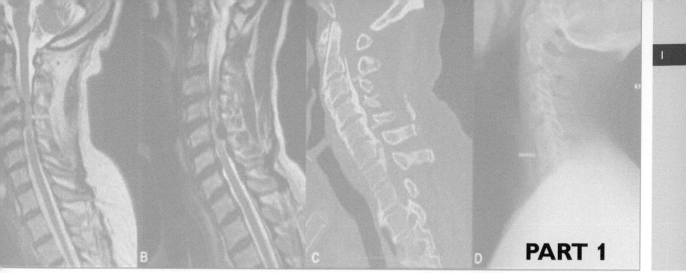

PART 1

AIRWAY, BREATHING, LUNGS

Chapter 1

Airway Fire

Pavel Balduyeu and Robert G. Loeb

Summary Page

Symptoms:

- Seeing a flash or flame
- Hearing a pop
- Smelling smoke

Differential Diagnosis:

- Nonairway patient fire
- Operating room fire

Introduction

An airway fire is a surgical fire that occurs in a patient's airway and may or may not include a fire in the attached breathing circuit.[1] According to estimates there are 217–650 operating room (OR) fires each year in the United States, with as many as 5–10% associated with serious injury or death.[2,3] Airway fires are particularly harmful to patients, constituting approximately 21% of all surgical fires and the majority of surgical fires that result in death.[4]

A fire requires three components known as the "fire triad" (Figure 1.1): an oxidizer (oxygen and/or nitrous oxide), an ignition source (electrosurgical device, laser, fiberoptic scope), and fuel (tracheotomy tube, tracheal tube, laryngeal mask, facemask, nasal cannula, sponges, gauze, drapes, alcohol-containing solutions).

Airway fires are completely preventable. Prevention should include fire safety education,[5] development and implementation of hospital protocols, and periodic OR fire drills during dedicated education time for all OR staff members.

All team members should discuss the risk of fire before the start of each surgical case (during briefing, time-out, or surgical pause). Risk factors include surgery above the xyphoid, use of laser or electrocautery, administration of open-source oxygen, and use of flammable surgical prep solutions.

Minimize high oxygen concentration near the surgical site to reduce fire risk. FiO_2 should be kept as low as clinically possible. Vacuum suctioning under the drapes or around the face prior to use of an ignition source can lower the oxygen concentration and reduce risk. See Box 1.1 for a list of procedures at higher risk of airway fire.

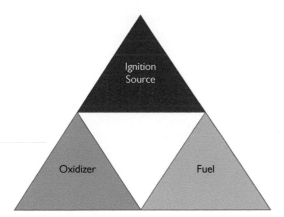

Figure 1.1 Fire triad.

BOX 1.1 PROCEDURES AT HIGHER RISK OF AIRWAY FIRE
Tracheostomy
Tonsillectomy
Laryngeal surgery, especially if laser is used
Surgeries involving the upper or lower airway
Procedures on the head or neck (increased risk with the use of an open oxygen source, i.e., nasal cannula/facemask)
Bronchoscopy
Eye surgery
Burr hole surgery for subdural hematoma
Temporal artery biopsy

Treatment

Note: The highest risk of airway fire occurs during surgery in the upper or lower airway (such as tonsillectomy, tracheotomy, and laryngeal surgeries) with a laser or electrocautery device. Airway fire can also occur during any surgery above the patient's xyphoid, including upper gastrointestinal endoscopy or bronchoscopy, especially when open oxygen administration is used.

Step by Step

1. **Verify diagnosis of airway fire (Figure 1.2).**
    Most common symptoms:
    *   Seeing a flash
    *   Hearing a pop
    *   Smelling smoke

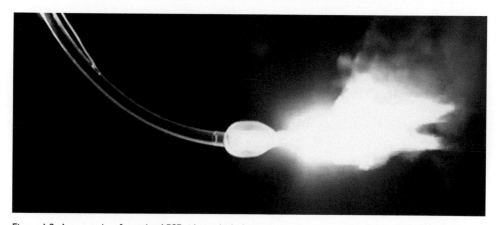

Figure 1.2 A screenshot from the APSF video, which demonstrates how a burning airway device produces heat, smoke, chemicals, and solid ash, which can cause damage to the distal airways. https://www.apsf.org/videos/or-fire-safety-video/

Source: Reprinted with permission, Copyright 2009, ECRI Institute. www.ecri.org. 5200 Butler Pike, Plymouth Meeting, PA 19462. 610-825-6000

2. **Notify surgeon and entire operating room team of suspected or confirmed fire.**
    In the event of a large fire, send for help and for a fire extinguisher, and call 911. Call for additional help.

3. **Immediately remove any airway device and simultaneously stop all flow of airway gases.**
    Remove any airway device present:
    *   Endotracheal tube (ETT)
    *   Supraglottic airway (SGA)
    *   Tracheotomy tube
    *   Nasal or oral airway
    *   Nasal cannula or facemask

Simultaneously stop the flow of airway gases: turn off the ventilator, fresh gas flow, and auxiliary oxygen. The fastest way is to disconnect the airway device from the breathing circuit or flowmeter and remove it.

>>**Tip on Technique:** Make sure not to place the burning material in the trash, where it can start a bigger fire. Place it on the open floor where others can extinguish it with water, an extinguisher, or smothering.

Caution!   The burning material can ignite a larger fire. The burning material could also injure other areas of the patient or OR personnel. Keep the burning material away from other highly flammable materials, such as alcohol prep solution.

Caution!   The patient will not be ventilated during this time and may begin to desaturate.

Save all involved materials and devices for further investigation.

4. **Pour water or saline into the patient's airway to extinguish any residual burning materials.**

Use direct vision when possible. Use enough fluid to extinguish the burning material, but not an excessive amount that could cause aspiration. For instance, use a laryngoscope to open the mouth, pour liquid into the airway, and then suction it out. Consider using a syringe or laryngeal spray device to irrigate the trachea, and then suction it out.

Caution!   The patient will not be ventilated during this time and may continue to desaturate.

Caution!   Pulmonary aspiration of burned material can occur.

---

5. **Reestablish ventilation and place a large-size endotracheal tube.**

Initially ventilate with air, avoiding supplemental oxygen and nitrous oxide. When replacing the ETT, a size 7.5 mm outer diameter (OD) or larger in an adult is recommended.

>>**Tip on Technique:** The breathing circuit may have been damaged and could still contain supplemental oxygen or nitrous oxide. Consider ventilating with a self-inflating rescue breathing device that is not connected to an oxygen tank while replacing the breathing circuit.

Caution!   Intubation may be difficult if the airway is swollen or bleeding—call for a difficult airway cart and additional assistance as needed (step 6).

---

6. **Call for help and additional equipment.**

At this point, assistance from outside the OR may be needed. Equipment may be needed for further management, such as a difficult airway cart. Consultants may be helpful, such as additional airway providers, otolaryngologists, and pulmonologists.

7. **Assess the upper and lower airways as soon as possible.**

The anesthesia provider, an otolaryngologist, or a pulmonologist should visualize the upper airway using direct or indirect laryngoscopy, looking for burned plastic fragments and soft tissue swelling. Bronchoscopy should be performed to assess the lower conducting airways for soot, smoke residue, redness, and edema. The patient should be ventilated with 100% oxygen to prevent desaturation during this time, and to displace carbon monoxide.

8. **Decide whether to cancel or proceed with the original surgical procedure.**

Weigh the emergent versus elective indication for the surgical procedure and severity of the airway burn. Once the airway is secured, emergent procedures may be completed with careful monitoring of respiratory mechanics and gas exchange, carbon monoxide levels, and hemodynamics. Elective surgery should be canceled.

9. **Postoperative care of the patient.**

Anticipate further swelling over the next 4–24 hours and the need to maintain an airway with an ETT or tracheostomy, and ventilatory support. Prolonged intubation and monitoring in an intensive care unit or burn unit may be required. A conservative approach (keeping the patient intubated in an intensive care unit) is safest for the patient and caregivers. Prophylactic antibiotics and steroids are not recommended for initial management of inhalation injury from heat and smoke, even though pneumonia and airway swelling may follow.

Consider consulting a burn specialist. Subsequent fluid shifts and organ damage may require specialized burn care. This may require transfer to a specialized center. If the airway fire happens in an outpatient facility, the patient should be transferred to a tertiary care hospital once stabilized.

Note: Swelling and edema of the airway are common after any degree of burn in the airway and can lead to life-threatening airway obstruction. Toxins released from burning plastics can also cause inhalation injuries and/or asphyxiation.

> **Caution!** Airway swelling/edema and lower airway injury may not be present immediately after a burn injury but can develop minutes to hours after the initial injury and extend beyond the site of the fire.

10. **Report the event to your risk management office and/or liability insurance carrier(s).**

Airway fires are reportable adverse events and considered totally preventable. The surgeon and anesthesiologist should disclose the event to the patient's family—risk management can be a resource in this process. Subsequent legal repercussions are likely.

Other Management Considerations

If the patient requires inspired oxygen concentration above 30% (due to certain comorbidities such as chronic obstructive pulmonary disease), use a sealed gas delivery device (ETT, SGA) instead of an open gas delivery device (nasal cannula, simple facemask) to reduce risk. Procedure drapes should be configured to minimize the accumulation of oxidizers (oxygen and nitrous oxide) under the drapes.

Control possible fuels:

- Flammable skin-prepping solutions should be given enough time to completely dry before draping.
- Gauzes/sponges should be moistened if located close to ignition source.

Consider the use of laser-resistant ETTs during laser airway surgery (appropriate for the surgery and for the type of laser) and inflate the tracheal tube cuff with saline tinted with methylene blue.[6] Consider apneic or jet ventilation techniques instead of an ETT during airway surgery.

Judicially manage possible ignition sources:

- Ignition devices should be activated only by the person using it and when the tips are in direct view.
- Sources should be turned off before leaving the surgical/procedure site and securely holstered each time when not in use.
- Proceduralist should notify anesthesiologist sufficiently in advance each time ignition source activation is anticipated in high-risk cases.
- Consider avoiding use of an ignition device in high-risk cases.

References

1. Apfelbaum JL, Caplan RA, Barker SJ, et al. Practice advisory for the prevention and management of operating room fires: an updated report by the American Society of Anesthesiologists Task Force on Operating Room Fires. *Anesthesiology*. 2013;118(2):271–290.
2. ECRI Institute. New clinical guide to surgical fire prevention. Patients can catch fire—here's how to keep them safer. *Health Devices*. 2009;38:314–332.
3. ECRI Institute. Preventing and fighting airway fires. Health System Risk Management 2016. https://www.ecri.org/search-results/member-preview/hrc/pages/surgan10
4. Clarke JR, Bruley ME. Surgical fires: trends associated with prevention efforts. *Pa Patient Saf Advis*. 2012;9:130.
5. Prevention and Management of Operating Room Fires Video. https://www.apsf.org/videos/or-fire-safety-video, APSF 2000
6. Sheinbein D, Loeb R. Laser surgery and fire hazards in ear, nose, and throat surgeries. *Anesthesiol Clin*. 2010;28(3):485–496.

Chapter 2

Bronchospasm

Joseph LaGrew II, Adam Chadwick, Sandra Gonzalez, and Sonia Mehta

Summary Page

Symptoms:

- Increasing peak airway pressures/ decreasing or absent tidal volumes
- Altered capnography
  - Upslope during plateau phase
  - Increasing or absent $EtCO_2$
- Signs of obstructed airway
  - Wheezing
  - Decreased compliance or inability to provide positive pressure ventilation
- Increased respiratory effort
  - Intercostal retractions
  - Paradoxical chest/abdominal movement
- Desaturation (decreasing SpO_2)
- Cyanosis
- Bradycardia or tachycardia
- Hypoxia
- Arrhythmia
- Hypotension
- Cardiac arrest

Differential Diagnosis:

- Endotracheal tube dysfunction
  - Kink
  - Mucus plug
  - Mainstem intubation
- Foreign body
- Aspiration
- Anaphylaxis
- Laryngospasm
- Supraglottic obstruction
- Tension pneumothorax

Introduction

Bronchospasm is a relatively common occurrence in the perioperative period with estimates as high as 20% in high-risk patients. Consideration of relative risk, disease severity and control, and examination and presentation on the day of surgery must be balanced with the response to short-acting beta agonists immediately before surgery and the need for surgery. Risk factors for bronchospasm are primarily modifiable and include poorly controlled or undiagnosed asthma, poorly controlled chronic bronchitis, smoking, current or recent upper respiratory tract infection, gastroesophageal reflux disease, insufficient anesthesia, and with endotracheal intubation, thoracic or abdominal surgeries. As inflammation and bronchoconstriction worsen, air trapping occurs, leading to rising airway pressures. Hypoxic pulmonary vasoconstriction can help to compensate initially, but increasing inflammation may obliterate this response. IV epinephrine in low doses helps to stabilize mast cells, preventing further inflammation, and acts as a bronchodilator. Epinephrine is the treatment of choice in bronchospasm with inadequate ventilation in addition to positive pressure ventilation with appropriate expiratory time. After successful treatment, identifying the underlying etiology of bronchospasm is helpful in preventing future episodes.

Treatment

Note: Treatment will vary depending on the timing at which bronchospasm occurs and the stability of the patient (Figure 2.1). If the patient is stable and already intubated, treatment will focus on pharmacological treatments (steps 10–12) to relieve bronchospasm. If the patient does not have a secure airway or is unstable, treatment begins with ensuring adequate ventilation, followed by intubation, while giving medications to reduce and treat the bronchospasm.

Step by Step

1. **Assess the patient's respiratory and hemodynamic status.**

    Assess the patient's blood pressure and heart rate. Auscultate the lungs and assess for lung compliance and adequate tidal volumes.

2. **Call for help and request to pause procedure, if applicable.**

    Alert the surgical team and operating room staff and call for additional help. Request to pause the procedure if the patient is unstable.

    In cases of bronchospasm refractory to treatment, consideration should be given to cancellation of elective cases. Once the patient is stabilized, length and type of surgery as well as patient comorbidities should be considered in discussions with the surgical team on the risk versus benefit of continuing with the case.

3. **Increase inhaled O_2 to 100%.**

4. **If patient is (pick one):**
    - Hemodynamically unstable: go to step 5.
    - Hemodynamically stable but ventilation is inadequate (<3 ml/kg tidal volume): go to step 7.
    - Hemodynamically stable with adequate ventilation: go to step 10.

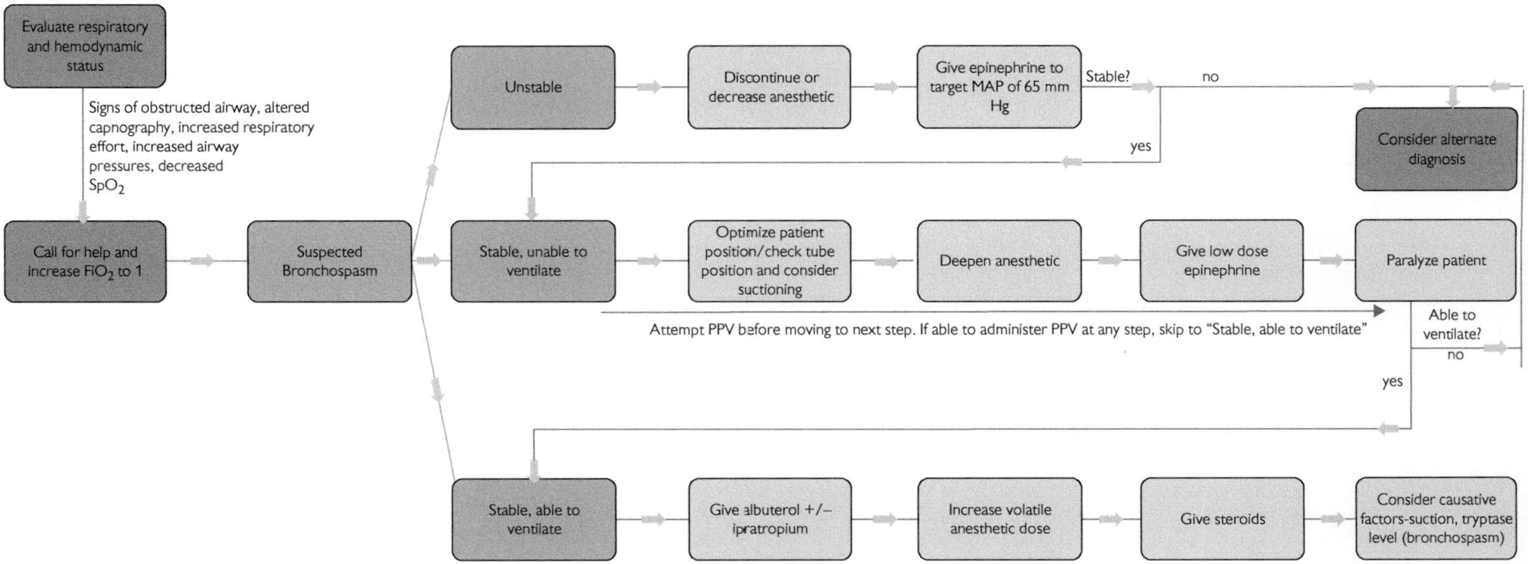
Evaluate respiratory and hemodynamic status
Signs of obstructed airway, altered capnography, increased respiratory effort, increased airway pressures, decreased SpO_2
Call for help and increase FiO_2 to 1
Suspected Bronchospasm
Unstable
Discontinue or decrease anesthetic
Give epinephrine to target MAP of 65 mm Hg
Stable?
no
yes
Consider alternate diagnosis
Stable, unable to ventilate
Optimize patient position/check tube position and consider suctioning
Deepen anesthetic
Give low dose epinephrine
Paralyze patient
Attempt PPV before moving to next step. If able to administer PPV at any step, skip to "Stable, able to ventilate"
Able to ventilate?
no
yes
Stable, able to ventilate
Give albuterol +/− ipratropium
Increase volatile anesthetic dose
Give steroids
Consider causative factors-suction, tryptase level (bronchospasm)

Figure 2.1 Algorithm for response to bronchospasm. PPV = positive pressure ventilation. MAP = mean arterial pressure.

5. **If the patient is hemodynamically unstable, discontinue or decrease anesthetic if possible and administer epinephrine IV.**

    Give epinephrine IV (pediatric: 1–4 mcg boluses; adult: 10–100 mcg boluses) with the goal to achieve a mean arterial pressure greater than 65 mmHg. IV epinephrine in low doses helps to stabilize mast cells, preventing further inflammation, and acts as a bronchodilator. Epinephrine is the treatment of choice in bronchospasm with inadequate ventilation in addition to positive pressure ventilation with appropriate expiratory time.

    If bradycardia or other arrhythmias occur, follow published advanced cardiac life support (ACLS) protocols.

6. **Attempt manual ventilation via mask or endotracheal tube.**

    If the patient is hemodynamically unstable and ventilation is unsuccessful, stop the procedure and consider differential diagnosis, such as aspiration, anaphylaxis, or tension pneumothorax.

    If the patient is hemodynamically stable but ventilation is unsuccessful, go to step 7.

    If the patient is hemodynamically stable and ventilation is successful, go to step 10.

7. **If patient is already intubated, go to step 10. If patient is hemodynamically stable but ventilation is inadequate and patient is not yet intubated, optimize patient positioning.**

    Optimize positioning (Figure 2.2) and attempt ventilation if the patient is not yet intubated. Proper patient positioning is key to the successful treatment of bronchospasm. The optimal head and neck position for patients is the "sniffing" position. This position optimizes the alignment of the oral, laryngeal, and pharyngeal axes to facilitate free movement of air in and out of the lungs as well as the most direct line of sight for endotracheal intubation.

    Supine positioning with the provider at the head of the bed is preferable. In infants and young children, ensure the head is in a neutral position (consider a towel or gel roll under the patient's shoulders) as the large occiput will lead to passive flexion of the neck, resulting in potential increased difficulty with mask ventilation. Adult patients are ideally placed in the sniffing position. For obese patients, placing them in reverse Trendelenburg position or raising the head of the bed to decrease abdominal pressure on the diaphragm will prevent further reduction in compliance.

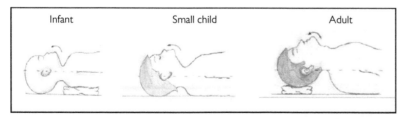

Figure 2.2 The optimal head and neck position for patients undergoing anesthesia with mask ventilation or oral intubation. In all cases the patient lies supine with the head oriented to the midline with the cervical spine extending (chin lifted cephalad). Patient positioning requires that padding be placed in different areas depending on age. Infants have a more pronounced occiput requiring padding behind the shoulders (A). Small children have a less pronounced occiput and require little to no padding (B). Adults require padding behind the occiput to achieve an optimal head and neck position (C).

8. **If unable to ventilate the patient, intubate the patient.**

    If intubation is difficult or impossible, follow published difficult airway algorithms such as the American Society of Anesthesiologists (ASA) Difficult Airway Algorithm. Also refer to Chapter 6 on management of the difficult airway. If the patient becomes hemodynamically unstable due to inability to intubate or ventilate, return to step 5.

9. **Confirm correct placement and position of the endotracheal tube in the trachea and consider suctioning the tube.**

> **Caution!** Suctioning should be considered only in patients with suspicion of mucus plugging of the endotracheal tube as suctioning can exacerbate bronchospasm.

10. **Give albuterol.**

    Give albuterol 8–10 puffs via metered dose inhaler (MDI) (80 mcg/actuation) or nebulizer (0.5%) through the inspiratory limb of the anesthesia circuit titrating to tachycardia. Consider combination treatment with ipratropium (Atrovent MDI 100 mcg albuterol/20 mcg ipratropium or 2.5 mg albuterol/0.5 mg ipratropium/3 ml nebulizer solution).

11. **Change/increase volatile anesthetic dose.**

    If using desflurane, switch to an alternate volatile agent, as desflurane can worsen bronchospasm. If using isoflurane or sevoflurane, consider increasing inspired partial pressure. Severe disease with minimal airflow will attenuate the efficacy of inhaled bronchodilators and volatile agents. Allowing sufficient expiratory time and manually ventilating through a definitive airway to assess compliance helps direct treatment.

12. **Give steroids.**

    Give dexamethasone 4–8 mg IV to reduce inflammation in the airway.

13. **Consider drawing tryptase levels to help discern mechanism/cause of bronchospasm within 6 hours of reaction if allergic reaction is suspected (preferably within 3 hours).**

    A broad differential must be considered both on presentation and when considering follow-up testing. Initially, intraoperative bronchospasm may be the presenting symptom of anaphylaxis, signaling impending hemodynamic collapse. See Chapter 23 on anaphylaxis for further details. Tryptase levels should be drawn and sent, preferably within 3 hours, though levels typically remain elevated for 3–6 hours. Referral for allergy testing may be a consideration depending on the likely cause of the episode.

Other Management Considerations

Management of bronchospasm starts preoperatively with optimizing risk factors. For patients with poorly controlled asthma (known recent hospitalizations, recent requirement for oral steroids, or increasing need of rescue inhaler) or chronic bronchitis with recent exacerbations, referral to the managing provider is warranted prior to surgery to optimize medical management when possible. Discontinuation of smoking for at least 2 months prior to surgery will reduce risk of perioperative bronchospasm. In patients with recent upper respiratory infection, surgery should be delayed when possible for 6 weeks following resolution of symptoms to decrease risk of bronchospasm.

After an event that is suspected to be IgE mediated, consideration should be given to referral for further evaluation in the case of suspected allergy (positive tryptase with suspected agent) or asthma (positive tryptase in patient with no previous diagnosis of asthma and no likely inciting medication).

Effective communication with available team members is critical in providing the most timely response to bronchospasm with inadequate ventilation. The ability of an individual to attempt continuous positive pressure ventilation or proceed to the next step in the response outlined above may be dependent upon the treating provider's ability to communicate with team members arriving on the scene to help. Specific delegation of actions and closed-loop communication from the treating provider will facilitate such a response.

References

1. Woods BD, Sladen RN. Perioperative considerations for the patient with asthma and bronchospasm. Br J Anaesth 2009; 103 (Suppl 1):i57–i65.
2. Kumeta Y, Hattori A, Mimura M, Kishikawa K, Namiki A. A survey of perioperative bronchospasm in 105 patients with reactive airway disease. Masui 1995; 44:396–401.
3. Schwilk B, Bothner U, Schraag S, Georgieff M. Perioperative respiratory events in smokers and nonsmokers undergoing general anaesthesia. Acta Anaesthesiol Scand 1997; 41:348–355.

Chapter 3

Foreign Bodies in the Airway and Esophagus

Lauren Moore, Tracy Wester, and Alison Ellis

Summary Page

Symptoms:

- Wheezing (especially unilateral)
- Diminished breath sounds on one side
- Cough
- Cyanosis
- Drooling
- Stridor
- Voice change, aphonia
- Decreased oral intake
- Dysphagia, emesis, vomiting

Differential Diagnosis:

- Airway foreign body
- Upper respiratory tract infection
- Lower respiratory tract infection/ pneumonia
- Esophageal foreign body
- Tracheomalacia
- Asthma
- Croup
- Acid reflux, esophagitis
- Epiglottitis

Introduction

Foreign body removal is a common emergency managed by the anesthesiologist, especially in pediatrics. Foreign bodies of the airway or esophagus occur purposefully or accidentally. Foreign bodies in the airway are risk factors for obstruction given the smaller size of pediatric airways and can cause a localized inflammatory reaction, making them harder to remove with the passage of time.[1] Large foreign bodies in the esophagus can impinge upon the trachea and cause stridor, retching, or anorexia. While foreign body aspiration is less common in adults, it remains an urgent concern because of airway reactions to the foreign body and concern for postobstructive pneumonia.

Aspirated foreign bodies are the leading cause of death in infants. They are usually seen in ages 6 months to 6 years. In adults the foreign bodies are usually related to food (i.e., fish or chicken bones). They often lodge in the right mainstem bronchus. The anatomy of the left main bronchus is such that there is a sharp left turn, making this less likely. In small pediatric airways, there is high risk for complete obstruction of a bronchus as well as potential for total obstruction of the trachea should the foreign body lodge at the cricoid cartilage.[2,3]

Regardless of age, local inflammatory reactions in the airway can cause granuloma formation, decreasing the airway diameter, increasing turbulent airflow, and increasing the chances of developing a postobstructive pneumonia (Figure 3.1). This is why foreign bodies in the airway must be removed in an urgent fashion. Most cases of foreign body aspiration have a convincing story for aspiration—the patient (or parent) can identify an episode of coughing and choking, possibly cyanosis, or wheezing, preceded by something having been in the mouth. Many airway foreign bodies are not seen on chest x-ray. However, hyperinflation of the affected lung on a lateral decubitus radiograph is very suspicious for a foreign body in the ipsilateral mainstem bronchus (see Figure 3.1). In adults and elderly patients with diseases leading to decreased gag reflexes (stroke, other neurologic disorders), aspiration can be much more likely, especially in patients who have indwelling objects in their mouth like dentures.

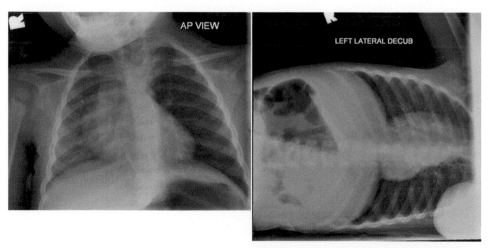

Figure 3.1 Anteroposterior (AP) and left lateral decubitus chest x-rays in an 8-year-old with peanut in the left main bronchus. Hyperinflation of the left lung is seen on AP chest x-ray and left-sided air trapping on subsequent lateral film. Image courtesy of the author with patient permission.

Treatment

Airway management should be planned in close collaboration with the proceduralist.[2] Be prepared for sudden desaturation or airway obstruction during the procedure, especially during manipulation of the foreign body.

Step by Step

1. **Assess the patient for airway, breathing, and circulation (ABCs).**

    Assess for airway patency, work of breathing, and adequate perfusion. Symptoms that indicate instability include cyanosis, severe retractions, or decreased consciousness. **If the patient is UNSTABLE, proceed directly to step 2.**

WARNING!! Respiratory failure causing hypoxia is the most common cause of cardiac arrest in infants and children. If there is doubt about adequate ventilation or oxygenation, it is important to call for help and be prepared to initiate advanced cardiac life support/pediatric advanced life support (ACLS/PALS) protocols.

If the patient is STABLE, provide supplemental oxygen if needed. Identify signs of dehydration (such as dry mucous membranes, sunken fontanelles in infants, decreased skin turgor, decreased urine output or wet diapers) and proceed to step 3.

Patients presenting with stridor may be sitting up to maintain airway patency, so be cautious when laying these patients supine.

2. **If the patient is UNSTABLE, treat per ACLS/PALS guidelines.**

    If the patient is **unconscious**:

    Check for pulse and breathing and call for help. Initiate chest compressions, rescue breaths, and ACLS/PALS algorithm as indicated, including preparation for ECMO if institutionally available. If the patient has required intubation or circulatory support (chest compressions, epinephrine), foreign body removal should be delayed until the patient has been stabilized. If they remain inadequately oxygenated or ventilated after intubation, consider ECMO as this will provide oxygenation and ventilation until the obstructive airway foreign body can be retrieved.

    If the patient is conscious but not breathing:

    For ADULTS and CHILDREN >1 YEAR, perform Heimlich maneuver.

    For INFANTS 1 YEAR and YOUNGER, provide alternating back slaps and chest presses on firm surface such as your forearm or lap until the object is dislodged or the infant loses consciousness (then treat as "Unconscious patient" above).

    If the patient is conscious and breathing but displays signs of respiratory distress (chest wall or suprasternal retractions), encourage cough if possible (this is more effective than the Heimlich maneuver). If minimal air movement is present, treat the patient as "conscious but not breathing."

    If the measures listed above result in foreign body removal, airway evaluation may still be necessary but should be delayed until the patient is sufficiently stable to tolerate an anesthetic. If the foreign body is still in place but the patient has been stabilized (conscious, oxygenating and ventilating well, appropriately resuscitated and requiring no support aside from supplemental oxygen), consider proceeding to step 3.

> **Caution!** While an advanced airway can help provide a secure airway for ventilatory support, attempting to place one in a child with a trachea-sized foreign body may result in the object becoming irrevocably lodged at the cricoid cartilage and complete airway obstruction.
>
> **Caution!** Blind finger sweep is not recommended due to the possibility of further advancing an unseen object.

>> **Tip on Technique:** After a round of back slaps and chest presses, you may open an infant's mouth to look for an object causing choking, but do not attempt to pull an object out unless you see it clearly.

3. **Obtain patient history/physical and review imaging.**

Note any patient comorbidities, allergies, or recent oral intake. Review chest x-ray with anteroposterior (AP) and lateral views if available and identify the type and location of the foreign body, if possible (see Figures 3.1 and 3.2).

>> **Tip on Technique:** Hyperinflation of the lower lung on a lateral decubitus x-ray is very suspicious for airway foreign body (see Figure 3.1).

> **Caution!** It is difficult to differentiate a foreign body in the esophagus versus the trachea with only a frontal view (AP or posteroanterior [PA]). Exam and history may be telling, but if this is the only available imaging it may be necessary to investigate both the trachea and esophagus in the operating room (OR). Chest x-ray can also give information about perforation (mediastinal free air) or postobstructive pneumonia from an airway foreign body.

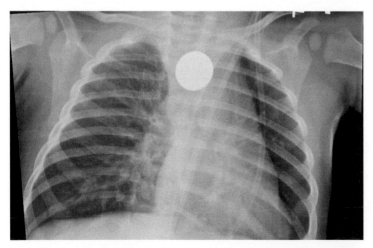

Figure 3.2 Chest x-ray of a coin in the esophagus of an 8-month-old (later found to be a penny), lodged at the thoracic inlet. Image courtesy of the author with patient permission.

4. **Obtain/confirm IV access.**

Obtain IV access, or if an IV is already present, confirm IV access is functioning properly (i.e., not infiltrated). While the expectation for large-volume blood loss is low, it is important to have reliable IV access in the event of an emergency (pneumothorax, esophageal perforation, cardiac arrest due to hypoxia or patient comorbidity).

> **Caution!** While obtaining IV access is important, it must be done with caution in small children with airway foreign bodies. Ideally, this is done in a controlled setting so as not to cause hysteria in the child, as this may lead to coughing and movement of the foreign body to potentially obstruct the entire trachea. Use of topical anesthetic creams can be helpful.

5. **Create a plan for removal with the proceduralist.**

Determine the urgency of the procedure and decide the best location for the procedure (OR, bronchoscopy suite, endoscopy suite). Make a plan for foreign body retrieval and, if in the airway, the need for spontaneous ventilation or endotracheal tube (ETT) placement (detailed airway plans are discussed in the following steps).

Options for removal of a foreign body in the airway include rigid bronchoscopy (cannot be performed with an ETT in place) or flexible fiberoptic bronchoscopy. Esophagoscopy would be performed for removal of an esophageal foreign body.

>> **Tip on Technique:** Airway and esophageal foreign body retrieval can be accomplished in non-OR settings such as bronchoscopy or endoscopy suites. The OR is frequently the preferred location given the proximity to the equipment and availability of help should it be needed. Rigid bronchoscopy is generally performed in the supine position, with or without a shoulder roll. It is important to maintain adequate depth of anesthesia during rigid bronchoscopy, especially if the patient is in suspension, as coughing in this position can cause cervical spine fractures.

6. **Create a plan for airway management.**

IV induction is strongly recommended. The location of foreign body (supraglottic, tracheal, mainstem, or distal airway) will guide airway management:

Spontaneous ventilation is preferred for supraglottic foreign bodies to reduce risk of advancement into the glottis with positive pressure ventilation and is also preferred if the location of the foreign body is unknown. The ETT can be placed after foreign body removal if indicated for ventilatory support.

Rapid sequence intubation is recommended for esophageal or distal airway foreign bodies as it allows for controlled ventilation and the use of a flexible bronchoscope via the ETT to retrieve it.

>> **Tip on Technique:** Foreign bodies at the glottic opening in children may completely obstruct the airway at the cricoid cartilage and necessitate an emergent surgical airway since pediatric airways are smaller. Air movement that may have been possible with spontaneous breathing might be lost with positive pressure. Foreign bodies located beyond the mainstem bronchi may be beyond the reach of rigid bronchoscopes but tend to have less effect on oxygenation and ventilation.

> **Caution!** Inhaled induction is reserved as a last resort, as children will frequently fight a mask placed on their face and potentially dislodge or move the foreign body and cause airway obstruction. Also, high-dose sevoflurane used in inhaled inductions may still cause apnea, necessitating positive pressure ventilation.
>
> **Caution!** Syndromes with difficult airways or altered cognition may make airway management and retrieval more challenging. Obtaining IV access and positioning may also be difficult in these patients. It is important to have a clear plan with contingencies and communicate constantly with the proceduralist.

7. **Obtain and set up necessary equipment.**

    Have multiple airway devices readily accessible and difficult airway equipment available if needed: age-appropriate laryngoscopes and tubes of various sizes, video laryngoscope, flexible fiberoptic bronchoscope, supraglottic airways, and surgical airway equipment.

    Note: Airway equipment should always be available even if intubation is not planned!

    The proceduralist should have their equipment immediately available and ready to use.

8. **Induce general anesthesia and secure the airway if planned.**

    Induce as planned with the proceduralist **present in the room** in case an emergent airway procedure is needed (surgical airway).

    If spontaneous ventilation is planned, consider:

    *   Midazolam 0.1–0.2 mg/kg IV (pediatric) or 2–5 mg IV (adult)
    *   Ketamine 0.25–1 mg/kg IV (pediatric) or 20–30 mg increments IV (adult)
    *   Dexmedetomidine 0.25–1 mcg/kg IV (pediatric) or 4–12 mcg IV (adult) bolus
    *   Propofol 0.25–1 mg/kg IV boluses titrated to effect

    >> **Tip on Technique:** A balanced anesthetic with sedatives that minimize respiratory depression (midazolam, ketamine, dexmedetomidine) in combination with inhaled sevoflurane and/or propofol can achieve general anesthesia while maintaining spontaneous ventilation.

    For rapid sequence intubation consider:

    *   Propofol 1–2 mg/kg IV (pediatric patients may require 2–4 mg/kg IV for adequate hypnosis) OR etomidate 0.2–0.6 mg/kg IV PLUS
    *   Succinylcholine 0.5–1 mg/kg IV (adult) or 1–2 mg/kg IV (pediatric) OR rocuronium 1.2 mg/kg IV

> **Caution!** IN INFANTS it is important to precede succinylcholine dose with a vagolytic medication because of bradycardia associated with this drug:
>
> *   Atropine 10–20 mcg/kg IV with minimum dose of 0.1 mg OR
> *   Glycopyrrolate 4–10 mcg/kg up to 0.1 mg/dose

>> **Tip on Technique:** If attempting airway foreign body removal with spontaneous ventilation, it is often useful to topicalize the vocal cords with local anesthetic (usually 2% lidocaine) to prevent laryngospasm:

- For infants and children: 2 mg/kg sprayed onto vocal cords
- For adults: 60–100 mg sprayed onto vocal cords (3–5 mL)

> **Caution!** Airway swelling may occur with foreign bodies in the airway or esophagus for prolonged periods of time. It may be necessary to use a smaller endotracheal tube to secure the airway, and multiple sizes should be available.

9. **Maintain adequate depth of anesthesia.**
   Consider the use of any of the following (or some in combination):
   - Propofol 100–300 mcg/kg/min IV infusion
   - Dexmedetomidine 0.25–1 mcg/kg IV (pediatric) or 4–12 mcg IV (adult) bolus; 0.2–1 mcg/kg/hr IV infusion
   - Ketamine 0.25–1 mg/kg IV (pediatric) or 20–30 mg increments IV (adult)
   - Midazolam 0.1–0.2 mg/kg IV (pediatric) or 2–5 mg IV (adult)
   - Remifentanil 0.02–0.2 mcg/kg/min IV infusion
   - Inhalational anesthesia (sevoflurane, isoflurane)

   >> **Tip on Technique**: Intravenous medications are often preferred after induction to maintain anesthesia with airway foreign bodies to allow adequate depth of anesthesia if an ETT is not used or must be removed during the procedure. If an airway is in place or a ventilating bronchoscope is being used, it is still possible to deliver inhaled anesthetic.

   If choosing muscle relaxation with controlled ventilation, an intermediate-acting relaxant is usually preferred given the brevity of the procedure.

   >> **Tip on Technique:** Consider glycopyrrolate 4 mcg/kg IV, max 0.1 mg (pediatric) or 0.1–0.2 mg IV (adult), as an antisialagogue to reduce secretions.

> **Caution!** If using ketamine, it is advisable to precede it with midazolam to prevent delirium, and with glycopyrrolate to reduce secretions. Remifentanil can blunt airway reflexes but can also lead to chest wall rigidity or apnea.

   >> **Tip on Technique:** It is possible to provide positive pressure ventilation through a rigid ventilating bronchoscope if needed. The anesthesia circuit can be connected directly to this piece of equipment. Tidal volumes and pressures should be watched closely to prevent barotrauma.

10. **Remove the foreign body.**
    Remain vigilant! Foreign body retrieval can be a constantly changing process, and airway foreign bodies may become esophageal because of dropping or manipulation.

Sudden airway obstruction or oxygen desaturation may occur, so communication between the anesthesiologist and proceduralist is imperative.

Extubation may be necessary if attempting airway foreign body removal via the ETT to facilitate foreign body retrieval, as it may not fit through the tube or can become lodged, causing obstruction. Foreign bodies and surgical manipulation are airway irritants that may cause coughing or patient movement that makes retrieval difficult or dangerous. Muscle relaxation may be preferred by a proceduralist to prevent this, but this preference must always yield to patient safety.

Sometimes a foreign body in the airway or esophagus may have migrated into the posterior pharynx or supraglottic area. If, during direct laryngoscopy, the foreign body is clearly visible, it may be removed with Magill forceps.

> **Caution!** When removing a foreign body, it is always possible that the proceduralist may drop it during removal. For an airway foreign body this may occur at the glottic opening or within an ETT if present and cause complete obstruction. Advancing the foreign body distally into the airway may temporarily relieve the obstruction (with a bougie or surgical instrument). For an esophageal foreign body, the presence of an ETT can protect the airway from iatrogenic airway foreign bodies.

>> **Tip on Technique:** Consider administering a single dose of dexamethasone (0.5 mg IV, max dose 10 mg) to avoid or treat airway swelling if there was considerable manipulation during airway foreign body removal, or in pediatric patients in whom a large esophageal foreign body has caused airway compression.

‼ **Potential Complications:** If an ETT is present, it is important to maintain the security of the ETT while the procedure is in progress, as this is a shared airway with the proceduralist and accidental extubation is possible.

> **WARNING!!** When an esophageal foreign body has been present for a prolonged period of time (especially a lithium disc battery), esophageal perforation is a distinct concern.[4] Blind passage of an orogastric or nasogastric tube is not recommended.

11. Emergence and extubation.

Assessment for airway swelling should be performed prior to consideration for extubation, and the proceduralist should participate in the extubation plan. The decision to extubate should also take postoperative disposition into consideration; the patient may be appropriate for discharge home or may need overnight admission based on hemodynamic status and/or airway injury/swelling. Equipment for reintubation and mask ventilation should be present before attempting extubation.

Criteria for extubation should include:

- Complete reversal of anesthetic agents (specifically neuromuscular blockers)
- Adequate ventilation and oxygenation
- Wakefulness and the ability to follow commands

12. Postoperative care and concerns.

It is important to consider recovery location. Communicate with proceduralists any concerns about oxygenation or ventilation as this may necessitate overnight admission or even intensive care unit (ICU) level of care. Patients with simple foreign body removals and no evidence of airway compromise may be discharged home from the postanesthesia care unit (PACU).

> **Caution!** Postoperative intubation and ICU level of care may be indicated if there is concern for airway edema, postobstructive pneumonia, negative pressure pulmonary edema from tracheal obstruction, and/or concerns for perforation of airway or esophagus.

Other Management Considerations

Airway foreign body aspiration typically occurs in a bimodal fashion, occurring in patients <4 years old and >75 years old. Mental status, dysphagia, and neuromuscular disorders can increase the likelihood of foreign body aspiration. Foreign bodies lodged in the esophagus are more common in the pediatric population than in adults and are most frequently coins, usually stuck at the thoracic inlet. In small children, a swallowed coin lodged in the esophagus can compress the airway as well as cause decreased oral intake and dehydration. In adults and patients with pathologies predisposing to esophageal stricture, food may often become lodged in the esophagus.

The aspiration of inorganic objects can lead to direct airway injury. However, organic objects may absorb fluid when aspirated and worsen the degree of obstruction over time. Aspiration of either object may create a localized inflammatory response. Antibiotics and steroids are not usually given for foreign body aspiration but may be indicated if evidence of respiratory tract infection or granulation tissue is present. With airway foreign bodies in the glottic opening or trachea, consider ECMO early as this takes time to set up and implement.

Further Reading

Pediatric Anesthesia Podcast of the Month—August 2018: Update on Button Battery Ingestion Guidelines (https://vimeo.com/284784072).

Fidkowski CW, Zheng H, Firth PG. The anesthetic considerations of tracheobronchial foreign bodies in children: a literature review of 12,979 cases. Anesthesia & Analgesia. October 2010; 111 (4): 1016–25.

References

1. Sodickson A, Hardy J. Mechanical airway disruption. In: McEvoy MD, Furse CM, Advanced Perioperative Management. 1st ed. New York, NY: Oxford University Press; 2014: 150–55.
2. Ezer SS, et al. Foreign body aspiration in children: analysis of diagnostic criteria and accurate time for bronchoscopy. Pediatric Emergency Care. 2011; 27(8): 723–26.
3. Hannallah R, Brown K, Verghese S. Otorhinolaryngologic procedures. In: Cote CJ, Lerman J, Anderson B, A Practice of Anesthesia for Infants and Children. 5th ed. Philadelphia, PA: Elsevier Saunders; 2013: 653–82.
4. Rosenfeld E, Sola Jr R, Yu Y, St Peter S, Shah S. Battery ingestions in children: variations in care and development of a clinical algorithm. Journal of Pediatric Surgery. 2018; 53: 1537–41.

Chapter 4

Laryngospasm

Joseph LaGrew II, Adam Chadwick, Sandra Gonzalez, and Sonia Mehta

Summary Page
Symptoms:

- Increasing peak airway pressures/ decreasing or absent tidal volumes
- Absent $EtCO_2$ waveform
- Signs of obstructed airway
  - Inspiratory stridor or absent breath sounds
  - Decreased compliance or inability to provide positive pressure ventilation
- Increased respiratory effort
  - Intercostal retractions
  - Paradoxical chest/abdominal movement
- Desaturation (decreasing SpO_2)
- Cyanosis
- Bradycardia or tachycardia
- Hypoxia
- Arrhythmia
- Hypotension
- Cardiac arrest

Differential Diagnosis:

- Endotracheal tube dysfunction
  - Kink
  - Mucus plug
  - Mainstem intubation
- Bronchospasm
  - Inadequate depth of anesthesia
  - Draining blood or secretions
  - Desflurane
  - Asthma exacerbation
- Drug reaction
- Foreign body
- Supraglottic obstruction
- Aspiration
- Tension pneumothorax
- Breath holding

Introduction

Laryngospasm has an estimated incidence of 0.78% and is found in higher proportions in the pediatric and neonatal populations, with certain types of surgeries and medical comorbidities. Infants, children, and those undergoing oropharyngeal, esophageal, and airway surgeries as well as hypospadias repair are associated with increased risk of laryngospasm. Nonmodifiable risk factors include obesity with obstructive sleep apnea (OSA), gastroesophageal reflux disease (GERD), recent or active upper respiratory tract infection (URI), passive cigarette smoke exposure, airway manipulation, volatile anesthetics, depth of anesthesia, use of supraglottic airway, and supraglottic secretions, blood, and tumors/masses. Effective screening and balancing the need for surgery against the risk of laryngospasm is critical to preoperative assessment. Modifiable risk factors should be optimized preoperatively. Treatment focuses on inhibiting the glottic reflex by removing stimulation, stimulating afferent relaxation of the cords, deepening anesthesia, or paralyzing the patient (Figure 4.1). While other methods may effectively treat laryngospasm, paralysis is the definitive treatment for laryngospasm for a patient refractory to other methods or who is in extremis. Identifying the underlying cause is critical once ventilation is restored to prevent recurrence.

Treatment

First, confirm the diagnosis of laryngospasm by auscultating for breath sounds. Absence of breath sounds, the presence of inspiratory stridor, greatly decreased compliance, or complete obstruction to ventilation are signs and symptoms of laryngospasm. Decreased oxygen saturation via pulse oximetry, increased airway pressures, and an altered capnography pattern may accompany these symptoms as well.

Partial laryngospasm or glottic spasm may present with stridorous breathing and minimal airflow but may be clinically indistinguishable and requires the same treatment as complete spasm.[1]

Step by Step

1. **Call for help and attempt to provide positive pressure ventilation while optimizing patient positioning.**

   Discontinue stimulating activities and ask the surgeons to pause the procedure, if applicable. Good mask seal and application of jaw thrust can maximize delivery of positive pressure.

   Supine positioning with the provider at the head of the bed is preferable. In infants and young children, ensure the head is in a neutral position (consider a towel or gel roll under the patient's shoulders) as a large occiput will lead to passive flexion of the neck, resulting in potential increased difficulty with mask ventilation (Figure 4.2A and B). Adult patients are ideally placed in the sniffing position (Figure 4.2C). For obese patients, placing them in reverse Trendelenburg position or raising the head of the bed to decrease abdominal pressure on the diaphragm will prevent further reduction in compliance.

   Proper and timely positive pressure ventilation are the most critical actions in the diagnosis and initial treatment of laryngospasm. The importance of patient position, mask seal, and proper jaw thrust technique are critical in assessing the efficacy of interventions and may obscure response to treatment if performed suboptimally. The

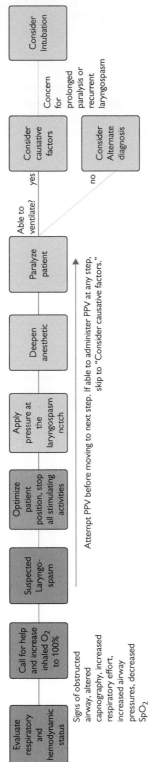

Figure 4.1 Response to bronchospasm/laryngospasm algorithm. PPV = positive pressure ventilation.

position that optimizes alignment of the oral, laryngeal, and pharyngeal axes to facilitate the free movement of air in and out of the lungs as well as the most direct line of sight for endotracheal intubation is ideal.

>>**Tip on Technique**: Consider a two-handed technique to deliver positive pressure breaths with a jaw thrust maneuver if mask ventilation is difficult (Figure 4.3). A two-handed mask technique with modification (placement of thumbs and thenar prominences along the lateral aspects of the mask with the fingers placed along the mandible) may provide ventilation in difficult mask situations. It is important when using this method to avoid applying pressure to the submental soft tissues with the fingers along the mandible and to avoid pushing the patient's chin downward rather than lifting it into the mask with a jaw thrust.

Note: Positive pressure ventilation should be attempted at every step (or continuously if possible) until ventilation is successful and/or laryngospasm resolves.

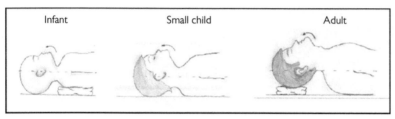

Figure 4.2 The optimal head and neck position for patients undergoing anesthesia with mask ventilation or oral intubation is the "sniffing position." Infants have a more pronounced occiput requiring padding behind the shoulders (A). Small children have a less pronounced occiput and require little to no padding (B). Adults require padding behind the occiput to achieve an optimal head and neck position (C).

2. **Increase inhaled oxygen to 100% to reduce the risk of hypoxia. Deepen anesthesia to reduce stimulation.**

    Deepen anesthesia with propofol 1–2 mg/kg and/or inhalational anesthetic. IV agents may be preferable as inhalational anesthetics require a patent airway.

Caution! Patients may become bradycardic with resultant hypotension as a result of hypoxia. If the patient becomes hemodynamically unstable at any point, paralysis with neuromuscular blockade is the definitive treatment to restore oxygenation and avoid cardiovascular collapse (step 4). Treat hemodynamics concurrently if needed.

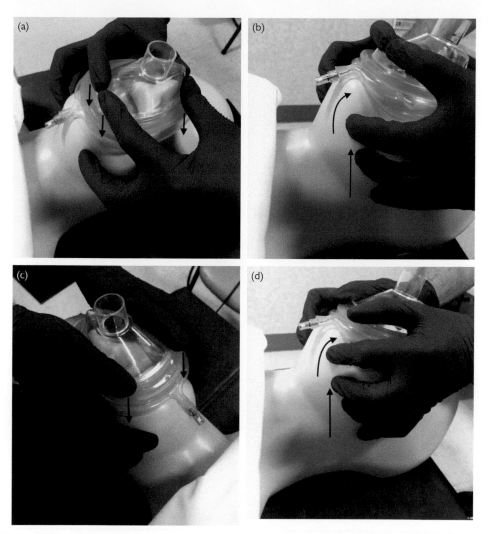

Figure 4.3 The classic two-handed masking technique using the C-E hand grip bilaterally (A–B). The index fingers and thumbs form the "C" holding the mask firmly on the face covering the patient's nose and mouth to create a seal. The third and fourth fingers are placed along the mandible with the fifth finger placed just posterior to the angle of the mandible forming the "E." The "E" fingers pull the patient's face into the mask with a jaw thrust maneuver, promoting airway patency (C–D).

3. Apply pressure at laryngospasm notch (Figure 4.4).

Firm pressure applied by the index or third fingers bilaterally in a medial and cephalad direction in the laryngospasm notch has been shown to break laryngospasm prior to the administration of muscle relaxants or sedatives.[2,3]

The laryngospasm notch is located behind the lobule of the pinna of each ear with borders as follows:

- Anterior: ascending ramus of the mandible
- Posterior: mastoid process, cranial: base of the skull

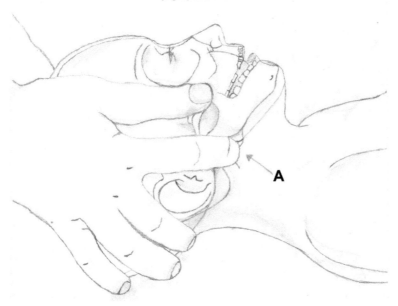

Laryngospasm Notch

Figure 4.4 Firm pressure applied by the index or third fingers bilaterally in a medial and cephalad direction in the laryngospasm notch (A) has been shown to break laryngospasm prior to the administration of muscle relaxants or sedatives. The laryngospasm notch is located behind the lobule of the pinna of each ear with borders as follows: anterior: ascending ramus of the mandible; posterior: mastoid process; cranial: base of the skull.

4. Give muscle relaxation to paralyze the patient.

Note: This is the ONLY definitive treatment and should be considered after step 2 in patients with hypoxia, especially in those with resultant bradycardia and hypotension.

Succinylcholine is the first choice and can be given via a variety of routes:

- 1–2 mg/kg IV
- 3–5 mg/kg IM
- 3 mg/kg intralingual or submentally

>>**Tip on Technique:** Consider administering atropine 20 mcg/kg IV or IM. Succinylcholine given without atropine may cause bradycardia, leading to hemodynamic instability in pediatric patients during or after treatment of laryngospasm.

>>**Tip on Technique:** Rocuronium is an alternative (dose 1.2 mg/kg IV); however, rocuronium may result in prolonged paralysis at the dose indicated above. Sugammadex, a reversal agent for rocuronium, is not Food and Drug Administration approved for use in children currently but can be used in adults to reverse prolonged relaxation.

Other Management Considerations

Once ventilation is restored, identifying the underlying cause is critical to prevent recurrence.

The patient is at risk for recurrence of laryngospasm after anesthetic agents and/or paralytic agents have worn off. If there is concern for prolonged muscle relaxation or recurrence, consider endotracheal intubation. Potential causes and risk factors for each individual should be reviewed to create the best plan for emergence, as laryngospasm is also a risk after extubation.

References

1. Hampson-Evans DA, Morgan P, Farrar M. Pediatric laryngospasm. Pediatric Anesthesia. 2008 Apr 1;18(4):303–307.
2. Larson P. Laryngospasm—the best treatment. Anesthesiology. 1998;89:1293–1294.
3. Johnstone RE. Laryngospasm treatment—an explanation. Anesthesiology. 1999;91:581–582.
4. Gavel G, et al. Laryngospasm in anaesthesia. Continuing Education in Anaesthesia Critical Care & Pain Journal. 2014;14:47–51.
5. Flick RP, et al. Risks factors for laryngospasm in children during general anesthesia. Pediatric Anesthesia. 2008;18(4):289–296.
6. Olsson GL, Hallen B. Laryngospasm during anaesthesia. A computer incidence study in 136,929 patients. Acta Anaesthesiologica Scandinavica. 1984;28:567–575.
7. Visvanathan T, Kluger MT, Webb RK, Westhorpe RN. Crisis management during anaesthesia: laryngospasm. BMJ Quality & Safety. 2005 Jun 1;14(3):e3.

Chapter 5

One-Lung Ventilation

Patricia Nwajuaku, Dustin L. Hegland, and Joseph C. Goldstein

Summary Page

Symptoms:

- Desaturation
- Hypercarbia
- Hemodynamic instability

Differential Diagnosis:

- Ventilation/perfusion (V/Q) mismatch
- Right-to-left shunt
- Diffusion impairment
- Hypoventilation
- Low FiO_2

Introduction

One-lung ventilation is required in a variety of thoracic, cardiac, gastrointestinal, and neurological spine surgeries. Knowledge of the tracheal-bronchial anatomy and its variations and a sound understanding of ventilation and perfusion concepts, as well as a methodical approach to troubleshooting, are required when faced with challenging clinical circumstances.

Indications for one-lung isolation include pulmonary hemorrhage, lung abscess or unilateral infectious process, broncho-pleural fistula, need for bronchial lavage, or video-assisted or robotic-assisted thoracoscopic surgery. Contraindications include patients who cannot tolerate one-lung ventilation or who depend on both lungs to ensure adequate oxygenation and ventilation.

Generally, double-lumen tubes (DLTs) are preferred for lung isolation. Advantages include independent access to either lung and a larger access lumen that improves lung deflation. In general, left-sided DLTs are placed for right-sided procedures and vice versa, with ventilation provided to the nonoperated lung (Figure 5.1).

Potential contraindications for DLT placement include airway/main bronchus size not adequate for available DLTs (e.g., pediatric patients), airway/facial trauma requiring a direct subglottic surgical approach, tracheostomy or stoma in place, or prohibitive airway pathology and difficult airway scenarios requiring nasal and/or awake fiberoptic intubation. Common problems include difficulties with placement of double-lumen tubes or endobronchial blocking devices with or without the added challenges of a difficult airway. During one-lung ventilation, hypoxemia (usually defined as desaturation with SpO_2 values of <90% and/or PaO_2 values of <60 mmHg), hypercarbia, and hemodynamic instability frequently require swift intervention to ensure optimal care.[1]

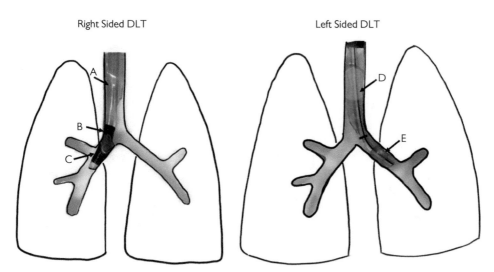

Right Sided DLT   Left Sided DLT

Figure 5.1 Schematic of right and left double-lumen tubes in situ. A and D: Tracheal cuffs. B and E: Bronchial cuffs. C: Bronchial lumen. When bronchial cuff is inflated and bronchial lumen is clamped, no ventilation is delivered to that lung. When tracheal lumen is clamped, ventilation is delivered to the isolated lung through the bronchial lumen.

Management

This chapter addresses management of the following procedures and issues associated with one-lung ventilation:

- Difficulties with Tube Placement, Use of Double-Lumen Tubes, and Inadequate Lung Isolation (Section A)
- Difficult Intubation (Section B)
- Converting from a Single-Lumen Endotracheal Tube to a Double-Lumen Tube (or vice versa) (Section C)
- Inability to Oxygenate or Ventilate (Section D)
- Hemodynamic Instability During One-Lung Ventilation (Section E)
- Surgical Field and Operative Lung Are Not Adequately Deflated for the Procedure (Section F)
- Extubation (Section G)

A. Difficulties with Tube Placement, Use of Double-Lumen Tubes, and Inadequate Lung Isolation

Step by Step

1. Choose the correct-sized tube.

Double-lumen tubes are larger than routinely used single-lumen tubes and can be more challenging to pass into the trachea and position correctly to allow lung isolation and ventilation of each lung separately. Choosing the optimal DLT size is important, as too small or too large DLTs pose different risks to the patient and might lead to repeated airway instrumentation. If you are unable to pass a double-lumen tube, consider placing a smaller-sized double-lumen tube.

>> **Tip on Technique.** Since it has been shown that DLT size cannot reliably and consistently be predicted by formulas, measuring tracheal and bronchial widths by computed tomography (CT) scan (usually available in patients presenting for lung reduction procedures) is the gold standard to determine optimal DLT size.[2–4]

> **Caution!** A DLT that is too small can result in inappropriate seating in the mainstem bronchus, likely will require higher cuff pressures, and may lead to repeated positioning attempts. In contrast, a DLT that is too large increases the risk of tracheal or bronchial injury and leads to a higher incidence of sore throat, as well as laryngeal complications such as arytenoid dislocation.

2. Consider placing a single-lumen tube and a bronchial blocker.

Fiberoptic guidance will aid placement and manipulation of the bronchial blocker to achieve lung isolation (Figure 5.2). Bronchial blocker placement may be preferred for pediatric patients or in the setting of a difficult airway, especially if there is a high likelihood of postoperative continued intubation. Other indications include lesions of the trachea or bronchial tree, esophageal surgery where a double-lumen tube may obstruct the surgical field, the presence of a tracheostomy or stoma, or minimally invasive cardiac surgery.[5]

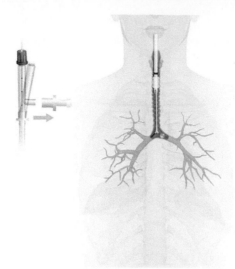

Figure 5.2 Image of bronchial blocker straddling carina. Ventilation can be provided via either lumen into the right or left main bronchus. In this image the left-sided balloon is inflated and only the right lung is being ventilated. Courtesy of Teleflex Medical, with permission.

>> **Tip on Technique:** Place the largest single-lumen endotracheal tube (ETT) possible. This will aid with ease of bronchoscopy and manipulation of the chosen endobronchial blocker.

Caution! A disadvantage with single-lumen tube lung isolation is reduced access to the nonventilated lung (e.g., for suctioning, inspection, continuous positive airway pressure [CPAP]).

3. **Consider placing a single-lumen ETT into the bronchus of the lung to be ventilated and intermittently withdrawing the ETT to ventilate both lungs.**

   Other options are to use extracorporeal membrane oxygenation (ECMO) or cardiopulmonary bypass.

4. **Reposition the tube, as needed, to ensure good lung isolation.**

   Most issues associated with poor lung isolation revolve around correct placement and repositioning.[6]

B. Difficult Intubation

Step by Step

1. **If the intubation is difficult, follow recommended difficult airway algorithms.[7,8]**

   Avoid repeated DLT intubation attempts, which can potentially result in airway edema, injury, or desaturation.

2. **Consider aborting attempts to place a DLT and use a single-lumen ETT plus a bronchial blocker or intermittent mainstem intubation for lung isolation.**

>>**Tip on Technique.** Consider using video laryngoscopy or flexible bronchoscopy to place a single-lumen ETT if visualization was difficult.

3. **Consider also converting from using a single-lumen ETT (once successfully placed) to a DLT (see below).**

C. Converting from a Single-Lumen ETT to a DLT (or vice versa)

Step by Step

1. **Ensure appropriate depth of anesthesia and consider the risks and benefits of paralysis.**
   These include abolishing spontaneous ventilation versus coughing, and laryngospasm.

2. **Consider video laryngoscopy–assisted exchange under direct vision.**

3. **Use an appropriate DLT-compatible exchange catheter.**
   Ensure the selected exchange catheter will fit through each lumen of the double-lumen tube.

4. **To convert a single-lumen tube to a DLT:**
   Place the exchange catheter through the single-lumen tube with fiberoptic guidance (to direct the exchange catheter into the left or right main bronchus). Remove the single-lumen tube under direct vision and advance the DLT over the exchange catheter into the trachea. Use fiberoptic guidance to confirm correct placement and lung isolation.

5. **To convert a DLT to a single-lumen tube:**
   Place an exchange catheter through the bronchial DLT lumen with fiberoptic guidance. Remove the tube under direct vision and place the single-lumen tube over the exchange catheter into the trachea.

>> **Tip on Technique:** Consider using two exchange catheters through each DLT lumen for increased safety in case one catheter becomes dislodged during the exchange.

D. Managing Inability to Oxygenate or Ventilate

Step by Step:

Note: The following steps may be performed in parallel as needed.

1. **Administer 100% FiO_2.**

2. **Communicate the problem to the surgical team and call for help early.**

3. **Initiate advanced cardiac life support (ACLS) if the patient is hemodynamically unstable.**

4. **Assess the need to return to two-lung ventilation.**
   Pulmonary pathology may result in desaturation despite all emergent issues being addressed.[1] Return to two-lung ventilation if needed by either deflating the bronchial cuff of the DLT or deflating the cuff of the bronchial blocker.

5. Perform manual ventilation and auscultate the lungs.

Evaluate for resistance and assess for bronchospasm. Confirm breath sounds to exclude pneumothorax and assess if the tube position is too deep (unilateral breath sounds would be present). Assess for wheezing/bronchospasm. Listen for rhonchi and suction the ETT if present.

If bronchospasm is present, consider treatment with bronchodilators:

- Albuterol 90 mcg/actuation (metered dose inhaler [MDI]), 8–10 puffs
- Ketamine 0.25–0.5 mg/kg IV
- Magnesium 30–50 mg/kg IV
- Lidocaine 0.5–1.5 mg/kg IV
- Epinephrine 2–100 mcg IV

6. Do a quick safety check and exclude machine-related issues.

Exclude machine-related issues such as valve malfunction, bellows or CO_2 absorber leak, scavenger system issues, or FiO_2 monitor malfunction. Consider using a backup self-inflating bag connected to an independent oxygen tank. Assess the anesthesia circuit, components, and connections and evaluate for kinks or bending of the DLT.

7. Perform a bronchoscopic examination.

Ensure optimal DLT or bronchial blocker position. Suction mucus AND consider bronchio-alveolar lavage to clear thick secretions.

8. Perform maneuvers to optimize oxygenation and ventilation.

Apply CPAP to the nonventilated lung and titrate positive end-expiratory pressure (PEEP) to the ventilated lung. Consider disconnecting from the ventilator if breath stacking is suspected. Consider recruitment maneuvers of the ventilated lung: with the patient off the ventilator, adjust the APL valve to 30 cmH_2O and hold for 30 seconds before resuming ventilation. Also consider a different mode of ventilation or adjusting tidal volumes. Increase the inspiration-to-expiration (I:E) ratio. Make sure to assess and monitor for air trapping or breath stacking. Consider frequent disconnects from the ventilator to reduce this risk.

Optimize perfusion to the ventilated lung by optimizing blood pressure and assessing volume status. Consider giving a fluid challenge. Optimize hypoxic pulmonary vasoconstriction (HPV).

Consider vasoactive infusions to raise blood pressure, such as:

- Phenylephrine 0.3–1 mcg/kg/min IV
- Vasopressin 1–2 unit(s)/hr IV

Caution! Consider minimizing HPV inhibiting agents, such as vasodilators (nitroglycerin, nitroprusside) and volatile anesthetics.

---

9. Involve the surgical team.

If the above maneuvers are unsuccessful and oxygenation is still inadequate, discuss with the surgeons any potential surgical interventions to increase oxygenation, such as temporary surgical clamping of the pulmonary artery or its branches to the nonventilated lung. If a pulmonary artery catheter is present in the pulmonary artery of the nonventilated lung, consider temporary inflation of the balloon.

10. If oxygenation improves, attempt to reestablish one-lung ventilation.

If the patient cannot tolerate one-lung ventilation despite maneuvers, consider intermittent two-lung ventilation or altering or aborting the procedure. More invasive options include extracorporeal membrane oxygenation (ECMO) or cardiopulmonary bypass if the procedure cannot be aborted or altered.

E. Hemodynamic Instability During One-Lung Ventilation

Step by Step

Determine the urgency of the situation and follow the steps below:

1. **In case of impending cardiovascular collapse initiate ACLS early and administer 100% FiO$_2$.**

2. **Call for help early and communicate with the surgical team.**

   Exclude surgical causes such as bleeding; surgical manipulation that could affect hemodynamics such as pressure to lungs due to inflation (i.e., during video-assisted thoracic surgery [VATS]), surgical instruments, or manual pressure; or arrhythmias secondary to surgical cardiac irritation.

3. **Consider rapid fluid administration and vasopressors for hypotension.**

   Give epinephrine, 10–100 mcg IV, or vasopressin, 1–2 units IV. Give crystalloid or colloid solutions as needed to maintain hemodynamics.

4. **Consider returning to two-lung ventilation.**

   Optimize oxygenation and address hypoxemia as a possible cause (consider initiating maneuvers described in the previous section). Deflate the bronchial cuff of the DLT or the bronchial blocker cuff and remove the clamp from the nonventilated lumen of the DLT.

5. **Consider increasing ventilation to address respiratory acidosis.**

   Note: Acidosis will affect vasopressor response. Consider administration of sodium bicarbonate 50–100 mEq IV if present.

6. **Consider tension pneumothorax of the ventilated lung.**

   Treat with intrathoracic or external needle decompression if needed.

7. **Consider "breath stacking," "over-PEEPing," or "air trapping."**

   Check the scavenging system (adequate suction level for flows) and disconnect the patient from the ventilator and observe the capnogram. Increase I:E ratio and optimize PEEP levels.

8. **Consider cardiac causes.**

   These could include surgical injury (tamponade or rupture), right ventricular failure (pulmonary hypertension or embolism), gas/air embolism, or myocardial ischemia.

F. Surgical Field and Operative Lung Are Not Adequately Deflated for the Procedure

Step by Step

1. **Communicate with the surgical team and assess the situation.**

   Ask if the lung isolation is inadequate for the procedure and if intervention is needed. If so, perform the following steps listed below.

2. **Increase FiO$_2$ to 100% and confirm adequate ventilation before performing any maneuvers.**

Doing so maximizes oxygenation and decreases the risk of desaturation.

3. **Assess the DLT for issues that may be preventing lung isolation.**

Suction the DLT or bronchial blocker port to rule out obstruction. Check for inadequate cuff inflation (consider the use of a manometer) and add 1–2 ml per cuff if appropriate and reevaluate. Perform bronchoscopic examination to rule out migration and/or malposition of the tube. If in doubt, check early that the DLT is in the correct position.

4. **Assess for causes of inadequate lung deflation.**

If there is inadequate deflation time, apply suction to the nonventilated lung to increase the deflation time. Consider surgical assistance to improve deflation, such as gentle lung manipulation, removing adhesions, or increasing insufflation pressure (if VATS procedure). Cuff rupture could also be a cause of inadequate lung deflation: consider use of a manometer to measure cuff pressure. If the cuff is ruptured, a DLT or bronchial blocker exchange will be required.

G. Managing Extubation

Extubation in the operating room is desired to avoid positive pressure mechanical ventilation, which puts stress on the fresh surgical anastomotic site(s). The postoperative plan should be discussed during the debriefing or conclusion of the procedure.

Step by Step

1. **Assess for contraindications to extubation with surgical team.**

Optimize the patient for extubation: fully reverse neuromuscular blockade and ensure normothermia, hemodynamic stability, and adequate postoperative analgesia. Suction the endotracheal tube and evaluate for cough reflex. Extubation may be contraindicated if there is concern for airway edema, hemodynamic instability, or inadequate oxygenation or ventilation.

2. **Prepare for noninvasive methods of airway and oxygen support after extubation.**

Additional support such as CPAP may be required after extubation. Consider the temporary use of an airway exchange catheter if difficult reintubation is anticipated. This catheter can be used for reintubation as well as for oxygenation.

Caution! There is a risk of barotrauma when ventilating through a small-bore airway exchange catheter.

---

3. **Prepare a reintubation plan and have equipment and medications readily available.**

This should be performed PRIOR to extubation, because if the patient fails extubation, reintubation may be required urgently. Have an airway cart and medications available to provide adequate conditions for reintubation, such as propofol and muscle relaxants. Vasopressors may also be needed if hemodynamic instability occurs due to inadequate oxygenation or ventilation.

4. If extubation criteria are not met, consider an exchange maneuver from a DLT to a single-lumen ETT.

If extubation is not planned, it is preferable to convert the DLT to a single-lumen tube for postoperative ventilation, as a single-lumen tube is more easily managed by intensive care unit staff and provides a larger lumen for suctioning and ventilation. See Section C for details on converting a DLT to a single-lumen tube. Plan for adequate sedation. Consider a mode of ventilation that allows for spontaneous ventilation to minimize positive pressure ventilation stress on surgical anastomotic site(s).

Further Reading

Ochroch E, Weiss SJ. Thoracic Anesthesia. In: Longnecker DE, Mackey SC, Newman MF, Sandberg WS, Zapol WM. eds. Anesthesiology, 3e. New York, NY: McGraw-Hill; 2017:888–938.

Anesthesia for Thoracic Surgery. In: Butterworth IV JF, Mackey DC, Wasnick JD. eds. Morgan & Mikhail's Clinical Anesthesiology, 6e. New York, NY: McGraw-Hill; 2018:553–582.

Mueller J. One-Lung Ventilation. In: Freeman BS, Berger JS, eds. Anesthesiology Core Review: Part Two Advanced Exam. New York, NY: McGraw-Hill; 2016:181–184.

References

1. Bartz RR, Moon RE. Chapter 3. Physiology of One-Lung Ventilation. In: Barbeito A, Shaw AD, Grichnik K, eds. Thoracic Anesthesia. New York, NY: McGraw-Hill; 2012:45–61.
2. Brodsky J, Macario A, Mark JB. Tracheal diameter predicts double-lumen tube size: A method for selecting left double-lumen tubes. Anesth Analg 1996; 82:861–864.
3. Hannallah M, Benumof JL, Silverman PM, Kelly LC, Lea D. Evaluation of an approach to choosing a left double-lumen tube size based on chest computed tomographic scan measurement of left mainstem bronchial diameter. J Cardiothorac Vasc Anesth 1997; 11:168–171.
4. Slinger P. Choosing the appropriate double-lumen tube: A glimmer of science comes to a dark art. J Cardiothorac Vasc Anesth 1995; 9:117–118.
5. Clayton-Smith A, Bennett K, Alston RP, et al. A comparison of the efficacy and adverse effects of double-lumen endobronchial tubes and bronchial blockers in thoracic surgery: A systematic review and meta-analysis of randomized controlled trials. J Cardiothorac Vasc Anesth 2015; 29:955–966.
6. Tuxen DV. Chapter 25. Independent Lung Ventilation. In: Tobin MJ, ed. Principles and Practice of Mechanical Ventilation, 3e. New York, NY: McGraw-Hill; 2013:1097–1101.
7. Collins S, et al. Lung isolation in the patient with a difficult airway. Anesth Analg 2018; 126:1968–1978.
8. Morris IR. Lung Separation in the Patient with a Difficult Airway. In: Hung OR, Murphy MF, eds. Hung's Difficult and Failed Airway Management, 3e. New York, NY: McGraw-Hill; 2018.

Chapter 6

Unanticipated Difficult Airway

Lauren C. Berkow

Summary Page

Symptoms:

- Hypoxemia
- Stridor
- Airway obstruction
- Hypotension
- Bradycardia
- Respiratory arrest
- Cardiac arrest

Differential Diagnosis:

- Tracheal foreign body
- Laryngospasm
- Bronchospasm
- Tension pneumothorax

Introduction

Difficulty with airway management in the perioperative setting remains a challenge for anesthesia providers. Prediction and recognition of risk factors for airway difficulty can allow advance planning and strategies to prevent unanticipated difficulty, but prediction remains a challenge. Once difficulty is encountered, efforts should focus on achieving and maintaining adequate oxygenation and ventilation, to allow time for alternate strategies or awakening the patient. In the emergent setting or a patient in extremis, usually awakening them is not an option, and airway access must be obtained. Supraglottic airway devices can often rescue failed mask ventilation and can also be used as a conduit for intubation after placement. The most experienced providers should perform airway maneuvers whenever possible. In the setting of failed direct laryngoscopy, videolaryngoscopy (VL) or flexible bronchoscopic intubation may be successful and should be considered if oxygenation is adequate. If ventilation and/or oxygenation are NOT adequate, it is important not to repeat airway interventions that have failed, and instead move on to another technique (Figure 6.1).[1] A surgical airway can be lifesaving and should be performed early before hemodynamic instability or cardiac arrest occurs.

Outside the operating room (OR), such as the intensive care unit (ICU) or the wards, patients requiring emergent airway management may have hemodynamic instability, a recent failed extubation, or poor oxygen reserves, putting them at higher risk for complications. Many have recently failed extubation or are hemodynamically unstable, putting them at increased risk of desaturation and airway complications. Space to manage the airway and airway resources may be limited in these environments, but the management steps are the same as in the OR.

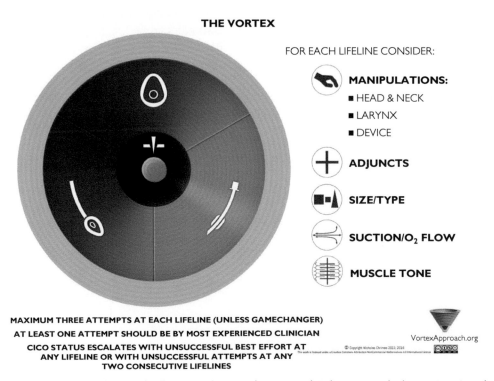

THE VORTEX

FOR EACH LIFELINE CONSIDER:

MANIPULATIONS:
- HEAD & NECK
- LARYNX
- DEVICE

ADJUNCTS

SIZE/TYPE

SUCTION/O_2 FLOW

MUSCLE TONE

MAXIMUM THREE ATTEMPTS AT EACH LIFELINE (UNLESS GAMECHANGER)
AT LEAST ONE ATTEMPT SHOULD BE BY MOST EXPERIENCED CLINICIAN
CICO STATUS ESCALATES WITH UNSUCCESSFUL BEST EFFORT AT
ANY LIFELINE OR WITH UNSUCCESSFUL ATTEMPTS AT ANY
TWO CONSECUTIVE LIFELINES

VortexApproach.org

Figure 6.1 The Vortex Cognitive Aid. This approach stresses that no more than three attempts by the most experienced provider should be performed, and if ventilation and laryngoscopy are unsuccessful, escalate to a cannot intubate, cannot oxygenate (CICO) rescue procedure such as a surgical airway. With permission from Dr. Nicholas Chrimes.

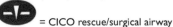 = CICO rescue/surgical airway

In a relatively stable patient who requires airway management outside the OR, if difficulty is suspected or encountered, consider moving them to the OR for management, where more resources are available.

Management

Step by Step

1. Recognize difficulty with airway management.

Call for help early. Alert the team in the OR that airway management is difficult or failed. Call for additional personnel as well as equipment, if needed. If a difficult airway cart is available, bring it to the room (Figure 6.2).

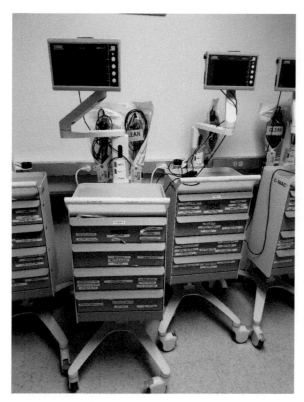

Figure 6.2 Example of a difficult airway cart.

Standardization of airway equipment into an airway cart allows availability and portability of emergency airway equipment whenever it is needed. The cart should contain at a minimum supraglottic airway devices, videolaryngoscopes, flexible intubation scopes, bougies, and equipment to perform a surgical airway (Figure 6.3).

```
┌─────────────────────────────────────────────────┐
│              Rigid laryngoscopes                  │
│                                                   │
│              Videolaryngoscopes                   │
│                                                   │
│   Tracheal tubes and guides (stylets, bougies)    │
│                                                   │
│         Supraglottic airway devices               │
│                                                   │
│       Flexible endoscopic intubation scopes       │
│                                                   │
│      Equipment to perform a surgical airway       │
│                                                   │
│         Exhaled carbon dioxide detector           │
└─────────────────────────────────────────────────┘
```

Figure 6.3 Recommended equipment to be included in a difficult airway cart. Adapted from Apfelbaum JL, Hagberg CA, Caplan RA. Practice guidelines for management of the difficult airway: an updated report by the American Society of Anesthesiologists Task Force on Management of the Difficult Airway. Anesthesiology 2013; 118(2): 251–70.

Airway difficulty can be any of the following:[2]
- Difficult or failed mask ventilation
- Difficult or failed laryngoscopy
- Inability to place the endotracheal tube (ETT) despite visualization of the vocal cords

Any of the above scenarios can result in:
- Hypoxemia: decreased oxygenation saturations due to lack of adequate ventilation
- Hypercarbia: due to inadequate ventilation and retained CO_2
- Hemodynamic instability: bradycardia and hypotension, then advancing to cardiac arrest

‼ Potential Complication: Inadequate oxygenation and/or ventilation can lead to arterial desaturations, which, when severe, can result in bradycardia, arrhythmias, brain damage, and cardiac arrest. These complications may require management in tandem with airway management. Successful resolution of these complications is dependent on achieving adequate oxygenation and ventilation.

WARNING‼　　If the patient becomes unstable with worsening hypoxia or vital signs at any point during airway management, proceed directly to step 6 (surgical airway) and commence advanced cardiac life support (ACLS) if necessary. A surgical airway can be lifesaving and should be performed early before hemodynamic instability or cardiac arrest occurs.

>> Tip on Technique: After difficulty is recognized, the ability to adequately mask ventilate and oxygenate will determine the next steps.

2. Attempt/confirm mask ventilation.
Attempt or confirm mask ventilation and deliver 100% oxygen.
If initial attempts fail, attempt one or more of the following:
- Place an oral airway and optimize head position.
- Attempt two-person mask ventilation (Figure 6.4).

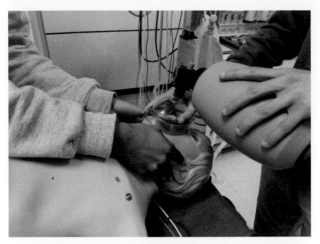

Figure 6.4 Picture depicting the two-person mask ventilation technique. One person performs bilateral jaw thrusts while the second person performs ventilation via bag-mask.

WARNING!! If at any point during this step the patient becomes hemodynamically unstable (rapidly dropping oxygen saturations, cardiac arrest), begin ACLS and perform a surgical airway (step 6).

If mask ventilation is inadequate or impossible, IMMEDIATELY proceed to step 3.

>> **Tip on Technique:** Consider ramping the patient for improved ventilation, or delivering supplemental oxygen via high-flow nasal oxygenation.[3] Ramping obese patients to align the ear with the sternal notch has been shown to improve both ventilation and laryngoscopy. High-flow nasal oxygenation has been proven to prolong apnea time and reduce desaturation during airway management.[3]

Light anesthesia can be a cause for difficult mask ventilation. If suspected, deepen anesthetic and consider giving a muscle relaxant if not already given.

Caution! Certain patients are at higher risk of oxygen desaturation during even short periods of apnea: morbid obesity, obstructive sleep apnea, pregnancy, chronic obstructive pulmonary disease, and other pulmonary diseases that impair oxygen exchange in the lungs.

---

3. Attempt supraglottic airway placement if mask ventilation fails or is inadequate.
Place a first- or second-generation supraglottic airway device and confirm adequate ventilation and oxygenation.

WARNING!! If at any point during this step the patient becomes hemodynamically unstable (rapidly dropping oxygen saturations, cardiac arrest), begin ACLS and perform a surgical airway (step 6). If ventilation is UNSUCCESSFUL, expect the patient to continue to desaturate and require a surgical airway.

If ventilation is successful, consider:[4]

- Awakening patient if an option (step 4)
- Using the supraglottic airway device for the case if appropriate
- If initial laryngoscopy was unsuccessful and a more secure airway is needed:
  - Consider an alternate intubation technique (step 5).
  - Consider intubation via the supraglottic airway (step 5).
  - Consider performing a surgical airway (step 6).

>> **Tip on Technique:** Select the appropriately sized device based on the weight of the patient to obtain an optimal seal. Second-generation devices contain an additional gastric port to allow decompression of the stomach.

!! **Potential Complication:** If edema or obstruction is present at the level of the vocal cords, placement of a supraglottic airway device may not result in successful ventilation.

WARNING!!   Supraglottic airway devices do not protect against aspiration in the setting of a full stomach. Weigh the risk of aspiration against the larger risk of inability to oxygenate or ventilate.

---

4. Consider awakening patient, if possible.

Caution!   Awakening the patient should ONLY be considered if the patient is stable and maintaining oxygen saturations via mask ventilation.

Allow anesthetic agents to wear off, and reverse opioids or benzodiazepines if appropriate:

- Naloxone 0.04 mg IV boluses to reverse opioids
- Flumazenil 1–2 mg IV to reverse benzodiazepines

If muscle relaxation was given, mask ventilate or assist the patient until it wears off. Consider giving sugammadex 16 mg/kg IV if rocuronium was given.

Caution!   Sugammadex as a strategy for the cannot-intubate, cannot-oxygenate scenario is NOT recommended.[5] Consider only if the patient is stable and can be ventilated to decrease the time to return of spontaneous ventilation.

Once patient is awakened, options include:

- Cancelling the case
- Performing awake intubation: proceed to step 7.

5. Attempt intubation with alternate technique.

WARNING!!   If at any point during these steps the patient becomes hemodynamically unstable (rapidly dropping oxygen saturations, cardiac arrest), begin ACLS and perform a surgical airway (step 6).

The MOST experienced provider should reattempt intubation.

The device chosen will depend on which initial device was unsuccessful. Do not repeat a failed technique! If direct laryngoscopy was unsuccessful, consider an alternate blade size or style, or attempt VL. VL can provide a more anterior view to the glottis compared to direct laryngoscopy.[6]

>> **Tip on Technique:** Consider using an angulated blade to obtain a more anterior view. Rigid stylets or flexible intubation scopes can be used in combination with VL to improve success. If difficulty with tube placement is encountered, retracting the VL blade out of the mouth can aid in tube advancement.

!! **Potential Complication:** Blind placement of the ETT during VL can result in soft tissue (palate, tonsil) injury.[7] Inserting the ETT into the mouth under direct vision can prevent this.

> **Caution!** Blood or secretions may obstruct the video camera and hinder view.

If VL was unsuccessful, consider flexible endoscopic intubation. Intubation can be performed via the oral or nasal route.

>> **Tip on Technique:** Jaw thrust may facilitate visualization of the vocal cords.

> **Caution!** Avoid the nasal route if the patient is anticoagulated due to risk of bleeding, or in the presence of nasal or basal skull fracture.

Another alternate technique is intubation via a supraglottic airway device. If a supraglottic airway device was placed for ventilation, this technique will allow ventilation via the supraglottic airway during the procedure as well. First, insert an Aintree Intubation Catheter (AIC) and flexible intubation scope via the supraglottic airway.[8] Then advance the AIC/scope combination through the vocal cords into the trachea until the carina is visualized. Remove the supraglottic airway device (deflate the cuff first) and flexible scope, leaving the AIC in place. Advance an ETT over the AIC into the trachea, remove the AIC, and confirm ventilation, end-tidal CO_2, and chest rise and fall.

>> **Tip on Technique:** The flexible scope can be reinserted through the AIC prior to removal to confirm placement of the ETT. In an emergency, ventilation can be performed via the AIC. If difficulty is encountered advancing the ETT, a jaw thrust or twisting the ETT can facilitate advancement.

!! **Potential Complications:** These include injury to the trachea from the AIC, inability to advance the ETT over the AIC into the trachea, and barotrauma due to overaggressive ventilation via the AIC.

6. Perform surgical airway.

The most experienced provider should perform the surgical airway!

Several options exist. An open or percutaneous cricothyrotomy is recommended in the emergent setting. An open cricothyrotomy is contraindicated in children younger than 12 years old, and a tracheostomy should be performed in these patients.

Jet ventilation can also be performed to provide emergent ventilation by placing an angiocath via the cricothyroid membrane but has a high risk of barotrauma.

> **Caution!** This is a temporizing measure until a cricothyrotomy or other successful method of ventilation can be achieved.

>> **Tip on Technique:** Open cricothyrotomy using a scalpel and a bougie has lower complication rates than the percutaneous technique, which is more time consuming and requires more steps.[4,9] Palpation or ultrasound can be used to locate the cricothyroid membrane[10] (Figure 6.5). Placement of a shoulder roll can facilitate surgical airway placement.

If a surgical airway is required to manage the airway, a discussion should then proceed as to whether to proceed or cancel the proposed surgery. In the emergent setting, surgery may need to proceed.

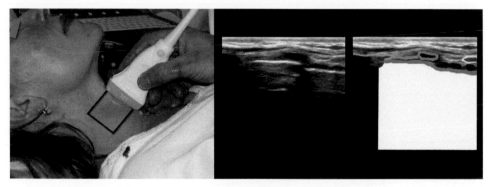

Figure 6.5 Identification of the cricothyroid membrane using ultrasound. Left panel: Placement of the ultrasound probe in the midsagittal plane over the trachea. Right panel: green line: thyroid cartilage; orange line: cricothyroid membrane; purple circle: cricoid cartilage; dark blue circles: anterior tracheal rings; yellow circle: isthmus of thyroid gland; light blue line: tissue/air border. White area below tissue/air border is artifact. From Kristensen MS, Teoh WH, Garumann O, Laursen CB. Ultrasonography for clinical decision-making and intervention in airway management: from the mouth to the pleura. Insights Imaging. 2014; 5: 253–279. (Open access)

7. If the patient was awakened, perform awake intubation.

Once the patient is awakened, intubation can be performed with the patient spontaneously breathing. This is also an option in patients with an anticipated difficult airway. Flexible endoscopic intubation via either the oral or the nasal route is the most commonly performed technique, but awake direct laryngoscopy or VL can also be performed. The sitting-up position can facilitate awake intubation.

> **Caution!** Avoid the nasal route if the patient is anticoagulated, due to risk of bleeding, or in the presence of nasal or basal skull fracture.
>
> **Caution!** Judicious sedation may be considered if the patient is anxious but can result in obtundation and airway obstruction. Additional sedation may not be required if the patient is still emerging from anesthesia.

>> **Tip on Technique:** Airway topicalization is usually required to allow the patient to tolerate awake intubation. Areas to be topicalized will depend on the route chosen.

The oral route requires topicalization of the tongue, oropharynx, vocal cords, and trachea.
The nasal route requires topicalization of the nasopharynx, posterior oropharynx, vocal cords, and trachea.
Options include:

- Topical administration of 2% lidocaine to tongue, oropharynx
- Nebulized 2% lidocaine
- 2% lidocaine ± nasal decongestant to bilateral nares (for nasal route)
- Airway blocks (all three should be performed for complete topicalization) (Figure 6.6):
- Glossopharyngeal nerve: inject 1–2 ml of 2% lidocaine bilaterally or apply topically to base of tonsillar pillars
- Superior laryngeal nerve: inject 1–2 ml of 2% lidocaine bilaterally at greater cornu of hyoid bone
- Recurrent laryngeal nerve: inject 1–2 ml of 2% lidocaine via cricothyroid membrane

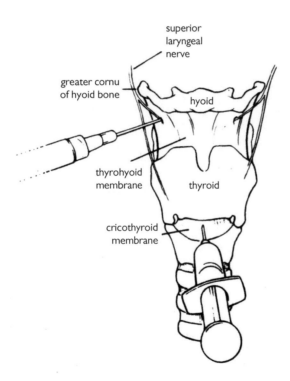

Figure 6.6 Locations to perform superior laryngeal nerve block (at greater cornu of hyoid bone) and recurrent laryngeal nerve block (via cricothyroid membrane). Figure courtesy of author.

8. Stabilize and reassess the patient.

Deliver 100% oxygen until oxygen levels are within normal parameters. Treat hemodynamics if necessary (hypotension, bradycardia, arrhythmias).

Discuss next steps and whether to proceed with the procedure. Whether or not to proceed will depend on the emergent nature of the procedure as well as the stability of the patient. If a surgical airway was performed, discuss with the surgical team if it should be converted to a formal tracheostomy.

9. **Assess for extubation and postoperative considerations.**

Whether or not to extubate a patient with a difficult intubation at the end of the procedure should be a carefully weighed decision. If airway edema is suspected, the ETT should be left in place postoperatively until the edema is resolved.[11] Have a high threshold for keeping the patient intubated. Consider steroids for airway edema (dexamethasone 4–8 mg IV), as well as close monitoring in an ICU postoperatively.

If extubation is performed, consider extubation to continuous positive airway pressure (CPAP), bilevel positive airway pressure (BiPAP), or high-flow nasal oxygen. Have difficult airway equipment available in the room for extubation in case of failure. If extubation fails and the patient is NOT making efforts to breathe spontaneously, **return IMMEDIATELY to step 1!**

If the patient is still making efforts to breathe spontaneously, apply jaw thrust and place a nasal airway and/or oral airway (nasal airways are better tolerated in patients with intact gag reflexes). Consider applying CPAP or placement of a supraglottic airway if previous maneuvers are unsuccessful.

Consider administration of naloxone (0.04 mg IV, repeat as needed) to reverse opioid medications if appropriate.

Consider additional doses of muscle relaxant reversal medications if appropriate:

- Sugammadex 2 mg/kg mg IV
- Neostigmine 0.07 mg/kg plus glycopyrrolate 0.04–0.08 mg IV

Other Management Considerations

Clearly document the difficult airway and airway management in the patient record. Consider placement of a difficult airway bracelet and difficult airway sign above the patient's bed to alert providers. Advise enrollment into Medic Alert Registry (www.medicalert.org) and discuss the difficult airway with the patient and family. Consider providing a difficult airway letter to the patient for future use.

References

1. http://vortexapproach.org/
2. Apfelbaum JL, Hagberg CA, Connis RT, Abdelmalak BB, Agarkar M, Dutton RP, Fiadjoe JE, Greif R, Klock Jr PA, Mercier D, Myatra SN. American Society of Anesthesiologists practice guidelines for management of the difficult airway. Anesthesiology. 2022 Jan;136(1):31–81.
3. Weingart SD, Levitan RM. Preoxygenation and prevention of desaturation during emergency airway management. Ann Emerg Med. 2012;59:165–75.
4. Frerk C, Mitchell VS, McNarry AF, Mendonca C, et al. Difficult Airway Society 2015 guidelines for management of unanticipated difficult intubation in adults. Br J Anaesth. 2015 Dec;115(6):827–48.
5. Naguib M, Brewer L, LaPierre C, Kopman AF, Johnson KB. The myth of rescue reversal in "can't intubate, can't ventilate" scenarios. Anesth Analg. 2016;123:82–92.
6. Berkow L, Morey T, Urdaneta F. The technology of videolaryngoscopy. Anesth Analg. 2018 May;126(5):1527–34.
7. Greer D, Marshall KE, Bevins S, Standlee A, et al. A review of videolaryngoscopy pharyngeal wall injuries. Laryngoscope. 2017;127:439–53.

8. Berkow L, Schwartz L, Kan K, Corridore M, Heitmiller E. Use of the laryngeal mask airway-Aintree Intubating Catheter-fiberoptic bronchoscope technique for difficult intubation. J Clin Anesth. 2011;23(7):534–39.

9. Higgs A, McGrath BA, Goddard C, Rangasami J, et al. Guidelines for the management of tracheal intubation in critically ill adults. Br J Anaesth. 2018;120(2):323–52.

10. Kristensen MS, Teoh WH, Garumann O, Laursen CB. Ultrasonography for clinical decision-making and intervention in airway management: from the mouth to the pleura. Insights Imaging. 2014;5:253–79.

11. Difficult Airway Society Extubation Guidelines Group, Popat M, Mitchell V, Dravid R, Patel A, Swampillai C, Higgs A. Difficult Airway Society guidelines for the management of tracheal extubation. Anaesthesia. 2012;67:318–40.

Chapter 7

Tracheostomy Complications

Matthew Hernandez and Arturo Torres

Summary Page

Symptoms:

- Hypoxemia/hypercarbia
- Bleeding
- Increased ventilatory pressures
- Airway loss

Differential Diagnosis:

- Tracheostomy versus laryngeal stoma
- Tracheostomy versus cricothyrotomy

Introduction

Tracheostomy is a surgically created airway midline through the neck and into the proximal trachea. This procedure is utilized in patients with prolonged mechanical ventilation and in patients with anticipated difficult airway access. The approach can be done open or percutaneously, or a combination of both. Both approaches can be done at the bedside, depending on local practices and surgical aptitude. If done in the operating room (OR), then it is commonly performed via an open approach. The choice of approach is usually related to patient body habitus, vascular anatomy, airway anatomy, positioning, or risk of bleeding.[1] In the emergent cannot-intubate, cannot-ventilate scenario, a cricothyrotomy may be performed via the cricothyroid membrane to provide ventilation. Once the patient is stabilized, a cricothyrotomy is sometimes revised to a formal tracheostomy.

Obesity can make landmark identification difficult. A concerning anatomical challenge is the inability to hyperextend the neck due to cervical immobility. This causes difficulty with both tracheal access and airway manipulation during an emergency. Tracheostomy in these patients is best done via an open approach in the OR. Patients with difficult bag-mask ventilation and laryngoscopy will also be challenging tracheostomy candidates. In this subset of patients, always have difficult airway equipment in the OR prior to starting surgery.

An important consideration prior to proceeding with a tracheostomy deals with timing and patient selection. The timing of a tracheostomy will depend on the need and patient setting. For intensive care unit (ICU) patients the ideal timing remains controversial. There is evidence supporting both early (7 days) and late (14 days) placement.[2] More importantly, the patient's condition will determine readiness. There are very few absolute contraindications for an elective tracheostomy (Table 7.1). It is important to realize that the patient cannot be in an actively decompensating status since respiratory insufficiency is always a possibility during insertion.

Table 7.1 Contraindications for Tracheostomy Placement

Absolute Contraindications	Relative Contraindications
Elevated intracranial pressure or cervical (neck) instability	Resolving hemodynamic instability
Respiratory failure or instability	Mild coagulopathy or thrombocytopenia
Shock	Increased secretion burden
Severe coagulopathy	Aberrant airway or vascular anomaly
Symptomatic pneumonia	

The preoperative examination needs to focus on the stability of the cardiopulmonary, neurological, and coagulation systems. Review previous laryngoscopy attempts in case emergent endotracheal tube (ETT) replacement due to either dislodgement or cuff damage is needed.

The two most dangerous complications are bleeding and loss of the airway. Risk factors for bleeding include platelet count <50,000, activated prothrombin time (APTT) >50 seconds, known bleeding disorders, and insertion of a large cannula size (>9 mm internal diameter).[3] Often, ICU patients are being actively anticoagulated with heparin. A reasonable approach prior to surgery is to stop the heparin infusion for 2 hours and check a thromboelastogram (TEG) to ensure the heparin effect is gone along with an APTT. Before a tracheostomy is attempted, there should be adequate advanced airway equipment and practitioners present who are trained in securing difficult airways.

Complications can occur both during tracheostomy placement and in patients with a tracheostomy already in place. Quick recognition is essential to prevent life-threatening complications. This chapter will discuss these two scenarios as separate sections.

Section 1—Treatment of Complications During Tracheostomy Insertion

The following complications will be discussed step by step:

A. How to reduce the risk of airway fire
B. How to prevent cuff damage during tracheostomy insertion
C. Management of cuff damage or loss of ETT cuff pressure and tidal volume
D. Management of the inability to ventilate after tracheostomy insertion
E. Management of sudden increase in airway pressure with cardiovascular collapse
F. Management of bleeding during dissection for tracheostomy placement

A. How to Reduce the Risk of Airway Fire

Airway fire risk is increased in patients requiring higher FiO_2 levels and with open tracheostomies due to electrocautery usage.

Step by Step

1. Communicate early with the surgeons if cautery will be used, and instruct them to inform you prior to usage.

If electrocautery is to be used, ensure that FiO_2 is decreased to <30% or lower if the patient can tolerate it. Discuss the use of electrocautery at the procedural timeout and the importance of communication to allow time to reduce oxygen levels prior to cautery usage.

2. If patient is unable to tolerate lower FiO_2 levels, request that the surgical team avoid using cautery.

Reduce the oxygen levels to as low as the patient will tolerate, and inform the surgeons of the risk of electrocautery. It may be possible to use cautery for very short periods and then raise the oxygen levels if the patient desaturates. Immediately prior to tracheostomy tube insertion, the FiO_2 can be increased to 100% in case of airway loss.

B. How to Prevent Cuff Damage During Tracheostomy Insertion

The majority of tracheostomies are performed in patients who already have an endotracheal tube in place. If the tube is not retracted properly above the site of the tracheostomy, it can be damaged during insertion. The following steps can be taken to prevent damage to the ETT cuff.

Step by Step

1. Ensure proper anesthetic depth and paralysis prior to manipulation to ensure there is no involuntary displacement and to optimize glottic view.

Consider hyperventilation and increasing FiO_2 to 100% with application of anesthetic prior to ETT manipulation. Confirm that muscle relaxation has been given and that the patient has an adequate level of anesthesia.

2. Retract the ETT prior to tracheostomy insertion.

Retract the ETT until the cuff is one-third through the glottis and ventilation is adequate. Note the distance the tube was retracted to view the cuff at the glottis. Slightly deflate the cuff while maintaining adequate tidal volumes. Communicate with the team that the tube has been retracted to a safe distance to avoid inadvertent cuff puncture.

>> **Tip on Technique:** Videolaryngoscopy can be used to facilitate retraction of the ETT to the ideal location to avoid cuff damage with either a knife or a needle. A flexible bronchoscope or ultrasound can also be used to retract the ETT (Figure 7.1) and can assist with needle and guidewire placement if a percutaneous technique is being used. The ideal placement is midline and between the 2–4 tracheal ring spaces.

> **WARNING!!** Airway/ventilation can be lost by retracting the cuff past the glottic opening, or extubation can occur due to blindly retracting the ETT. You must be prepared to resecure the airway if it is lost at any point during retraction.

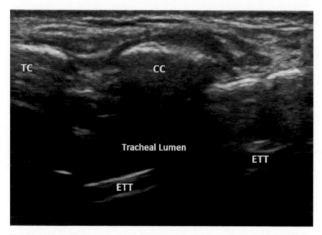

Figure 7.1 Sagittal image of anterior neck showing relevant sono-anatomy. The relation between the cartilages and tracheal rings can be seen. Orientating the probe in a transverse manner allows for scanning of blood vessels that may be encountered during a tracheostomy. TC: thyroid cartilage; CC: cricoid cartilage; ETT: endo-tracheal tube. Photo courtesy of author.

C. Management of Cuff Damage or Loss of ETT Cuff Pressure and Tidal Volume

If the cuff is damaged with initial tracheal access with needle or knife penetration, it can present as a decrease or loss of tidal volume and oxygen desaturation if there is a significant leak.

Step by Step

1. Immediately alert the surgeons to stop the procedure.

> **WARNING!!** You may have difficulty mask ventilating the patient in the event there is loss of the airway and there is a surgical incision in the neck/trachea. Have the surgical team occlude the surgical incision as best as possible and resecure the airway quickly.

2. If the cuff is ruptured, exchange the ETT.

Add air to the cuff to assess cuff integrity. If the cuff is ruptured, exchange the ETT via a bougie or remove and replace the ETT under direct vision via direct laryngoscopy or videolaryngoscopy.

>>**Tip on Technique:** ETT replacement should be with a smaller-size tube to prevent further glottic trauma.

3. If unable to replace the ETT, ensure adequate ventilation via bag-mask or place a supraglottic airway (SGA).

Provide mask ventilation with 100% oxygen. If unable to mask ventilate, place an SGA.

Caution! It may be difficult to resecure the airway via direct laryngoscopy. Ensure you are familiar with previous laryngoscopy attempts in case a new ETT is needed. In a patient with a known difficult airway, ensure that difficult airway equipment is readily available.

---

4. After replacement, pull back the ETT via laryngoscopy until the cuff is at the glottis.

Once the ETT is replaced and the patient is stable, tracheostomy placement can proceed.

D. Management of the Inability to Ventilate After Tracheostomy Insertion

Step by Step

1. Immediately alert the surgical team that you are unable to ventilate.

2. Check for malposition of the tracheostomy.

The most common cause of inability to ventilate after tracheostomy insertion is malposition of the tracheostomy (Figure 7.2). Confirm malposition by absence of capnography or via bronchoscopy (tracheostomy tube will not be visualized in the trachea). If the tracheostomy is malpositioned, remove it and go to step 3.

WARNING!! Do not attempt further positive pressure breaths via the tracheostomy while ensuring adequate anesthesia. Continuing positive pressure attempts with a malpositioned tracheostomy can cause a pneumothorax or subcutaneous emphysema.

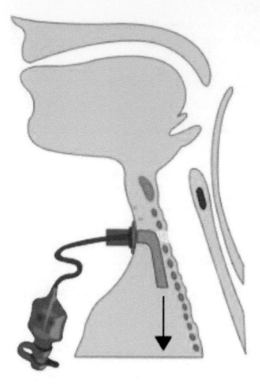

Figure 7.2 Malpositioned tracheostomy placement in a false track. Black arrow indicates airflow to the subcutaneous or pretracheal tissues. This may lead to anterior neck disfigurement from subcutaneous emphysema or a pneumothorax. With permission from the National Tracheostomy Safety Project, www.tracheostomy.org.uk.

3. Advance the preexisting ETT from its retracted position.

The preexisting ETT should be advanced from its retracted position past the insertion site until capnography is confirmed with adequate tidal volumes (Figure 7.3).

>> **Tip on Technique:** Know the position of the ETT tip. It should be at or above the cricoid cartilage. Hence, if the newly placed tracheostomy tube is malpositioned, advancing the ETT past the intended insertion site allows for ventilation (see Figure 7.3).

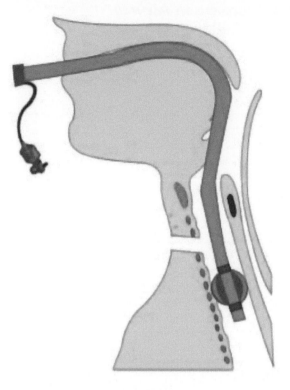

Figure 7.3 With any difficulty with tracheostomy tube insertion, remove the tube and advance the ETT past the insertion site to reestablish ventilation as demonstrated in the figure. With permission from the National Tracheostomy Safety Project, www.tracheostomy.org.uk.

4. If still unable to ventilate after advancing the ETT, perform bronchoscopy.

If ventilation is difficult or impossible after ETT advancement, consider either the presence of a pneumothorax or mainstem placement of the ETT. Bronchoscopy will confirm the location of the ETT. If the ETT is too deep, guide the ETT to a position just above the carina using the bronchoscope. Perform a chest x-ray to rule out pneumothorax.

!! **Potential Complication:** Not being able to advance the ETT in a malposition situation can result in loss of the airway. If the preexisting ETT cannot be advanced past the insertion site, bronchoscopy should be performed immediately.

5. Once ventilation is reestablished, reattempt tracheostomy placement.

Once ventilation is re-established, request that the surgical team reattempt insertion of the tracheostomy using bronchoscopic guidance via the ETT.

E. Management of Sudden Increase in Airway Pressure with Cardiovascular Collapse

Step by Step

1. Initiate cardiopulmonary resuscitation (CPR) and advanced cardiac life support (ACLS), if indicated.

> **WARNING!!**   Initiate CPR and ACLS immediately if the patient is in cardiac arrest regardless of the cause. Tension pneumothorax can quickly lead to cardiovascular collapse with delayed recognition and treatment. Deliver 100% oxygen and treat hemodynamics as needed.
>
> **WARNING!!**   Cease ventilation if subcutaneous emphysema develops with positive pressure.

2. Ensure proper positioning of the ETT and rule out pneumothorax.

Suspect a pneumothorax at any point in the procedure if loss of ventilation or increases in airway pressure occur. Ensure proper positioning of the existing ETT and confirm the diagnosis with a combination of auscultation, x-ray, and/or ultrasound and inform the surgical team of suspicion. Avoid further ventilation attempts until the pneumothorax is evacuated.

Note: Risk factors for pneumothorax during a tracheostomy include abnormal tracheal anatomy, short neck, chronic obstructive pulmonary disease, and difficult dissection to the anterior tracheal wall.

3. Perform needle thoracostomy (see Chapter 13 on tension pneumothorax for more details).

Have a low threshold for needle thoracostomy followed by chest tube insertion even if the diagnosis is not fully confirmed. Verify placement of the tracheostomy after chest tube insertion, since malposition could have contributed to the pneumothorax.

>> **Tip on Technique:** Needle decompression is only a temporizing measure and needs subsequent chest tube placement to ensure evacuation of a pneumothorax. Pretracheal fascia is continuous with the mediastinum; hence, the risk of pneumothorax and subcutaneous emphysema is always present with any tracheostomy.

!! **Potential Complication:** Further lung injury can be caused with both needle and tube thoracostomy by inexperienced hands.

F. Management of Bleeding During Dissection for Tracheostomy Placement

Step by Step

1. Maintain communication with surgeon and monitor surgical field for bleeding.

2. Maintain ventilation and hemodynamics.

Provide hemodynamic and respiratory support while the surgeon attempts surgical hemostasis with sutures or electrocautery. Control tachycardia/hypertension if it develops. Confirm adequate ventilation as a clot can potentially obstruct the airway.

> **WARNING!!** If cautery is needed for bleeding control, make sure to decrease FiO_2 to a minimum to maintain saturations >90% to decrease the risk of airway fire.
>
> **WARNING!!** With a percutaneous technique, if bleeding persists after application of pressure, surgical exploration may be required.

3. Perform anterior neck ultrasound.

Perform ultrasound to assess for aberrant vascular anatomy (Figure 7.4) and identify anterior neck vasculature.

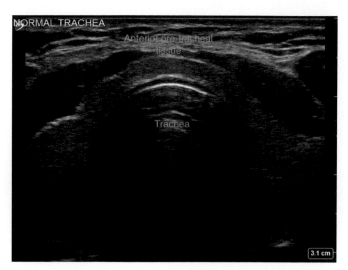

Figure 7.4 Scanning the trachea from the cricoid cartilage to the sternal notch in a transverse manner with ultrasound prior to incision will allow identification of any blood vessels in the anterior pretracheal tissue. This allows for identification of any aberrant vasculature that can lead to unexpected hemorrhage. Photo courtesy of author.

4. Ensure the patient is not coagulopathic.

Check coagulation factors and TEG and confirm the presence of type and screen or send one if necessary. With significant blood loss, assume an artery may have been lacerated and transfusion may be required.

5. Perform bronchoscopy after bleeding is controlled.

With excessive bleeding, after the source is controlled, bronchoscopic exploration should be performed to clean the distal airways and remove any clots if found.

!! **Potential Complication:** Significant bleeding into the airway can lead to airway plugging and inability to adequately oxygenate and ventilate the patient. In a patient with a short neck, tracheostomy insertion below the fourth tracheal ring increases the risk of innominate artery injury.

Section 2—Complications in Patients with a Preexisting Tracheostomy

The following complications will be discussed step by step:

G. Identifying whether the patient has a tracheostomy or a laryngectomy stoma

H. Management of the inability to ventilate via an existing tracheostomy

I. Management of accidental decannulation of a preexisting tracheostomy

> **WARNING!!** It is essential to know how old the tracheostomy is. For open-approach tracheostomies the tract is considered mature at 4 days. For percutaneous approaches the recommendation is 7–10 days. The definition may vary among institutions.

Pearl: All fresh tracheostomy patients should have a warning sign in their room indicating "difficult airway" for at least 7 days to prevent any accidental decannulation with unnecessary manipulation.

G. Identifying Whether the Patient Has a Tracheostomy or a Laryngectomy Stoma

Step by Step

1. Determine if the patient has a laryngectomy stoma or a tracheostomy.

It is important not to confuse a laryngectomy stoma with a temporary or permanent tracheal stoma. The former is present in patients after a laryngectomy. There is no longer a connection from the naso- or oropharynx with the glottis (Figure 7.5). Always inquire when a stoma is encountered to determine if it is a permanent laryngectomy stoma or a tracheostomy stoma.

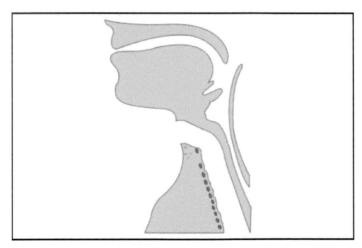

Figure 7.5 Laryngectomy. Notice there is NO connection between the glottis and pharynx. With permission from the National Tracheostomy Safety Project, www.tracheostomy.org.uk.

For laryngectomy stomas, an ETT can be passed into the stoma for ventilation.

> **Caution!** The only way to ventilate laryngectomy patients is through the stoma. Laryngoscopy should not be attempted.

2. If a tracheostomy is present, identify the tracheostomy type.

Identify the type (cuffed versus uncuffed, fenestrated versus nonfenestrated; Figure 7.6) and the age of the tracheostomy (determines how mature the track is). If the tracheostomy is 5 days old or less, ensure that it is sutured in place and has trach ties for securement.

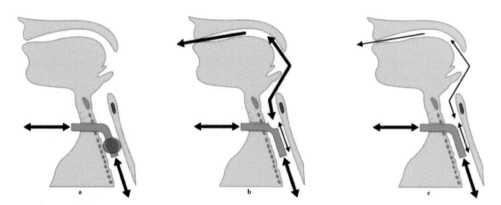

Figure 7.6 Airflow patterns shown in black arrows with different types of tracheostomy tubes. A: Nonfenestrated cuffed. B: Fenestrated and uncuffed. C: Nonfenestrated and uncuffed. With permission from the National Tracheostomy Safety Project, www.tracheostomy.org.uk.

3. Confirm that the inner cannula can connect to the anesthesia circuit and maintain positive pressure ventilation (PPV).

If the procedure requires paralysis, a cuffed nonfenestrated tube will be needed. It may be difficult to reliably deliver PPV via an uncuffed tube. Suction the tracheostomy and clean/replace the inner cannula prior to OR transport if needed. For transport have an extra tracheostomy kit of similar size and a 6.0 ETT in case the current tube is dislodged.

>> **Tip on Technique:** If tracheostomy exchange is needed to be compatible with the anesthesia circuit, there are two options. If the patient is spontaneously breathing and not tracheostomy dependent, bedside exchange for a cuffed tracheostomy is an option if the site is mature (older than 7 days). For tracheostomy-dependent patients (older than 7 days), tracheostomy exchange in the OR is recommended. Ensure adequate muscle relaxation prior to exchange.

!! **Potential Complication:** Mucous occlusion of the inner cannula or bleeding during tracheostomy exchange can occur.

> **WARNING!!** Ensure the tracheostomy is patent and there are no signs of increasing peak ventilatory pressure suggesting tube obstruction, which is most commonly from secretions. There is a significant difference between a mature (>7 days old) and immature stoma/tracheostomy. If a fresh tracheostomy is dislodged, there is high risk for inability to replace it or creation of a false passage with blind reinsertion.

H. Management of the Inability to Ventilate via an Existing Tracheostomy

Step by Step

1. Inform the surgeons to halt the current operation and avoid further positive pressure breaths.

Immediately alert the surgeons that there is an issue with ventilation and proceed to steps 2 and 3.

2. Deflate the tracheal tube cuff (if present) and remove the inner cannula to assess for obstruction.

Attempt gentle ventilation after removal of the inner cannula. If this was not the source of the obstruction and ventilation is still not adequate, go immediately to step 3.

3. Provide oxygenation via the upper airway while occluding the tracheostomy tube.

Deliver 100% oxygen via the upper airway. Occlude the tracheostomy tube site to prevent a leak. If unable to ventilate from above, insert a supraglottic airway or attempt laryngoscopy. Knowing previous successful laryngoscopy attempts can be useful.

> **Caution!** Patients with laryngectomies no longer have upper airway patency (see Figure 7.5). The only way to ventilate is through their stoma. Fresh laryngectomies usually have a transparent tube within them. Pass a suction catheter to clean any occlusion. An ETT can also be placed inside the stoma to establish ventilation with persistent obstruction.

4. Once ventilation is reestablished, insert a suction catheter through the tracheostomy to assess for tube occlusion.

If a suction catheter passes, suspect partial occlusion. If the catheter is unable to pass, suspect complete occlusion or decannulation and remove the tracheostomy tube and inspect the stoma for occluding sources. A bronchoscope can also be inserted through the stoma to assess the track for patency. If bronchoscopy is not available and the tracheostomy is more than 7 days old, insert a bougie through the existing stoma and reinsert a new tube over it. Reconfirm adequate ventilation via the new tube with capnography to ensure proper placement.

‼ **Potential Complication:** If capnography is not seen with initial ventilation, do not keep providing positive pressure since the tube may be in a false track (see Figure 7.2) and can cause a pneumothorax.

I. Management of Accidental Decannulation of Preexisting Tracheostomy

Step by Step

1. Inform surgeons and halt the operation.

Immediately alert the surgeons that there is an issue with ventilation and that the tracheostomy may have been dislodged.

2. Provide oxygenation via the upper airway.

Deliver 100% oxygen via the upper airway.

>>**Tip on Technique:** If unable to provide ventilation via the upper airway, cover the stoma with either an SGA or pediatric facemask to ventilate.

3. If the tracheostomy is older than 7 days, reinsert the tracheostomy blindly with or without the use of a guidance tool (e.g., obturator or bougie).

> **Caution!** Do not reinsert tracheostomy tube blindly if tract is <7 days old. Instead, provide oxygenation above the glottis via SGA or another adjunct airway device.

4. If unable to ventilate from above or reinsert tracheostomy, insert SGA or attempt laryngoscopy.

Knowing previous successful laryngoscopy attempts can be useful. With reestablishment of ventilation, inform the surgical team that the tracheostomy site may need exploration prior to reinsertion.

!! **Potential Complication:** Respiratory arrest can occur from delayed reestablishment of the airway.

>>**Tip on Technique:** Consider placing a flexible bronchoscope through the newly placed ETT from above to guide reinsertion of the tracheostomy into the correct position. The bronchoscope can also be placed through the stoma and track to ensure patency and for possible reinsertion of tracheostomy tube.

>> **Tip on Technique:** Always carry a bougie or tracheal obturator while dealing with patients with preexisting tracheostomies. Similar-sized and smaller-sized extra tracheostomy tubes should also be available for transport.

Other Management Considerations

Many ICU patients have percutaneous tracheostomies performed at the bedside without anesthesia providers. Yet, in patients with known difficult airways, an anesthesia provider may be consulted. Unlike the controlled OR setting, the ICU has many variables beyond the control of the anesthesia provider. Limitation of space, unfamiliarity of staff, and equipment variation are some examples. When performing the procedure at the bedside, it is paramount to plan ahead and communicate with all the members to identify their roles and how best they can assist you. It is also prudent to bring your own airway equipment and medication if possible.

Potential for airway loss remains a threat with all tracheostomy-dependent patients. Long-term complications include bleeding and tracheal stenosis. If a patient remains dependent on a tracheostomy and mechanical ventilation for over a week, the risk of cuff erosion and fistula formation increases. A trach-innominate fistula is the most feared complication with chronic tracheostomies. It usually presents with a sentinel bleed (approximately 10 ml of bright red blood). The bleeding is copious and requires emergent tamponade with surgical control. It is important to assess all tracheostomy patients for bleeding before proceeding to the OR for any procedure.

Subglottic stenosis is a known complication of any tracheostomy regardless of the length of insertion. Any patient who previously had a tracheostomy can be at risk for subglottic stenosis. The preoperative airway exam should note if there is a history of a tracheostomy and comment on the reason for placement and duration. Regardless of their upper airway exam, a regular-sized ETT may be difficult to insert if subglottic stenosis is present. Always have smaller-sized ETT tubes available for elective procedures involving previous tracheostomy patients.

Further Reading

National Tracheostomy Safety Project: http://www.tracheostomy.org.uk/
An indispensable resource for all matters related to tracheostomy care and management. Provides free informatics regarding routine and emergent care of tracheostomies and permanent laryngeal stomas.

References

1. Cipriano A, Mao ML, Hon HH, et al. An overview of complications associated with open and percutaneous tracheostomy procedures. *Int J Crit Illn Inj Sci*. 2015;5(3):179–188. doi:10.4103/2229-5151.164994.
2. Huang H, Li Y, Ariani F, Chen X, Lin J. Timing of tracheostomy in critically ill patients: a meta-analysis. Salluh JIF, ed. *PLoS ONE*. 2014;9(3):e92981. doi:10.1371/journal.pone.0092981.
3. Simon M, Metschke M, Braune SA, Püschel K, Kluge S. Death after percutaneous dilatational tracheostomy: a systematic review and analysis of risk factors. *Crit Care*. 2013 Oct 29;17(5):R258. doi:10.1186/cc13085.
4. Ziyaeifard M, Totonchi Z. Real-time ultrasound guided the new standard technique for percutaneous dilatational tracheostomy (PDT). *Anesth Pain Med*. 2015 Jun 22;5(3):e24653. doi:10.5812/aapm.24653v2.

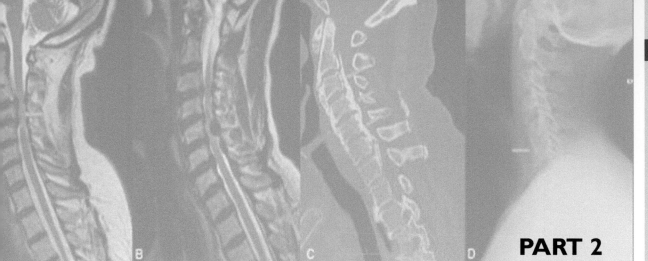

PART 2

CARDIAC

Chapter 8

Arrhythmias

Loren R. Francis and Eric W. Nelson

Summary Page

Symptoms:

- Low heart rate
- High heart rate
- Hypotension
- Chest pain
- Dizziness
- Fainting
- Sweating

Differential Diagnosis:

- Sinus bradycardia
- First-degree atrioventricular (AV) block
- Second-degree AV block
  - Type I Wenckebach
  - Type II
- Third-degree AV block
- Sinus tachycardia
- Atrial tachycardia
- Atrial fibrillation
- Atrial flutter
- Ventricular tachycardia
- Ventricular fibrillation

Introduction

Arrhythmias are a common perioperative complication. How a patient tolerates an arrhythmia depends on the heart rate, how long the arrhythmia lasts, and if the patient has coexisting cardiac disease. Arrhythmias may present as a previously known comorbidity or as a new condition. They may be the result of inadequate anesthesia, a surgical cause, or a myocardial abnormality. Some arrhythmias, such as certain bradycardias, heart block, and atrial arrhythmias, do not require immediate treatment if the patient is hemodynamically stable. On the other hand, there are arrhythmias that cause hemodynamic instability and require urgent intervention with medication, electrical and mechanical support, or advanced cardiac life support (ACLS). It is important as an anesthesiologist to quickly diagnose, identify the cause, and treat any arrhythmia that may occur during the perioperative period.

Arrhythmias occur in the perioperative period most commonly in patients who already have underlying heart disease. Electrolyte and acid-base disorders predispose patients to arrhythmias in the perioperative period. Patients undergoing endocrine surgery may be at risk for arrhythmias due to thyrotoxicosis or pheochromocytoma. Intracranial bleeds may also put a patient at risk for an arrhythmia due to mass effect.

In the intraoperative period, factors such as hypoxemia, hypercarbia, and hypothermia may all predispose a patient to an arrhythmia. Volatile anesthetics also can lead to arrhythmias, as can an inadequate depth of anesthesia. Surgical factors predisposing to arrhythmias include peritoneal traction, carotid sinus stimulation, extraocular muscle movement, and direct mechanical stimulation of the heart. While most arrhythmias seen perioperatively are self-limiting or benign in nature, tachyarrhythmias can lead to increased myocardial oxygen demand and hypotension.

A stable ventricular tachycardia may also degrade into an unstable ventricular tachycardia or ventricular fibrillation.

When treating an arrhythmia, always try to find and correct the underlying cause of the arrhythmia. Comorbidities such as chronic obstructive pulmonary disease, hypoxia, coronary artery disease, myocardial ischemia, mitral valve disease, pericardial disease, hyperthyroidism, sepsis, electrolyte imbalances, and drug use can precipitate atrial arrhythmias. Atrial fibrillation is the most common cardiac arrhythmia and is often a complication of cardiac surgery.

Bradyarrhythmias and tachyarrhythmias will be discussed separately.

Bradyarrhythmias

Treatment

WARNING!! For any of the following arrhythmias, if the patient is hemodynamically unstable, call for help and begin ACLS immediately.[1]

For diagnosis and management of bradyarrhythmias, first determine which type of bradyarrhythmia is present (Table 8.1):

Table 8.1 **Types of Bradyarrhythmias**

Bradyarrhythmia Type	ECG Findings	Section
Sinus Bradycardia	HR < 60 bpm	Go to Section A
First-Degree AV Block	P-R interval > 200 ms	Go to Section B
Second-Degree AV block	Progressive P-R prolongation with a dropped beat (Type 1) Constant P-R interval with a dropped beat (Type 2)	Go to Section C
Third-Degree AV Block	Regular P waves and QRS complexes with two separate and different rates	Go to Section D

A. Diagnosis and Treatment of Sinus Bradycardia

1. Evaluate vital signs for hemodynamic instability.

> **WARNING!!** If the patient is hemodynamically unstable, call for help and begin ACLS.

Sinus bradycardia is defined as heart rate <60 beats per minute (bpm) (Figure 8.1).

If the patient is hemodynamically stable, correct any identifiable, underlying causes while ruling out ischemia. Consider cancelling surgery for further workup if the arrhythmia is new.

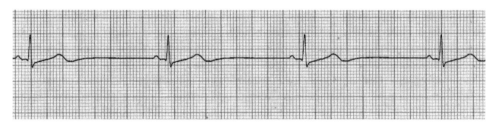

Figure 8.1 Sinus bradycardia. Source: litfl.com with permission.

2. Treat with medications or pacing if necessary.

Titrate glycopyrrolate to heart rate (0.2–1 mg IV) if necessary. If the bradycardia is refractory, consider atropine (0.5–1mg IV).

If the bradycardia is refractory to other measures and the patient becomes hemodynamically unstable, begin ACLS. Transcutaneous pacing via a defibrillator or placement of a transvenous pacer wire may be necessary.

>> **Tip on Technique**: Transcutaneous pacing is simple and quickly achieved via a defibrillator and defibrillation pads. Transvenous pacing wires may be placed via a venous introducer. The internal jugular vein is typically the most convenient; however, a subclavian approach may also be used.

> **WARNING!!** Patients often require deep sedation or general anesthesia for transcutaneous pacing due to discomfort.

3. Treat the underlying cause.

Causes of sinus bradycardia include vagal stimulation, abdominal insufflation, perioperative myocardial infarction, undersensing, and pacemaker dysfunction in patients with an internal pacemaker.

B. Diagnosis and Treatment of First-Degree Atrioventricular Block

First-degree atrioventricular (AV) block presents with a P-R interval >200 ms (Figure 8.2).[2] Usually no treatment is necessary, but if the P-R interval is >300 ms, patients may become symptomatic. Patients with first-degree block may also become symptomatic with exercise or surgical stress as the P-R interval does not shorten along with R-R interval shortening with increasing heart rate.

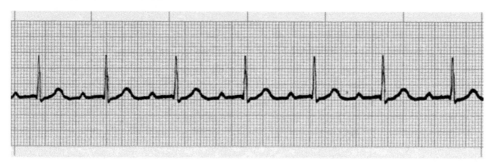

Figure 8.2 First-degree block. Source: litfl.com with permission.

C. Diagnosis and Treatment of Second-Degree Atrioventricular Block

1. Determine whether the second-degree AV block is Mobitz Type 1 (Wenkebach) or Mobitz Type 2.

Mobitz Type 1 AV block (Wenkebach) is defined as a progressive P-R prolongation with a dropped beat (Figure 8.3) and often does not require treatment.[2]

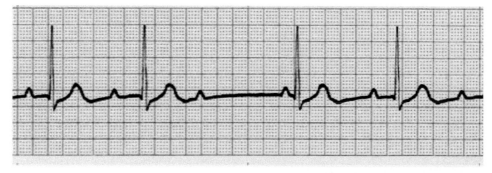

Figure 8.3 Type 1 second-degree block Wenckebach. Source: litfl.com with permission.

Mobitz Type 2 second-degree AV block is defined as a constant P-R interval with a dropped beat (Figure 8.4). This arrhythmia may lead to complete heart block and if so is an indication for permanent pacemaker placement. If it occurs intraoperatively, transcutaneous or transvenous pacing may be necessary if the patient is unstable.

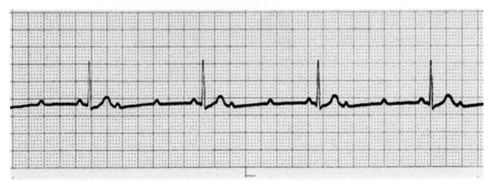

Figure 8.4 Type 2 second-degree block. Source: litfl.com with permission.

>> **Tip on Technique:** Looking for regular P-P intervals and irregular R-R intervals can aid in the diagnosis of Type 1 versus Type 2 block.

D. Diagnosis and Treatment of Third-Degree Atrioventricular Block

1. Evaluate vital signs for hemodynamic instability.

WARNING!! If the patient is hemodynamically unstable, call for help and begin ACLS.

Regular P waves and QRS complexes are seen with third-degree AV block, but they have two separate and different rates (Figure 8.5). This arrhythmia is also known as complete heart block, in which the atria and ventricle are electrically separated from one another.

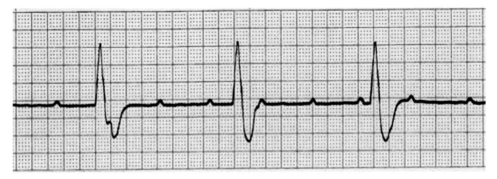

Figure 8.5 Third-degree block. Source: litfl.com with permission.

2. Treat the underlying cause and consider pacing, if needed.

If the patient is hemodynamically stable, correct any identifiable, underlying causes while ruling out ischemia. Consider cancelling surgery for further workup if the arrhythmia is new.

> **WARNING!!**   Patients with complete heart block often require pacing support.

!! Potential Complication: Hypotension can occur due to AV desynchrony.

Tachyarrhythmias

> **WARNING!!**   For any of the following arrhythmias, if the patient is hemodynamically unstable, call for help and begin ACLS immediately.

For all of the tachyarrhythmias described below, if the patient is hemodynamically stable, then correct any identifiable, underlying causes while ruling out ischemia. Consider cancelling surgery for further workup if the arrhythmia is new.

For diagnosis and management, first determine which type of tachyarrhythmia is present (Table 8.2):

Table 8.2 **Types of Tachyarrhythmias**

Tachyarrhythmia Type	ECG Findings	Section
Sinus Tachycardia	HR 100–160 bpm	Go to Section E
Supraventricular Tachycardia	Regular but abnormally fast atrial rate of 150–250 bpm	Go to Section F
Atrial Flutter	Rapid regular atrial depolarizations at a rate of 250–300 bpm with regularly conducted ventricular beats, usually at an even ratio like 2:1 or 4:1	Go to Section G
Atrial Fibrillation	Irregularly irregular pulse with a rate of 400–600 times/min	Go to Section H
Ventricular Premature Beats	QRS > 120 ms and altered morphology followed by a compensatory pause	Go to Section I

Treatment

E. Diagnosis and Treatment of Sinus Tachycardia

1. Evaluate vital signs for hemodynamic instability and diagnose rhythm as sinus tachycardia.

> **WARNING!!**   If hemodynamically unstable, call for help and begin ACLS.

Sinus tachycardia presents with a heart rate in the range of 100–160 bpm (Figure 8.6).

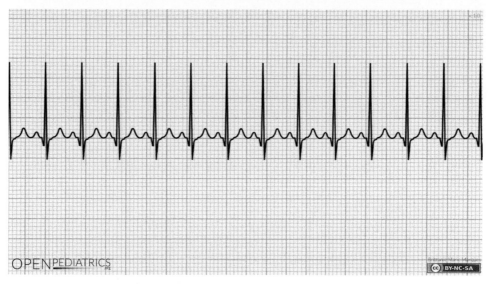

Figure 8.6 Sinus tachycardia. Source: litfl.com with permission.

>> **Tip on Technique:** An electrocardiogram (ECG) will show P waves with normal morphology preceding each QRS, a fixed P-R interval, and a shortened QT interval.[2]

2. Treat with medications if needed.

Sinus tachycardia is generally well tolerated, but be vigilant for signs and symptoms of myocardial ischemia. If present, administer a beta blocker such as metoprolol 2.5–5 mg IV until tachycardia resolves.[3]

!! **Potential Complication:** Sinus tachycardia causes increased myocardial oxygen demand and can precipitate myocardial ischemia in patients with coronary artery disease.

WARNING!! Sinus tachycardia allows less time in diastole, which can decrease cardiac filling, decrease cardiac output, and decrease peripheral perfusion. Decreased diastolic time also decreases time for coronary perfusion, potentially worsening myocardial ischemia.

---

3. Treat underlying causes.

Consider differential diagnoses for sinus tachycardia:

- General: anxiety, pain, stress, anemia
- Cardiac: myocardial ischemia, heart failure, cardiogenic shock, pericarditis
- Pulmonary: respiratory distress, pulmonary embolism
- Infectious: fever, sepsis
- Endocrine: hyperthyroidism
- Drug related: adrenergic drugs, caffeine, alcohol, illicit drugs

Offer pain relief and supplemental oxygen as needed, and provide a relaxed environment.

F. Diagnosis and Treatment of Supraventricular Tachycardia

1. Evaluate vital signs for hemodynamic instability.

> **WARNING!!** If patient is hemodynamically unstable, call for help and begin ACLS. Go IMMEDIATELY to step 2.

Supraventricular tachycardia (SVT) on ECG will show a regular but abnormally fast atrial rate from 150 to 250 bpm. The P wave might be hidden by the preceding T wave if the heart rate is very fast (Figure 8.7). Conduction to the ventricles can vary. Symptoms may include shortness of breath, palpitations, dizziness, sweating, and fainting.

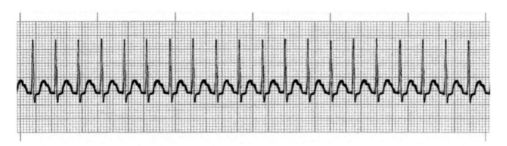

Figure 8.7 Supraventricular tachycardia. Source: litfl.com with permission.

!! **Potential Complication:** Decreased time for diastole impairs ventricular filling and increased heart rate increases myocardial oxygen consumption, which can cause angina, heart failure, and myocardial ischemia.

2. PROCEED DIRECTLY TO DEFIBRILLATION OR ELECTRICAL CARDIOVERSION IF PATIENT IS UNSTABLE.

Perform defibrillation (200 biphasic) or synchronized cardioversion (120J biphasic, increasing output if necessary) depending on the stability and vital signs of the patient.

3. Consider maneuvers to abort the SVT.

Potential maneuvers include:

- Valsalva maneuver: a moderately forceful attempted exhalation against a closed airway
- Carotid sinus massage: find the place on the patient's neck approximately 4 cm caudad to the angle of the jaw on each side and press firmly for 5–10 seconds
- Drug therapy:
  - Adenosine 6 mg IV, repeat with 12 mg IV if rhythm doesn't convert
  - Verapamil 0.075–0.015 mg/kg IV over 2 minutes
  - Diltiazem 0.25 mg/kg IV
- Synchronized cardioversion (120J biphasic, increasing output if necessary), or defibrillation (200 biphasic) if patient becomes hemodynamically unstable

> **Caution!** Administration of adenosine can cause a short systolic pause.

> **Caution!** Carotid sinus massage should not be used in elderly patients or those with known carotid disease. Risks of carotid sinus massage include stroke, reflex bradycardia, and ventricular arrhythmias.[2]

4. Consider differential diagnosis and correct any reversible causes.

Causes may include:

- Use of caffeine, stimulants (cocaine, methamphetamine), marijuana, medications (asthma medications, cold and allergy medications)
- Electrolyte imbalance, hypoxia, stress, lack of sleep
- Myocardial infarction, cardiomyopathy, valvular heart disease
- Wolff-Parkinson-White syndrome
- Digoxin toxicity

G. Diagnosis and Treatment of Atrial Flutter

1. Evaluate vital signs for hemodynamic instability.

> **WARNING!!** If hemodynamically unstable, call for help and begin ACLS. Go IMMEDIATELY to step 2.

Atrial flutter presents as rapid regular atrial depolarizations at a rate of 250–300 bpm with regularly conducted ventricular beats, usually at an even ratio like 2:1 or 4:1, so the pulse may feel normal (Figure 8.8). Symptoms include palpitations, shortness of breath, fatigue, and dizziness.

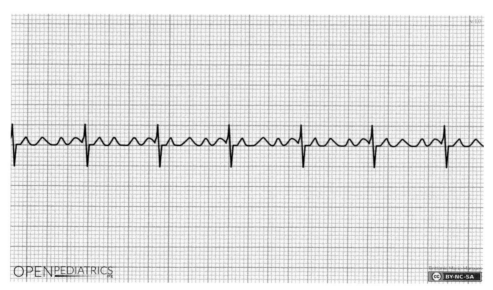

Figure 8.8 Atrial flutter. Source: litfl.com with permission.

>> **Tip on Technique:** ECG will show atrial activity in a sawtooth P wave pattern. This arrhythmia originates from a single atrial focus with circuit reentry.

2. PROCEED DIRECTLY TO ELECTRICAL CARDIOVERSION IF PATIENT IS UNSTABLE.

Perform synchronized cardioversion at 120J biphasic (increase if necessary), synchronized to the R wave of the QRS complex. Repeat as needed.

> **Caution!** The faster the ventricular rate, the more dangerous the arrhythmia.

3. Control the ventricular rate and convert to sinus rhythm.

The goals are to control the ventricular rate and convert to normal sinus rhythm. This can be accomplished with diltiazem 0.25 mg/kg IV followed by infusion at 5–15 mg/hour (to control rate) and/or synchronized cardioversion as described above in step 2.

Other medications can also be given to control rate and rhythm:

- Ibutilide 1 mg IV over 10 minutes[3]
- Procainamide 100 mg slowly IV until arrhythmia is suppressed: infuse 2–6 mg/min to a maximum total dosage of 17 mg/kg[3]

> **Caution!** Avoid procainamide in patients with AV block, thrombocytopenia, or myasthenia gravis.

It is important to maintain sinus rhythm to prevent thrombus and embolism. Radiofrequency catheter ablation may be required if other treatments are unsuccessful.

Prolonged atrial flutter requires anticoagulation.

> **WARNING!!** There is a risk of thrombus formation in the left atrium and left atrial appendage with a subsequently increased risk of embolization and stroke. If the patient has been in atrial flutter for more than 48 hours, cardioversion is contraindicated unless the patient has been adequately anticoagulated.

H. Diagnosis and Treatment of Atrial Fibrillation

1. Evaluate vital signs for hemodynamic instability.

> **WARNING!!** If hemodynamically unstable, call for help and begin ACLS. Go IMMEDIATELY to step 2.

Atrial fibrillation presents as an irregularly irregular pulse with ectopic impulses in the atria that fire at a rate of 400–600 times/min causing the atria to quiver instead of contracting.[2] Symptoms include palpitations, weakness, fatigue, and shortness of breath. Determine the ventricular rate, as a ventricular response >100 bpm is considered uncontrolled.

>> **Tip on Technique:** ECG will show irregularly irregular QRS complexes without distinct P waves.

2. PROCEED DIRECTLY TO ELECTRICAL CARDIOVERSION IF PATIENT IS UNSTABLE.

Perform synchronized electrical cardioversion (120J biphasic, higher if this does not work), synchronized to the R wave of the QRS complex.

3. Control rate and convert to sinus rhythm.

Monitor blood pressure carefully, ideally with an arterial line.

Rate control is viewed as more important than maintaining sinus rhythm. The goal is to keep the ventricular rate <100 bpm. Medication options for rate control include:

- Diltiazem 0.25 mg/kg IV followed by infusion at 5–15 mg/hr
- Esmolol 500 mcg/kg IV bolus followed by 50 mcg/kg/min infusion
- Metoprolol 2.5–5 mg IV bolus
- Amiodarone 150 mg IV

Convert to sinus rhythm with either electrical cardioversion (see step 2) or pharmacologic cardioversion: ibutilide 1 mg IV over 10 minutes, can repeat once.

WARNING!!   Though ibutilide is the best agent available for acute cardioversion of atrial fibrillation, it has a 4% risk of causing torsades de pointes.[3]

!! Potential Complication: Cardiac output is reduced with a lack of atrial kick and there is an increased risk of thrombus formation in the left atrium and left atrial appendage.

Caution!   If the patient has been in atrial fibrillation for longer than 48 hours, cardioversion is contraindicated unless the patient has been adequately anticoagulated to minimize risk of embolization.

---

4. Correct underlying causes and rule out ischemia.

Once the patient is hemodynamically stable, correct any identifiable, underlying causes while ruling out ischemia. Consider cancelling surgery for further workup if the arrhythmia is new.

I. Diagnosis and Treatment of Ventricular Premature Beats

1. Evaluate vital signs for hemodynamic instability.

WARNING!!   Ventricular premature beats (VPBs) can lead to more serious arrhythmias such as ventricular tachycardia or ventricular fibrillation.

VPBs are commonly seen in routine ECGs, with QRS >120 ms and altered morphology followed by a compensatory pause.[4] They may result in an irregular pulse if frequent. The heart beat associated with a VPB may be weaker than a normal heart beat.

2. If symptomatic, consider pharmacologic treatment to offer relief.

Pharmacologic treatments can include:

- Beta blockers
- Calcium channel blockers

- Procainamide
  - Inject 100 mg slowly IV until arrhythmia is suppressed
  - Infuse 2–6 mg/min
  - Maximum total dosage is 17 mg/kg[3]
- Amiodarone
  - Give 150 mg IV over 5 minutes, followed by
  - Infusion of 1 mg/min × 6 hours, followed by
  - 0.5 mg/min × 18 hours
  - 800–1600 mg PO daily in divided doses[3]
- Lidocaine
  - Administer 1–1.5 mg/kg as an IV bolus
  - Can repeat every 5 minutes up to 300 mg total in 1 hour
  - IV infusion to follow at 1–4 mg/min[3]

Caution! Avoid procainamide in patients with AV block, thrombocytopenia, or myasthenia gravis.

Caution! Long-term oral therapy with amiodarone can cause bradycardia, heart block, pulmonary fibrosis, thyroid dysfunction, or elevated liver function tests.

Caution! Watch out for development of seizures as that may indicate lidocaine toxicity.

Other Management Considerations

Patients with internal pacemakers and/or defibrillators should be allotted special consideration. If there is concern for electromagnetic interference during the procedure (such as monopolar cautery above the umbilicus), the pacemaker should be placed in an asynchronous mode to avoid undersensing and the implantable cardioverter-defibrillator (ICD) should be disabled to prevent oversensing.

Pacemakers should be interrogated within 12 months and defibrillators within 6 months prior to surgery. It is important to note if the patient is pacemaker dependent and has had any recently treated tachytherapies. It is also important to note whether electromagnetic interference such as monopolar electrocautery will be used above the umbilicus during surgery. If so, pacemaker-dependent patients should have their devices reprogrammed to an asynchronous mode and ICDs should be programmed off or a magnet placed over the ICD to disable tachytherapies.

>> **Tip on Technique**: If using a magnet on an ICD, take the magnet off so the patient's ICD may respond appropriately if necessary to the diagnosed arrhythmia. If a patient is pacemaker dependent and becomes bradycardic, ascertain that electromagnetic interference isn't causing pauses in the pacemaker.

Standard American Society for Anesthesiologists (ASA) monitors are required for patients with an implantable pacemaker or ICD; however, invasive monitoring is not indicated unless the surgery or the patient dictates. It is imperative to turn a patient's device back to its original settings postoperatively and to monitor the patient continuously if their ICD tachytherapies are programmed off, until they are programmed back on again.

Any symptomatic bradyarrhythmia is a primary indication for permanent pacing. Both Mobitz Type 2 and third-degree heart block are primary indications for permanent pacing regardless of symptoms.

Further Reading

Cheng A, et al. Cardiac electrophysiology: Diagnosis and treatment. In: Kaplan MD, Joel A, Reich MD, David L, Savino, Joseph S, Kaplan's Cardiac Anesthesia: The Echo Era: Expert Consult Premium. 6th ed. St. Louis, Missouri: Elsevier; 2011: 74–95.

References

1. Panchal AR, et al. Part 3: Adult Basic and Advanced Life Support: 2020 American Heart Association Guidelines for Cardiopulmonary Resuscitation and Emergency Cardiovascular Care. Circulation. 2020; 142(16_suppl_2): S366–S468.
2. Coviello JS. *ECG interpretation made incredibly easy!* Lippincott Williams Wilkins; 2016.
3. Marino PL. *Marino's the ICU book.* Lippincott Williams Wilkins; 2015.
4. Manolis AS. Ventricular premature beats. https://www.uptodate.com/contents/ventricu lar-premature-beats?topicRef=961&source=see_link. Updated 2018. Accessed 09/22/18.

Chapter 9

Cardiac Tamponade

Matthew M. Andoniadis

Summary Page

Symptoms:

- Dyspnea
- Tachypnea
- Cough
- Chest pain
- Nausea
- Dysphagia
- Fatigue
- Tachycardia
- Hypotension
- Diaphoresis
- Syncope
- Mental status changes
- Cyanosis
- Pulsus paradoxus
- Elevated jugular venous pressure with jugular venous distension
- Muffled heart sounds
- Peripheral edema

Differential Diagnosis:

- Myocardial infarction
- Valvular heart disease
- Aortic dissection
- Pneumothorax
- Septic shock
- Cardiogenic or neurogenic shock
- Congestive heart failure
- Constrictive pericarditis
- Pulmonary embolism
- Hypoxemia

Introduction

Cardiac tamponade may occur insidiously or suddenly. Acute tamponade can be induced from postcardiac surgical bleeding, chest trauma, myocardial infarction, myocardial wall rupture, or aortic dissection. Chronic causes of cardiac tamponade may be secondary to pericarditis caused by bacterial, fungal, or viral infections; autoimmune and connective tissue diseases; malignancy; hypothyroidism; uremia; and Still disease (a multisystem inflammatory disorder).[1] Acute iatrogenic causes are numerous and include interventional cardiology procedures, electrophysiological procedures, transcatheter valve replacements, central line and chest tube insertion mishaps, and pacemaker and implantable cardioverter-defibrillator lead manipulations. Pneumopericardium may also result in cardiac tamponade.[2] Post–cardiac surgery, large pericardial effusions are more common after valve surgery and are commonly associated with anticoagulation. A high index of suspicion is crucial to allow for prompt diagnosis and treatment. Hemopericardium secondary to iatrogenic causes has increased in frequency as more cardiac interventional procedures are performed each year. Worldwide, the most common causes of pericardial tamponade are infectious.

Specific comorbidities that may complicate the treatment of a patient with cardiac tamponade may include extremes of age, preexisting pulmonary disease, pulmonary hypertension, morbid obesity, difficult airway, coagulopathy, and preexisting low cardiac output states.

Table 9.1 summarizes the various causes of cardiac tamponade.

Cardiac tamponade should be considered in any patient who suddenly complains of dyspnea and orthopnea accompanied by physical examination findings of hypotension, jugular venous distension (JVD), and muffled heart sounds, which is also known as Beck's Triad. Tachycardia, altered mental status, and pulsus paradoxus frequently are associated signs of cardiac tamponade.[3,4] Transthoracic echocardiography (TTE) will confirm the diagnosis by visualizing pericardial fluid and abnormal right ventricular diastolic wall motion.[5] Emergent drainage in these patients is via a surgical pericardial window or echocardiographic catheter pericardiocentesis. The anesthetic management of a patient with cardiac tamponade physiology varies from being prepared for a hemodynamically unstable orthopneic patient who can only tolerate local anesthetic and vocal support to administering a full general anesthetic with the placement of a double-lumen endotracheal tube, one-lung ventilation, and transesophageal echocardiography (TEE) guidance to a loculated pericardial fluid collection. The most severe anesthetic management error fails to recognize an acute tamponade and proceeds to routine general anesthesia induction, leading to hemodynamic collapse. Determining which anesthetic plan will be required is accomplished by performing a timely and thorough preoperative evaluation and discussing the surgical and anesthetic management with the cardiovascular surgical attending.

Table 9.1 Etiology of Cardiac Tamponade

Common Acute Causes
Idiopathic
Malignancy, neoplasm
Post-op cardiac surgery, mediastinal hemorrhage
Hemopericardium
Iatrogenic (interventional cardiology, electrophysiological ablation, transcatheter valve replacement, central line, chest tube, pacemaker and implantable cardioverter-defibrillator procedures)
Uncommon Acute Causes
Chest trauma
Myocardial infarction
Myocardial wall rupture
Aortic dissection
Pneumopericardium
Purulent pericarditis
Common Chronic Causes
Pericarditis
TB in developing countries
Uremia
Uncommon Chronic Causes
Fungal infection
Bacterial infection in developed countries
Viral infection
Still disease
Collagen vascular diseases (systemic lupus erythematosus, rheumatoid arthritis, Sjogren's and scleroderma)
Post radiation
Hypothyroidism
Chylopericardium

Management

This case ideally should be covered by anesthesiologists trained in cardiac anesthesia, with a perfusionist present in the operating room (OR) in case cardiopulmonary bypass is needed. However, for patients in extremis, any available anesthesiologist may provide supportive care for an emergent pericardiocentesis. A routine general anesthesia set up to include medications to treat hemodynamics should be sufficient.

Step by Step

1. Evaluate the patient and determine if tamponade is acute versus chronic.

The normal pericardium holds up to 50 ml of serous fluid. Chronic pericardial effusions may slowly get to a volume of up to 2,000 ml before becoming clinically significant. In contrast, an acute cardiac tamponade with hemopericardium, for example, will become symptomatic at only 10% of that value.[6]

> **Caution!** It is essential to quickly determine if the patient has an acute, rapidly accumulating tamponade versus a chronic tamponade.

A critically ill cardiac tamponade patient will appear completely different at the initial encounter: sitting up, tachypneic, barely able to converse, often with diaphoresis, cyanosis, and the classic Beck's triad findings of hypotension, JVD, and muffled heart sounds. These are the true emergencies, and patients may present with shock, cyanosis, and altered mental status due to compression of the cardiac chambers.

In contrast, the chronic pericardial effusion patient with an extensive effusion on TTE may present for a pericardial window operation supine, alert, in no apparent distress, without supplemental oxygen, normotensive, and with a regular heart rate. Patients with chronic tamponade have more slowly increasing intrapericardial pressure and more benign symptoms.

Signs and symptoms of tamponade include dyspnea, tachypnea, orthopnea, tachycardia, hypotension, jugular venous distension, and elevated pressures (Figure 9.1), as well as pulsus paradoxus (a drop in systolic blood pressure of >10 mmHg with inspiration), decreased QRS voltage on electrocardiogram (ECG), and electrical alternans (a beat-to-beat shift in the QRS amplitude and axis)[7] (Figure 9.2).

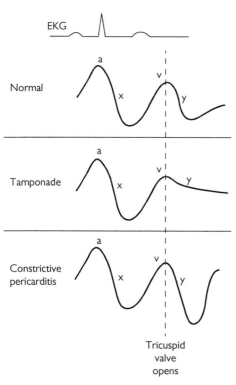

Figure 9.1 Elevated CVP with loss of normal early diastolic Y descent on the venous waveform.
Source: Spodick DH. Acute cardiac tamponade. *N. Engl. J. Med.* 2003;349(7):684–690. With permission.

> **>> Tip on Technique:** Confirm elevated jugular venous pressures by the presence of a loss of the typical early diastolic "y" descent on central venous pressure waveform (see Figure 9.1)

Chest x-ray may reveal globular cardiomegaly and clear lungs in patients with chronic pericardial effusions. TTE will reveal the size and location of the pericardial effusion accumulation.

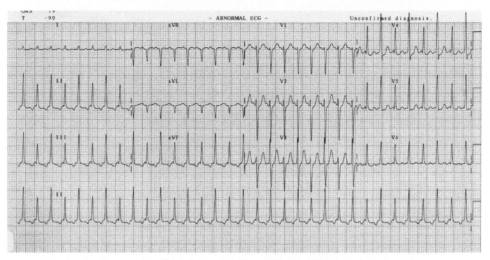

Figure 9.2 Electrical alternans is a beat-to-beat shift in the QRS amplitude and axis secondary to anterior-to-posterior swinging of the heart within the effusion-filled pericardium. Source: Available at: https://i1.wp.com/lifeinthefastlane.com/wp-content/uploads/2012/01/Electrical-alternans.jpg. Accessed July 7, 2018.

Visualize hemodynamic compromise on the echocardiogram via early diastolic collapsing of the right ventricle, late diastolic collapse of the right atrium, large tricuspid and mitral valve inflow respiratory variations, right-to-left bulging of the interventricular septum, and inferior vena cava dilation (Figure 9.3).

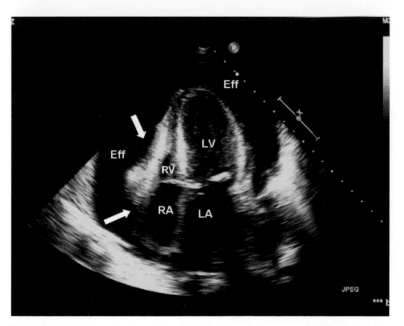

Figure 9.3 Transthoracic echocardiography showing a large pericardial effusion causing tamponade and collapse of the right ventricle. Source: Armstrong WF, Schilt BF, Helper DJ, Dillon JC, Feigenbaum H. Diastolic collapse of the right ventricle with cardiac tamponade: an echocardiographic study. *Circulation* 1982;65(7):1491–1496. With permission.

2. **Determine the best location to manage the patient.**

Once the cardiac tamponade diagnosis has been made, ideally, the cardiac surgical team is notified, and the goal is to bring the patient to the OR within 30 minutes. The team should consist of a cardiovascular surgeon, an anesthesiologist, a perfusionist, and specially trained cardiac nurses and surgical technicians. However, subxiphoid pericardial drainage may need to be urgently managed in non-OR anesthesia locations and necessitate only local anesthetic and minimal sedation if the patient is so hemodynamically decompensated that they will not survive until the entire team arrives.

On rare occasions, the cardiac tamponade patient may present as a STAT call to the cardiac catheterization lab, and upon arrival, the cardiologist requests anesthesia standby for an emergent pericardiocentesis.[8] The anesthesia provider must recognize the urgency of the situation and provide supportive care as needed in this non-OR environment, sometimes without an anesthesia machine. Provide oxygen, monitor the patient, and request airway equipment from the crash cart to be ready to intubate if required. Know when to call for further help: morbid obesity, difficult airway, cardiac or respiratory arrest, or another complication during the pericardial drainage. Usually, the patient will not tolerate any narcotics or sedatives until after the cardiologist has done the pericardiocentesis under local anesthesia.

> **Caution!** Severely orthopneic patients may prefer a reverse Trendelenburg positioning for respiratory comfort. This may also help with hemodynamics.

> **WARNING!!** If the patient is in extremis, proceed quickly to the next steps! Patients in extreme distress should have a pericardiocentesis or subxiphoid drainage under monitored anesthesia care (MAC) with only mild to moderate sedation or straight local anesthetic.

3. **Obtain additional IV access and place invasive lines.**

> **WARNING!!** If the patient is in extreme extremis, skip this step and go directly to step 4.

If general anesthesia is anticipated and time permits, insert an arterial line and large-bore IV access on a blood administration set before induction. If unable to obtain a large-bore IV, consider placement of a central line before induction.

> **Caution!** Infuse a fluid bolus with caution because this may increase the likelihood of postdrainage pulmonary edema. Consider the use of inotropes to maintain hemodynamic stability such as phenylephrine 50–100 mcg IV bolus or ephedrine 5–10 mg IV bolus.

4. **Management of the patient in extremis: Pericardiocentesis or subxiphoid drainage under MAC.**

> **Caution!** This should be performed as quickly as possible if the patient is hemo-dynamically unstable.

Minimal sedation and local anesthetic may be the safest anesthetic. If sedation is given, maintain spontaneous ventilation and consider judicious dosing of sedatives such as midazolam 0.5 mg IV, fentanyl 25 mcg IV, or ketamine 10 mg IV. Be prepared to treat hemodynamic changes.

5. **Consider induction of general anesthesia if the patient is hemodynamically stable.**

If the patient is in distress but NOT in extremis, have the surgeon scrub in before induction to expedite drainage of the cardiac tamponade. Preoxygenate the patient during awake prep and drape.

> **WARNING!!** For patients in distress, general anesthesia should NOT be induced until the surgeon is ready to make an incision.

The goal of general anesthesia is to avoid myocardial depression. Consider induction medications with less myocardial depressant effects such as etomidate 0.2 mg/kg IV or ketamine 1–2 mg/kg IV plus muscle relaxation (rocuronium 0.6 mg/kg IV if patient is NPO, succinylcholine 1 mg/kg IV if patient has a full stomach).[9]

Be prepared to treat postinduction hypotension. Ephedrine 5–10 mg IV is preferred over phenylephrine 40–100 mcg IV because cardiac output is heart rate dependent. Also consider administration of IV fluid boluses for postinduction hypotension.

Place a TEE only if the patient is more stable, usually in the setting of chronic pericardial effusions without tamponade. The cardiac surgeon will want to visualize the pericardial effusion's size and location and its resolution, especially if it was loculated.

>>**Tip on Technique:** Positive pressure ventilation may compromise preload and cardiac output, and some clinicians may prefer maintaining spontaneous ventilation postinduction until the pericardial fluid has been drained.

Pearl: Spontaneous ventilation may not provide an optimal surgical field. Controlled ventilation with low tidal volumes and peak airway pressures should maintain hemodynamics and provide enhanced surgical conditions.

If the surgeon prefers a thoracotomy approach or a video-assisted thoracoscopic pericardiectomy, be prepared for one-lung ventilation. A double-lumen endotracheal tube plus the bronchoscopy cart should be in the OR before induction.

6. **Prepare to manage and treat hemodynamic instability after fluid drainage.**

The blood pressure usually improves once the pericardial fluid is drained from the pericardium, but injury to heart or coronary vessels can occur.

> **WARNING!!** Injury to heart and coronary vessels during pericardial window may require emergency sternotomy and possible cardiopulmonary bypass for surgical repair.

> **Caution!** Postdecompression syndrome can also occur after pericardial drainage. Signs include sudden onset of right or left ventricular failure, possibly secondary to stunned myocardium or acutely augmented preload. This can result in a dilated right ventricle or a leftward shift of the interventricular septum and left ventricular failure. Early diagnosis by TEE is necessary so supportive inotropic treatment guided by pulmonary artery catheter monitoring can be initiated.[10,11]

7. Assess the patient for extubation.

> **Caution!** If the patient was in severe distress before induction, they will most likely not meet extubation criteria on emergence.

Plan on postoperative mechanical ventilation. To facilitate postoperative ventilator weaning, consider multimodal pain control with local anesthetic wound infiltration as well as nonsteroidal anti-inflammatory drugs such as acetaminophen 1000 mg IV, and low doses of opioids.

> **Caution!** If ketorolac is used, reduce the dose if over 65 years old and avoid if renal impairment exists.

>> **Tip on Technique:** Patients should be transferred with oxygen and monitors to a cardiac intensive care unit for postoperative care.

Other Management Considerations

Pericardial fluid collections causing tamponade can be treated surgically either via pericardiocentesis or via a pericardial window (Figures 9.4 and 9.5). Recovery and postoperative

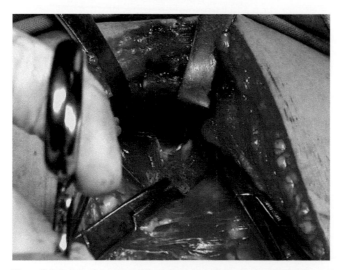

Figure 9.4 Image of a pericardial window, to make a communication between the pericardium and the pleural cavity. Source: Available at: http://www.trauma.org/images/image_library/. Image listing: 11176402815vps_negativa_mejorada.jpg. Accessed November 19, 2018.

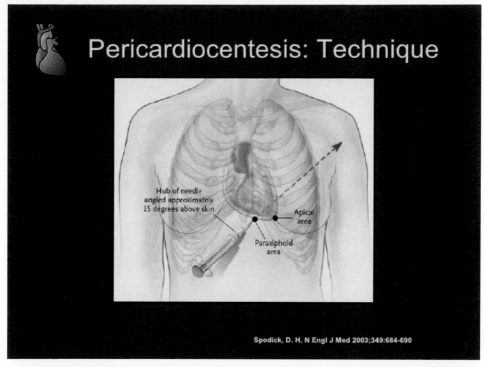

Spodick, D. H. N Engl J Med 2003;349:684-690

Figure 9.5 Pericardiocentesis procedure performed with an 18-gauge spinal needle inserted 30 to 45 degrees to the skin at the left sternal costal margin. It is then directed toward the left shoulder, ideally done with transthoracic echocardiography or ultrasound to the most extensive pericardial fluid collection. Source: Spodick DH. Acute cardiac tamponade. *N. Engl. J. Med.* 2003;349(7):684–690. doi:10.1056/NEJMra022643, with permission.

pain control are less complicated after a subxiphoid approach, but effusion recurrence may be higher than after a thoracotomy approach.

Further Reading

Glenn P. Gravlee, Andrew D. Shaw, Karsten Bartel. Hensley's Practical Approach to Cardiothoracic Anesthesia, sixth edition, published 2018, Lippincott Williams & Wilkens.

References

1. Parvez N, Carpenter JL. Cardiac tamponade in Still disease: a review of the literature. *South. Med. J.* 2009;102(8):832–837. doi:10.1097/SMJ.0b013e3181ad4847.
2. Cummings RG, Wesly RL, Adams DH, Lowe JE. Pneumopericardium resulting in cardiac tamponade. *Ann. Thorac. Surg.* 1984;37(6):511–518. doi:10.1016/S0003-4975(10)61146-0.
3. Guberman BA, Fowler NO, Engel PJ, Gueron M, Allen JM. Cardiac tamponade in medical patients. *Circulation* 1981;64(3):633–640. doi:10.1161/01.CIR.64.3.633.
4. Adler Y, Charron P, Imazio M, et al. 2015 ESC guidelines for the diagnosis and management of pericardial diseases: The Task Force for the Diagnosis and Management of Pericardial Diseases of the European Society of Cardiology (ESC) Endorsed by: The European Association for

Cardio-Thoracic Surgery (EACTS). *Eur. Heart J.* 2015;36(42):2921–2964. doi:10.1093/eurheartj/ehv318.

5. Armstrong WF, Schilt BF, Helper DJ, Dillon JC, Feigenbaum H. Diastolic collapse of the right ventricle with cardiac tamponade: an echocardiographic study. *Circulation* 1982;65(7):1491–1496.

6. O'Connor CJ, Tuman KJ. The intraoperative management of patients with pericardial tamponade. *Anesthesiol. Clin.* 2010;28(1):87–96. doi:10.1016/j.anclin.2010.01.011.

7. Spodick DH. Acute cardiac tamponade. *N. Engl. J. Med.* 2003;349(7):684–690. doi:10.1056/NEJMra022643.

8. Desikan S. Abstract PR016. *Anesth. Analg.* 2016;123:28. doi:10.1213/01.ane.0000492426.72648.75.

9. Aye T, Milne B. Ketamine anesthesia for pericardial window in a patient with pericardial tamponade and severe COPD. *Can. J. Anaesth.* 2002;49(3):283–286. doi:10.1007/BF03020528.

10. Sunday R, Robinson LA, Bosek V. Low cardiac output complicating pericardiectomy for pericardial tamponade. *Ann. Thorac. Surg.* 1999;67(1):228–231. doi:10.1016/S0003-4975(98)01143-6.

11. Chung J, Ocken L, Wolo E, Herman CR, Goldhammer JE. Acute right ventricular failure after surgical drainage of pericardial tamponade: A case report of pericardial decompression syndrome and review of the literature. *J. Cardiothorac. Vasc. Anesth.* 2019;33(3):768–771.

Chapter 10

Myocardial Ischemia

Alberto Bursian and Basma Mohamed

Summary Page

Symptoms:

- Chest pain, nausea and vomiting, diaphoresis (awake patient)
- ST-segment elevation or depression
- New T-wave inversion
- Hemodynamic instability
- New arrhythmia such as left bundle branch block
- New pathological Q waves on electrocardiogram
- Bradycardia or tachycardia
- Hypotension
- New wall motion abnormalities seen on transesophageal echocardiogram
- New or worsened valvular dysfunction
- Respiratory distress
- Asymptomatic (or absent symptoms due to analgesia around the time of surgery)
- Rising and falling pattern of values of cardiac troponins.

Differential Diagnosis:

- Aortic dissection
- Pneumothorax
- Musculoskeletal
- Pneumonia
- Gastroesophageal reflux disease
- Pericarditis
- Nonischemic causes of elevated cardiac enzymes:
  - Pulmonary embolism
  - Arrhythmia
  - Chronic kidney disease
  - Sepsis
  - Cardioversion

Introduction

Perioperative myocardial ischemia or myocardial infarction (MI) is the most common cause of perioperative cardiac complications in patients undergoing noncardiac surgery. Perioperative cardiac complications include cardiac death, heart failure, ventricular tachycardia, and nonfatal myocardial infarction. These complications occur in up to 5% of noncardiac surgery patients. Also, there is a larger group of patients who have a rise in troponin, a biomarker of cardiac injury, but no symptoms and no evidence of myocardial ischemia on electrocardiogram. In this chapter, we will focus on the evaluation and management of perioperative myocardial ischemia or infarction in patients undergoing noncardiac surgery. The etiology of perioperative myocardial ischemia can be plaque rupture versus supply-demand mismatch as a result of different factors including the stress of surgery and hemodynamic changes. Plaque rupture as a result may present as ST-elevation MI (STEMI), and this would warrant urgent involvement of the cardiologists for a possible intervention. Perioperative non-ST-elevation MI (NSTEMI) may result from supply-demand mismatch. This would need modification of risk factors perioperatively and can extend to postoperative care that includes observation and possible intervention. As a result of the high risk of perioperative cardiac morbidity, patients are better screened using different risk assessment tools, and referred to preoperative assessment based on their risk factors and the risk of surgery. It is advised to be proactive in the management of patients at high risk of perioperative major adverse cardiac events.

Treatment

Risk factors for perioperative MI include high-risk surgery (intrathoracic, vascular supra-inguinal, and intraperitoneal), history of ischemic heart disease, congestive heart failure, cerebrovascular disease, insulin-dependent diabetes, or a creatinine > 2mg/dl. [1]

High-risk patients[2-5] and scenarios include:

- Recent coronary intervention or myocardial ischemia <3 months
- Early interruption of dual antiplatelet therapy (DAPT)
- Systolic left ventricular (LV) dysfunction including global hypokinesis as a result of MI
- Patients with a positive stress test who are not candidates for coronary interventions
- Patients with confirmed multivessel disease
- Emergency surgery in the setting of unclear history of coronary artery disease (CAD)

Myocardial infarction and ischemia can be difficult to diagnose in the perioperative setting. Most patients present with atypical symptoms and not necessarily typical chest pain. This might be due to multiple comorbidities (e.g., diabetic patients with neuropathy and geriatric patients usually present with silent ischemia) or due to the use of narcotics and other pain medications. Physiological signs in the intraoperative phase that are consistent with MI are common and nonspecific, which usually results in delay until the diagnosis is confirmed, and the pursuit of supportive measures instead of the specific management of MI. Once the diagnosis of MI is suspected or confirmed, the focus should be on maintaining hemodynamic stability and preventing further ischemia.

Step by Step

>> **Tip on Technique:** All of the following steps could be done simultaneously when other team members are available for help.

1. **Suspect myocardial ischemia.**

   Signs/symptoms of myocardial ischemia include chest pain, nausea, and vomiting; diaphoresis (in an awake patient); ST-segment elevation or depression on electrocardiogram (ECG); new T-wave inversions; bradycardia or tachycardia; hemodynamic instability; and hypotension.

New wall motion abnormalities on transesophageal echocardiogram (TEE) or new pathological Q waves on ECG are strongly suggestive of acute myocardial infarction. Arrhythmias including left bundle branch block, ventricular tachyarrhythmias, and ventricular fibrillation can also occur.

Any hemodynamic instability in high-risk patients should raise the suspicion for MI.

2. **Call for help and notify the surgeon.**

Strongly consider halting or aborting surgery if possible. Call for a code cart. Consider having a code cart in the operating room (OR) at the beginning of surgery for high-risk patients.

3. **Perform ABCs of resuscitation.**

Airway and breathing: Deliver 100% O_2 at high flow. Confirm airway is patent and that the patient is breathing. Intubate the patient if needed (if not already under general anesthesia).

Circulation: Place defibrillation pads on the patient. If the patient is unstable and has a shockable rhythm, initiate cardiopulmonary resuscitation (CPR) and perform defibrillation per advanced cardiac life support (ACLS) protocols (see Chapter 12 on VF/VT). If the patient is in pulseless electrical activity (PEA) or asystole, start CPR and initiate ACLS protocols (see Chapter 11 on PEA/asystole).

If the patient is tachycardic and hypotensive, consider synchronized cardioversion if indicated.

4. **Confirm the diagnosis.**

Once the patient is stabilized, obtain a 12-lead ECG on the anesthesia monitors and check the ECG for ST-segment changes and arrhythmias (Figure 10.1). Consider transthoracic or transesophageal echocardiography (TTE or TEE) to look for wall motion abnormalities. Place an arterial line and obtain labs: arterial blood gas, troponins.

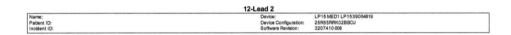

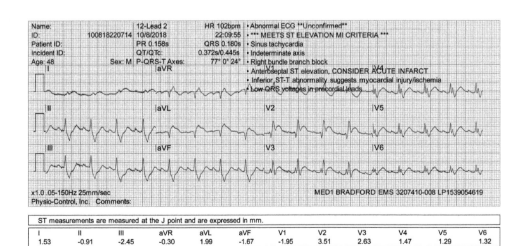

Figure 10.1 12-lead electrocardiogram showing non-ST-elevation MI.

5. Modify risk factors and prevent further ischemia.

The goals of treatment are to minimize the risk of myocardial supply-demand mismatch through decreasing the workload on the heart (treat tachycardia and hypertension, avoid light anesthesia, and optimize perioperative analgesia) and optimize oxygen-carrying capacity (increase FiO_2, treat hypotension to improve coronary perfusion pressure, and optimize blood loss anemia).

If the patient is hypotensive, give phenylephrine 50–100 mcg IV boluses if tachycardic or ephedrine 5–10 mg IV if bradycardic (heart rate below 60).

Caution! Avoid the use of high-dose phenylephrine infusion in patients with global hypokinesis or low left ventricular ejection fraction.

If the patient is hypertensive, confirm it is not related to pain or light anesthesia, and then deepen anesthetic. Consider labetalol 5–20 mg IV or nitroglycerin 50–100 mcg IV; also consider starting nitroglycerin infusion at 5 mcg/min (increase by 5 mcg/min up to effect).

If the patient is tachycardic and hypotensive, consider synchronized cardioversion if indicated. If no hypotension, consider esmolol 10–30 mg IV and titrate to effect. If tachycardia continues, treat with metoprolol 1–5 mg IV, titrating to effect.

WARNING!! Avoid phenylephrine if the patient is in cardiogenic shock. Avoid beta blockers and nitroglycerin if the patient is hemodynamically unstable.

Caution! Prophylactic nitroglycerin is of no benefit in high-risk patients. Starting a nitroglycerin infusion in patients with suspected perioperative MI should be done with caution due to hemodynamic instability associated with this condition.

---

6. Treat arrhythmias.

WARNING!! If hemodynamically unstable, follow the ACLS algorithm[6].

Place defibrillation pads (if not already in place) if an arrhythmia is confirmed. If hemodynamically stable, for bradycardia give atropine 0.2–0.4 mg IV or glycopyrrolate 0.1–0.2 mg IV, titrating to effect. Consider transvenous pacing if significant atrioventricular block.

> **Caution!** Confirm the diagnosis of perioperative MI prior to starting specific medications (nitroglycerin, beta blocker, heparin, or DAPT). Do not start beta blocker preoperatively if the patient was not already on it.[1] Left ventricular function should be evaluated prior to starting a negative inotropic medication such as a beta blocker. Titrate carefully due to risk of worsening cardiogenic shock. Start with the lowest dose of beta blocker or nitroglycerin and titrate to patient's response or stop if the patient becomes unstable.

Consider other medications to prevent further ischemia:
- Aspirin 81–325 mg and atorvastatin (PO, PR, or via a feeding tube)
- Heparin and DAPT can be started per cardiology. Use of anticoagulation or antiplatelet therapy should be discussed with cardiology and surgeons before initiating.
Transfuse packed red blood cells if anemia is suspected.

7. **Consult cardiology.**

Discuss the risks and benefits of antiplatelet therapy and percutaneous coronary intervention against the risk of bleeding. A high level of communication is recommended between the anesthesiologist, the surgeon, and the cardiologist. Coordination may be needed for emergency transfer to the cardiac catheterization suite while discussing with the cardiologist.

Based on the patient's presentation and the most likely pathophysiology, early intervention is advised (Figure 10.2).
- If ECG shows ST depression, the most likely pathology is Type 2 NSTEMI, which results from supply-demand mismatch. This could be optimized through improving oxygen-carrying capacity and improving the cardiac workload.
- If ECG shows ST elevation, the most likely underlying pathophysiology is STEMI. An emergency consultation with the cardiologist and an expedited transfer to the cardiac catheterization laboratory should follow the current recommendations regarding the time to revascularization.

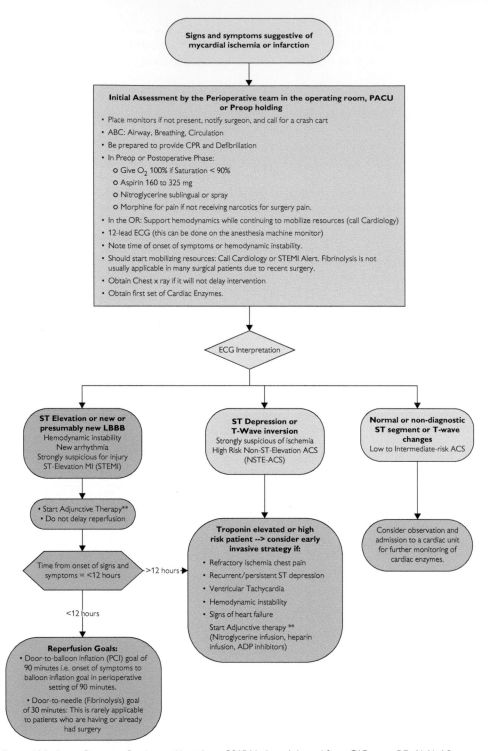

Figure 10.2 Acute Coronary Syndrome Algorithm—2015 Update. Adapted from O'Connor RE, Al Ali AS, Brady WJ, et al. Part 9: Acute coronary syndromes: 2015 American Heart Association guidelines update for cardiopulmonary resuscitation and emergency cardiovascular care. *Circulation*. 2015;132(18 suppl 2):S483–S500.

8. **Advanced care.**

   Consider central venous line placement to facilitate delivery of vasopressors and inotropic drug infusions. Consider intra-aortic balloon pump or transvenous pacing if other
maneuvers do not resolve hypotension or arrhythmias. Transfer to cardiac intensive
care unit for further management once stabilized.

Other Management Considerations

Management of perioperative myocardial ischemia is similar to acute coronary syndrome in and
out of the operating room setting with the following considerations[5]:

Patient in preoperative phase:

   Patients who are being evaluated for an elective surgery and who are high risk for
perioperative MI should receive a comprehensive preoperative evaluation that includes
risk stratification and further evaluation and management by cardiology if they show
signs or symptoms of acute coronary syndrome.

Postoperative MI in recovery room:

   Patients who develop signs or symptoms of acute MI should receive the above algorithm of care (see Figure 10.2). It might be difficult to identify patients with chest pain
due to the use of pain medications. Clinicians in the postoperative phase should have a
high index of suspicion in high-risk patients.

Further Reading

Books

- Barash PG, Cullen BF, Stoelting RK, et al. Preoperative Patient Assessment and Management.
  In *Clinical Anesthesia*. 8th ed. Philadelphia, PA: Wolters Kluwer; 2017. 23:591.
- Hines RL, Marschall KE, eds. *Stoelting's Anesthesia and Co-Existing Disease*. 7th ed. Philadelphia,
  PA: Elsevier; 2018.

Guidelines

Fleisher LA, Fleischmann KE, Auerbach AD, et al. 2014 ACC/AHA guideline on
   perioperative cardiovascular evaluation and management of patients undergoing
   noncardiac surgery: a report of the American College of Cardiology/American Heart
   Association Task Force on practice guidelines. *Journal of the American College of
   Cardiology* 2014;64(22):e77–e137.

References

1. Ford MK, Beattie WS, Wijeysundera DN. Systematic review: prediction of perioperative
   cardiac complications and mortality by the revised cardiac risk index. *Annals of Internal
   Medicine* 2010;152(1):26–35.
2. Gualandro DM, Campos CA, Calderaro D, et al. Coronary plaque rupture in patients with
   myocardial infarction after noncardiac surgery: frequent and dangerous. *Atherosclerosis*
   2012;222(1):191–195.
3. Fleisher LA, Fleischmann KE, Auerbach AD, et al. 2014 ACC/AHA guideline on
   perioperative cardiovascular evaluation and management of patients undergoing
   noncardiac surgery: a report of the American College of Cardiology/American Heart
   Association Task Force on practice guidelines. *Journal of the American College of Cardiology*
   2014;64(22):e77–e137.

4. Hines RL, Marschall KE, eds. *Stoelting's Anesthesia and Co-Existing Disease*. 7th ed. Philadelphia, PA: Elsevier; 2018.

5. Reed-Poysden C, Gupta K. Acute coronary syndromes. *BJA Education* 2015;15(6):286–293.

6. O'Connor RE, Al Ali AS, Brady WJ, et al. Part 9: Acute coronary syndromes: 2015 American Heart Association guidelines update for cardiopulmonary resuscitation and emergency cardiovascular care. *Circulation* 2015;132(18 suppl 2):S483–S500.

Chapter 11

Pulseless Electrical Activity (PEA) and Asystole

Claudia Sotillo and Basma Mohamed

Summary Page
Symptoms:

- Unconsciousness (if not already anesthetized)
- Normal sinus rhythm, bradycardia, or absent rhythm on electrocardiogram
- Pulselessness for 10 seconds
- Persistent hypotension prior to arrest
- Loss of end-tidal CO_2
- Loss of plethysmograph
- Resistance to vasopressors

Differential Diagnosis:

- Hypovolemia
- Hypoxia
- Hydrogen ions (acidosis)
- Hypo-/hyperkalemia
- Hypothermia
- Hypoglycemia
- Malignant hyperthermia
- Hypervagal response
- Toxins
- Tamponade
- Tension pneumothorax
- Thrombosis: pulmonary embolism or coronary
- Trauma
- QT prolongation
- Pulmonary hypertension

Introduction

Cardiac arrest in the perioperative setting is caused by multiple etiologies and pathologies that are different from the non-perioperative setting. Cardiac arrest in the operating room (OR) is unique in that it is witnessed by providers who are familiar with the patient's comorbidities, the event is usually preceded by hemodynamic instability, and the underlying etiology can be rapidly identified. Early identification of patients in crisis can prevent further progression to cardiac arrest and preclude the initiation of advanced cardiac life support (ACLS). In turn, this directly affects prognosis by allowing the anesthesiology team to provide focused, etiology-based resuscitative efforts and early mobilization of advanced levels of care.

Causes of cardiac arrest in the perioperative setting are quite different compared to out-of-hospital or in-hospital arrest. Cardiac causes can be related to anesthetic sympatholytic effects, vagotonic effects of surgical manipulation, severe hypovolemia in bleeding patients, or blockade of cardiac accelerator fibers associated with neuraxial anesthesia. Respiratory causes of cardiac arrest can be related to hypoxia that is associated with difficult airway management or bronchospasm. As a result, management of cardiac arrest in the perioperative setting should focus on certain differentials related to the anesthetic and surgical causes of arrest. This chapter will focus on the common causes of pulseless electrical activity (PEA)/asystole in the perioperative period and will provide the anesthesiology team with a step-by-step guide to help predict, prevent, and manage PEA/asystole in these patients.

Unfortunately, nonperfusing rhythms are common arrhythmias in the perioperative setting. PEA is the most common initial rhythm[1,2] and accounts for approximately 37.4% of arrest events in the perioperative setting, versus 38.5% for asystole.[3] Of note, asystole in the OR and postanesthesia care unit (PACU) is associated with better survival than arrests in other locations, indicating that shorter times to implementation of therapy directly improve survival and neurological outcomes.[3] As such, the immediate presence and availability of skilled care in the OR, PACU, and intensive care unit (ICU), coupled with readily available resources, may significantly modify and positively impact factors that influence outcomes from PEA arrest and asystole.

Management

It is sometimes difficult for the anesthesiology team to recognize that the patient is hemodynamically unstable and to initiate ACLS for cardiac arrest in a timely fashion. Under general anesthesia, respiration is controlled and the patient is under surgical drapes, making it difficult to assess mental status and check for apnea or respiratory distress. False alarms outnumber real events with OR monitors. Bradycardia is a common occurrence and is often associated with hypotension under anesthesia during routine cases. Monitor failure is also common (i.e., asystole could be electrode failure or lead disconnect) and it may be difficult if not impossible to obtain adequate monitoring in hypothermic, hypovolemic, burn, or morbidly obese patients, and in patients with peripheral vascular disease.

PEA manifests as electromechanical dissociation of the heart where an organized electrocardiogram (ECG) waveform presents without the generation of an effective left ventricular stroke volume, resulting in the absence of a palpable pulse or measurable blood pressure.[4–6]

Unlike the "shockable" rhythms (i.e., pulseless ventricular tachycardia [VT] or ventricular fibrillation [VF]), PEA is associated with poor survival rates and, if left untreated, can quickly progress to asystole within minutes.[2,7] When either PEA or asystole is present in the perioperative setting, both are defined as nonperfusing rhythms that require the immediate initiation of ACLS protocols.

Note: The first four steps can be started simultaneously.

> **Caution!** START CHEST COMPRESSIONS IMMEDIATELY IF NO PALPABLE PULSE FOR 10 SECONDS WHILE CALLING FOR HELP AND NOTIFYING THE SURGEON.

Step by Step

1. **Verify the diagnosis: Recognize that the patient is in PEA/asystole and rule out monitor failure.**

   If a PEA arrest is suspected, first check for a carotid pulse for 10 seconds. Concurrently, assess for the trend in blood pressure and the ECG rhythm. Evaluate for lead placement and possible disconnected ECG leads or malposition without causing any delay in starting the appropriate interventions (ACLS). Other indications of a pending cardiac arrest include decreased $EtCO_2$ and/or a decrease in or loss of pulse oximetry.

   Note: A cardiac rhythm without a palpable pulse is diagnostic of PEA. Asystole is the absence of both pulse and cardiac rhythm (Figure 11.1).

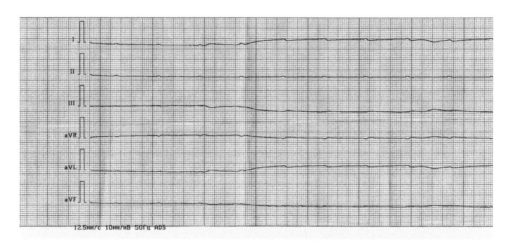

Figure 11.1 ECG tracing showing asystole. Source: https://www.shutterstock.com/image-photo/emergency-cardiology-resuscitation-ecg-tape-ventricular-1021721578; https://www.dreamstime.com/emergency-cardiology-resuscitation-ecg-ventricular-asystole-emergency-cardiology-resuscitation-ecg-tape-image110143126.

   >> **Tip on Technique:** A palpable carotid pulse is associated with a systolic blood pressure of 70–80 mm Hg. Based on the type of surgery and accessibility, femoral artery palpation might be an alternative but not an accurate one depending on the patient's position, the surgical field, and the patient's body habitus.

2. **Call for help and notify the surgeon and the team.**

   Once PEA arrest is suspected, notify the surgeon and call for help. Halt or abort surgery and call for a code cart and a defibrillator. Place defibrillation pads in case of return to a shockable rhythm.

Hold or decrease anesthesia if possible, decrease or stop volatile anesthetics, discontinue intravenous anesthesia if possible, and stop opioid infusions. Check with the surgeons if surgical manipulation or arterial bleeding is the cause of hemodynamic instability.

Caution! Patients with implanted pacemakers and defibrillators should not have defibrillation pads placed directly over their device! Instead, external defibrillation pads should be placed as close to their normal position as possible or in an anterior-posterior placement (where the left chest automated external defibrillator pad marked with a heart remains on the left chest and the pad that normally is placed on the right chest beneath the collarbone is instead moved to the left side of the back).

Caution! Check the patient for medication patches as the nonadhesive backing can have a metallic component that can contribute to thermal injury if the patient regains a shockable rhythm requiring defibrillation.

---

3. **Start cardiopulmonary resuscitation (CPR) immediately.**

Once CPR is started, minimize interruptions in chest compressions. Chest compressions should be at a rate of 100/min and the compression-to-ventilation ratio should be 30:2 if the patient is not intubated. If the patient is intubated, maintain a respiratory rate of 10–12 breaths/min without interruptions in compressions. During chest compression, maintain a depth of 2 inches and allow full compression and recoil with real-time feedback. Clinicians should titrate CPR to a goal diastolic pressure of 40 mmHg (preferably measured via arterial line) or $EtCO_2$ of 20 mmHg. Switch compressors every 2 minutes to avoid fatigue.

>> **Tip on Technique:** Place a hard backboard under the patient to optimize compressions. Supine positioning on a hard backboard is ideal for CPR.

WARNING!! Turning a prone patient supine in an emergency can risk loss of the airway, increased bleeding, unstable spine (if a neurosurgical patient), and disconnection of vascular catheters.

WARNING!! Do not stop CPR unnecessarily! Capnography is a more reliable indicator of effective CPR and return of spontaneous circulation (ROSC) than carotid or femoral arterial pulse palpation.[8] A low $EtCO_2$ indicates low cardiac output generated by chest compressions, provided that other causes of low $EtCO_2$ are ruled out (e.g., bronchospasm, mucous plug in the endotracheal tube [ETT]). $EtCO_2$ measurements <10 mmHg immediately after intubation and 20 minutes after initiation of resuscitative efforts are associated with poor chances for ROSC and survival. $EtCO_2$ may be considered as one component in a multimodal approach to decisions regarding ending resuscitative efforts. It should not be used in isolation. An increase in $EtCO_2$ above 20 mmHg after 20 minutes of resuscitation is associated with improved survival.

4. **Oxygenate, ventilate, and intubate.**

Ventilate using 100% O_2 at a rate of 10 breaths/min (1 breath every 6 seconds) and avoid hyperventilation. Achieving visible chest rise indicates adequate tidal volume. If the patient is not intubated, clinicians may proceed by placing an advanced airway (either an ETT or a supraglottic airway [SGA] device). Call for a difficult airway cart in anticipation of difficult airway. If the patient is already intubated, confirm the position and function of the airway device, assess oxygen source and circuit, and follow the capnography to monitor adequate resuscitative efforts.

>>**Tip on Technique:** If it is difficult to place an advanced airway device, consider an SGA or continue mask ventilation until ROSC. If mask ventilation is adequate, it is reasonable to delay advanced airway placement until after the second round of CPR.

Caution! Minimize interruptions in compressions while placing an advanced airway device.

WARNING!! Excessive ventilation has been associated with worse outcome. Increased intrathoracic pressure can decrease venous return and cardiac output specifically in patients with hypovolemia or obstructive airway disease.

5. **Volume resuscitation.**

Ensure adequate IV access and run IV fluids wide open. Activate massive transfusion protocols if the patient is in hemorrhagic shock.

6. **Give epinephrine IV.**

As part of the ACLS protocol, give epinephrine 1 mg IV every 3–5 minutes. The pediatric dose is 10 mcg/kg every 3–5 minutes. If there is not IV access, epinephrine can be given intraosseous or via the ETT. Note that early administration of epinephrine ("time to epinephrine" within 3 minutes) is associated with improved in-hospital survival and neurologically intact survival.

Note: Vasopressin has been removed from the algorithm in the 2015 American Heart Association Guidelines on Adult Advanced Cardiac Life Support as it was not shown to be superior to epinephrine.[8] Also avoid adenosine, cardiac pacing, and defibrillation as these are ineffective with nonperfusing, nonshockable rhythms.

7. **Continue CPR and IV epinephrine until either ROSC or a shockable rhythm occurs. Perform pulse and rhythm checks every five cycles of CPR or 2 minutes.**

After 2 minutes of CPR, assess the rhythm and ROSC.

Limit interruptions for pulse checks to 10 seconds or less.

8. **Assess rhythm and ROSC.**

If no ROSC occurs and the patient continues to be in PEA/asystole, continue ACLS and investigate the underlying etiology for PEA and asystole. If there is no ROSC and the rhythm has returned to a shockable rhythm (VT or VF), then proceed with ACLS, perform defibrillation, and continue to look for the underlying etiology for VT and VF.

If ROSC occurs, then proceed with post–cardiac arrest plan including transfer to an ICU.

Note: Elevated EtCO$_2$ is a strong indicator of adequate cardiac output and possible ROSC. Also, return of pulsatile flow on an arterial blood pressure tracing with cessation of CPR indicates ROSC.

Knowing when to cease resuscitative efforts can be challenging. Factors influencing the decision to stop further resuscitation include:[9–12]

- EtCO$_2$ <10 mmHg following prolonged resuscitation (>20 minutes)
- Duration of resuscitative effort >30 minutes without a sustained perfusing rhythm
- Unwitnessed arrest with prolonged time lapse between estimated time of arrest and initiation of CPR
- Elderly patient with severe disease comorbidities
- Absent brainstem reflexes
- No ROSC after third administration of 1 mg IV epinephrine

9. **Look for the underlying etiology of PEA/asystole.**

The differential diagnosis including 8Hs and 8Ts is shown in Table 11.1. Reversible causes of PEA/asystole once identified should be treated.

Table 11.1 Differential Diagnosis of PEA: The 8Hs and 8Ts

Hs	Ts
• **H**ypovolemia (hemorrhage)	• **T**oxins (anesthetics and anaphylaxis)*
• **H**ypoxia	• **T**amponade
• **H**ydrogen ions (acidosis)	• **T**ension pneumothorax
• **H**ypo-/**H**yperkalemia	• **T**hrombosis—pulmonary
• **H**ypothermia	• **T**hrombosis—coronary
• **H**ypoglycemia	• **T**rauma
• Malignant **H**yperthermia	• Q**T** prolongation
• **H**ypervagal response	• Pulmonary hyper**T**ension

* Indicates toxicity from anesthetic drugs or anaphylaxis in response to perioperative drugs such as antibiotics and neuromuscular blocking agents. This is different from the "Toxins" per the AHA guidelines—which refer to substance use related toxicity in the perioperative setting.

Specific considerations:

For hemorrhage: Activate massive transfusion protocols. Prime the rapid infuser with 250 ml of IV crystalloids and resuscitate with IV crystalloids until arrival of the packed red blood cells for transfusion. Administer vasopressors as needed: phenylephrine 50–100 mcg IV boluses followed by infusion at 0.5 mcg/kg/min or norepinephrine infusion at 0.02 mcg/kg/min. Consider placement of a central venous catheter for delivery of vasopressors or inotrope infusion(s) in addition to volume resuscitation.

For hypoxia: Deliver 100% oxygen via mask ventilation or an advanced airway. Consider bronchodilators, steroids, and suctioning of the ETT while continuing to identify causes of hypoxia. Confirm the placement of any advanced airway already in place, rule out pneumothorax, and manage laryngospasm if it is the main etiology. Rule out aspiration of gastric contents and rule out a hypoxic gas mixture.

Blood chemistry aberrations: Manage hyperkalemia, hypokalemia, and acidosis based on laboratory results.

Temperature: Cool or rewarm the patient as needed. Treat malignant hyperthermia if suspected or present.

Toxins: Review recently administered medications and stop the offending agent and treat appropriately (local anesthetics, anaphylaxis).

Tamponade: Perform catheter pericardiocentesis or open surgical drainage with or without pericardial window.

Tension pneumothorax: In addition to clinical suspicion, clinicians may use point-of-care ultrasound to rule out a tension pneumothorax. Intraoperative chest x-ray can be performed if available. Perform needle thoracostomy at the second intercostal space, midclavicular line of the affected hemithorax.

Thrombosis: Proceed with anticoagulation or thrombectomy.

Trauma: Identify the source of bleeding and proceed with hemodynamic resuscitation and stabilization.

> **Note:** Transesophageal or transthoracic echocardiography may be useful to evaluate for cardiac causes.

10. Consider placement of invasive monitoring.

Central venous line placement is indicated in patients with PEA/asystole as a measure to treat reversible causes in the form of fluid resuscitation, vasopressors, and inotrope drug administration. Ultrasound may be used for central venous line placement. In addition, the use of transthoracic or transesophageal echocardiography can be utilized as additional diagnostic tools.

11. Arrange for post–cardiac arrest care once ROSC achieved.

Patients post-ROSC will need to be admitted to the ICU with considerations for the option of extracorporeal membrane oxygenation (ECMO) with the surgical team.

Other Management Considerations

Other causes of PEA/asystole that might be encountered in patients receiving anesthesia include inhalational or intravenous anesthetic overdose, neuraxial anesthesia, local anesthetic systemic toxicity, and malignant hyperthermia. Other respiratory causes while the patient is under general anesthesia include auto positive end-expiratory pressure (auto-PEEP) and bronchospasm. Cardiac etiology could be the result of vasovagal and oculocardiac reflexes, intraoperative bleeding, air or pulmonary embolism, increased intra-abdominal pressure, transfusion and anaphylactic reactions, pacemaker failure, prolonged QT syndrome, and electroconvulsive therapy.

For pregnant patients, CPR providers must take the gravid uterus into consideration when following ACLS protocols. Several recommendations include relief of aortocaval compression with manual left uterine displacement, immediate notification of the obstetric team for perimortem cesarean section within 4–5 minutes of onset of compressions, and evaluation for local anesthetic systemic toxicity.[13–16]

See Figure 11.2 for the current 2020 American Heart Association Comprehensive Algorithm for Perioperative Advanced Cardiac Life Support including PEA/asystole.

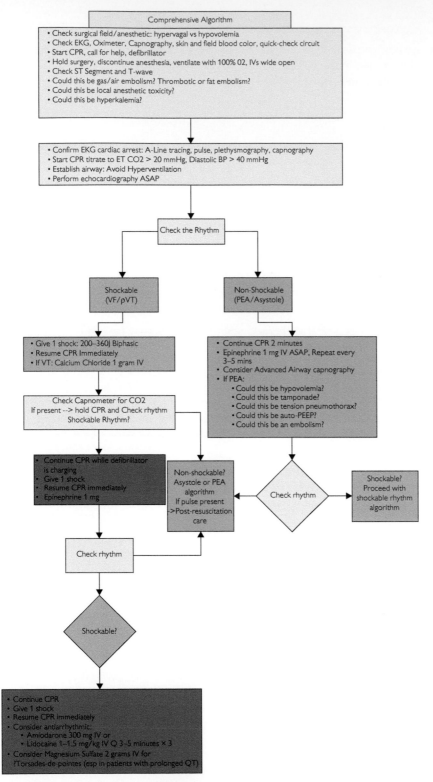

Figure 11.2 Adult Cardiac Arrest Algorithm. Adapted from American Heart Association 2020 Updated Guidelines: Panchal AR, Bartos JA, Cabañas JG, et al. Part 3: Adult Basic and Advanced Life Support: 2020 American Heart Association Guidelines for Cardiopulmonary Resuscitation and Emergency Cardiovascular Care. *Circulation*. 2020;142(16 Suppl 2). doi:10.1161/CIR.0000000000000916

References

1. Bergum D, Nordseth T, Mjølstad OC, Skogvoll E, Haugen BO. Causes of in-hospital cardiac arrest - incidences and rate of recognition. *Resuscitation*. 2015;87:63–68. doi:10.1016/j.resuscitation.2014.11.007

2. Parish DC, Dane FC, Montgomery M, Wynn LJ, Durham MD, Brown TD. Resuscitation in the hospital: relationship of year and rhythm to outcome. *Resuscitation*. 2000;47(3):219–229. doi:10.1016/S0300-9572(00)00231-8

3. Ramachandran SK, Mhyre J, Kheterpal S, et al. Predictors of survival from perioperative cardiopulmonary arrests: a retrospective analysis of 2,524 events from the Get with the Guidelines-Resuscitation registry. *Anesthesiology*. 2013;119(6):1322–1339. doi:10.1097/ALN.0b013e318289bafe

4. Engdahl J, Bång A, Lindqvist J, Herlitz J. Factors affecting short- and long-term prognosis among 1069 patients with out-of-hospital cardiac arrest and pulseless electrical activity. *Resuscitation*. 2001;51(1):17–25. doi:10.1016/S0300-9572(01)00377-X

5. Mehta C, Brady W. Pulseless electrical activity in cardiac arrest: electrocardiographic presentations and management considerations based on the electrocardiogram. *Am J Emerg Med*. 2012;30(1):236–239. doi:10.1016/j.ajem.2010.08.017

6. Littmann L, Bustin DJ, Haley MW. A simplified and structured teaching tool for the evaluation and management of pulseless electrical activity. *Med Princ Pract*. 2014;23(1):1–6. doi:10.1159/000354195

7. Andrew E, Nehme Z, Lijovic M, Bernard S, Smith K. Outcomes following out-of-hospital cardiac arrest with an initial cardiac rhythm of asystole or pulseless electrical activity in Victoria, Australia. *Resuscitation*. 2014;85(11):1633–1639. doi:10.1016/j.resuscitation.2014.07.015

8. Link MS, Berkow LC, Kudenchuk PJ, et al. Part 7: adult advanced cardiovascular life support: 2015 American Heart Association guidelines update for cardiopulmonary resuscitation and emergency cardiovascular care. *Circulation*. 2015;132(18 Suppl 2):S444–S464. doi:10.1161/CIR.0000000000000261

9. Jabre P, Bougouin W, Dumas F, et al. Early identification of patients with out-of-hospital cardiac arrest with no chance of survival and consideration for organ donation. *Ann Intern Med*. 2016;165(11):770–778. doi:10.7326/M16-0402

10. Levine RL, Wayne MA, Miller CC. End-tidal carbon dioxide and outcome of out-of-hospital cardiac arrest. *N Engl J Med*. 1997;337(5):301–306. doi:10.1056/NEJM199707313370503

11. Jeejeebhoy FM, Zelop CM, Lipman S, et al. Cardiac arrest in pregnancy: a scientific statement from the American Heart Association. *Circulation*. 2015;132(18):1747–1773. doi:10.1161/CIR.0000000000000300

12. Panchal AR, Bartos JA, Cabañas JG, et al. Part 3: adult basic and advanced life support: 2020 American Heart Association guidelines for cardiopulmonary resuscitation and emergency cardiovascular care. *Circulation*. 2020;142(16 Suppl 2):S366–S468. doi:10.1161/CIR.0000000000000916

13. Moitra VK, Gabrielli A, Maccioli GA, O'Connor MF. Anesthesia advanced circulatory life support. *Can J Anaesth*. 2012;59(6):586–603. doi:10.1007/s12630-012-9699-3

14. Vanden Hoek TL, Morrison LJ, Shuster M, et al. Part 12: cardiac arrest in special situations: 2010 American Heart Association guidelines for cardiopulmonary resuscitation and emergency cardiovascular care. *Circulation*. 2010;122(18 Suppl 3):S829–S861. doi:10.1161/CIRCULATIONAHA.110.971069

15. Drukker L, Hants Y, Sharon E, Sela HY, Grisaru-Granovsky S. Perimortem cesarean section for maternal and fetal salvage: concise review and protocol. *Acta Obstet Gynecol Scand*. 2014;93(10):965–972. doi:10.1111/aogs.12464

16. Jeejeebhoy F, Windrim R. Management of cardiac arrest in pregnancy. *Best Pract Res Clin Obstet Gynaecol*. 2014;28(4):607–618. doi:10.1016/j.bpobgyn.2014.03.006

Chapter 12

Management of Ventricular Tachycardia and Ventricular Fibrillation

Amanda Redding, Marc Hassid, and Ryan Smith

Summary Page
Symptoms:

- Palpitations/arrhythmias
  - Wide, regular QRS >150 bpm
  - Rapid, irregular rhythm with variability in morphology and amplitude
- Hypotension
- Ischemic chest discomfort
- Syncope
- Pulseless cardiac arrest

Differential Diagnosis:

- Ventricular tachycardia
  - Stable or asymptomatic
  - Unstable or symptomatic
- Torsade de pointes
- Ventricular fibrillation
- Atrial fibrillation with aberrancy
- Supraventricular tachycardia with prolonged conduction (see Chapter 8 on Arrhythmias)
- Equipment malfunction

Introduction

While intraoperative arrhythmias are common, ventricular tachycardia (VT) and ventricular fibrillation (VF) are potentially life-threatening arrhythmias that originate in ventricular structures. VT is defined as three or more consecutive ventricular premature contractions (VPCs) with a rate of at least 100 beats per minute, and may present with stable or unstable physiology. It is considered sustained if it persists for at least 30 seconds. Stable or asymptomatic VT affords the caregiver time for diagnosis, consultation, and formulation of a treatment plan, while unstable or symptomatic VT requires emergent intervention. Unstable VT is diagnosed by signs of decreased cardiac output and will typically present with a heart rate of at least 150 beats per minute. VF and pulseless VT should be treated immediately with defibrillation and advanced cardiac life support (ACLS) to try to achieve return of spontaneous circulation (ROSC).

Stable patients who present with VT are managed less urgently than unstable patients with VT or VF. It is important to quickly determine if a patient is stable or unstable. Measure blood pressure, organ perfusion (capillary refill, end-tidal CO_2), and level of consciousness. A stable patient should have a systolic blood pressure (SBP) >90 mmHg and an $EtCO_2$ >30 mmHg if intubated. SBP <90 mmHg, an $EtCO_2$ <30 mmHg if intubated, chest discomfort, or a confused or unarousable patient is usually considered unstable.

Management of stable versus unstable patients with VT will be discussed separately. VF is always considered an unstable rhythm.

A. Treatment of Unstable Ventricular Tachycardia and Ventricular Fibrillation

Step by Step

1. Check for pulse and assess hemodynamics. If no pulse, start cardiopulmonary resuscitation (CPR).

Palpate the carotid or femoral pulse in adults (use the brachial artery in infants).

> **WARNING!!** When no obvious pulse can be detected within 10 seconds, there is no pulse! START CPR IMMEDIATELY.

If there is no pulse and VT or VF is present on ECG (Figure 12.1 and 12.2), IMMEDIATELY START CPR. Call for a defibrillator simultaneously while starting CPR.

Compress the chest to a depth of 2 inches (5 cm) with an ideal rate of 100–120 compressions/min.

Adequate chest compressions are essential for providing blood flow. Effectiveness of compressions can be monitored using end-tidal CO_2 capnography (goal $EtCO_2$ >10 mmHg). Perform CPR for 2-minute cycles followed by a pulse check.

> **WARNING!!** Minimize pauses (interruptions should be <10 seconds) in chest compressions. CPR should ideally be performed supine (consider placement on a backboard). Nonsupine positions make CPR difficult, but not always impossible. A stretcher or bed should always be in close proximity to prone patients in case they must be turned supine for emergency treatment.

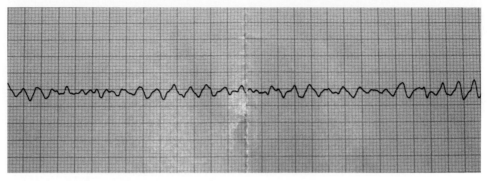

Figure 12.1 Ventricular fibrillation—chaotic, irregular ECG tracing; patient will not have a pulse.

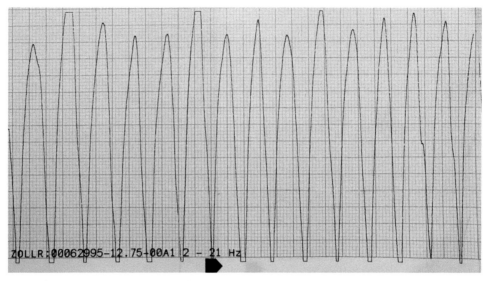

Figure 12.2 Ventricular tachycardia—regular rhythm with a wide QRS.

Do not spend too much time assessing hemodynamics as it may delay initiation of ACLS. Do not spend too much time troubleshooting a loose electrocardiogram (ECG) lead that may actually be unstable VT.

> **Caution!** In a patient with a left ventricular assist device (LVAD), pulsatility may be minimal and it may be very difficult to find a pulse. Consider expert consultation for unstable patients with VADs. Traditional noninvasive blood pressure measurement may not work. Consider an invasive arterial line or ultrasound to detect a pulse. Ultrasound examination of arterial blood flow while slowly releasing the pressure on a manual blood pressure cuff will determine the patient's mean arterial blood pressure ("return to flow"). VAD patients are at elevated risk for VT/VF; however, only a minority of these patients will become hemodynamically compromised.

If a pulse is present but the patient is in unstable VT, go to step 6.

2. Call for help and maximize ventilation while continuing CPR.

Immediately call a code and obtain the crash cart. Notify the surgeon and all the members of the team. Turn off any inhalational or IV anesthetic gases, as they can worsen hemodynamics. If the patient is already intubated, ensure delivered FiO_2 is 100%.

Caution! Avoid excessive ventilation (no more than 8–10 breaths per minute) with an established airway in place. If the patient is not intubated, start bag-mask ventilation with 100% oxygen.

---

3. Perform asynchronous defibrillation ASAP.

CONTINUE CPR while preparing the defibrillator. Do not stop CPR until immediately before delivering the shock. Deliver an initial dose of 120–200 J (Figures 12.3A–C) in adults. For neonates, infants, and children deliver 2 J/kg and increase to 4 J/kg if unsuccessful. The resuscitation will have a higher chance of success if pauses in CPR are minimized.

Sequence to follow to perform defibrillation:

- Apply defibrillator pads or paddles to the patient: left-sided posterolateral chest.
- Turn on the defibrillator and charge to 120–200 J (based on manufacturer recommendations).
- Ensure no one is in contact with the patient and clearly state "all clear."
- Press and hold the defibrillate button until a shock is delivered.
- Resume CPR cycles immediately after the shock is delivered.

>> **Tip on Technique:** If manufacturer recommendations are unknown, charge to the maximum joules available for the initial defibrillation. Subsequent shocks should be equivalent or higher than previous shocks, up to 360 J.

WARNING!! Do not delay defibrillation in order to provide a cycle of CPR. The best chance for survival occurs when defibrillation is within 3–5 minutes of cardiac arrest.

>> **Tip on Technique:** Self-adhesive pads are useful if available. The chest may need to be shaved if body hair prevents adhesion of pads.

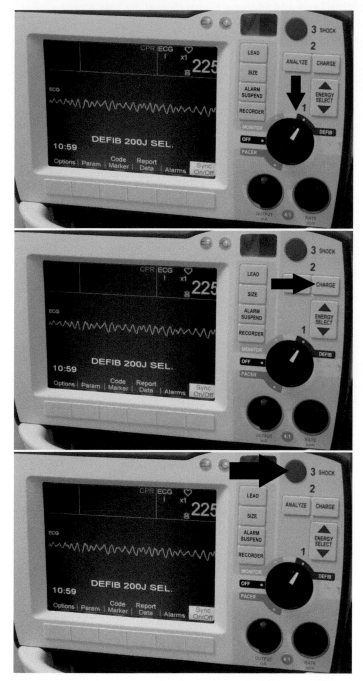

Figure 12.3 A–C. Sequence to defibrillate ventricular fibrillation—A: defibrillation step 1: activate defibrillation mode. B: defibrillation step 2: charge. C: defibrillation step 3: shock.

4. Administer epinephrine (and amiodarone when repeating this step, see Figure 12.4).

Epinephrine 1 mg IV/intraosseous (IO) should be administered every 3–5 minutes until pulse and ROSC occurs. If no IV is present, epinephrine 1 mg can be given IO every 3–5 minutes or by the first available route. If no IV or IO route is available, 2–2.5 mg diluted in 10 ml normal saline can be given intratracheally.

>> Tip on Technique: Amiodarone 300 mg IV can be considered as an alternative if VF/VT persists after the first shock and dose of epinephrine. If a second dose of amiodarone is needed, give 150 mg IV once, 3–5 minutes after the first dose.

WARNING!! Vasopressin has recently been removed from American Heart Association recommendations.

>> Tip on Technique: Several emergency medications such as epinephrine, atropine, lidocaine, and naloxone can be administered via the endotracheal tube. In certain situations, it may be far quicker for the anesthesia team to intubate an arresting patient than to secure venous access. The appropriate dose is generally twice the IV dose, and the drug must be diluted to a volume of approximately 10 ml.

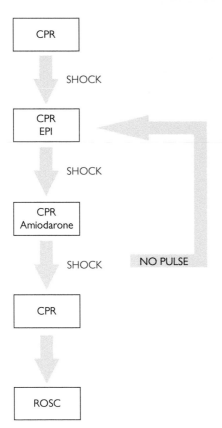

Figure 12.4 Treatment algorithm for pulseless VT and VF.

5. Check rhythm and pulse.

A pulse should be checked at the end of every 2-minute cycle of CPR. If pulseless VT or VF is still present, resume CPR and repeat steps 3 and 4 until pulse and ROSC return. IF VT (possible torsades de pointes) or VF is refractory to CPR/defibrillation, consider administering magnesium 1–2 g IV.

If a pulse is present and ROSC is confirmed, go to step 7.

Signs of ROSC include sinus rhythm on ECG with pulse present, a measurable blood pressure, a sustained increase in EtCO$_2$ (>30 mmHg) (if the patient is not paralyzed, spontaneous respirations may also return), and patient movement (if not paralyzed).

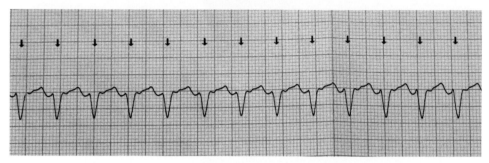

Figure 12.5 Unstable ventricular tachycardia—regular rhythm with a wide QRS.

6. If a pulse is present but the patient is in unstable VT (SBP <90 mmHg), perform synchronized cardioversion (Figure 12.5).

An unstable patient with VT who has a pulse will have a SBP <90 mmHg and be unarousable or confused (if not under anesthesia).

Do the following if not done previously (i.e., this is the initial presentation of VT):

- Notify the surgeon and all the members of the team.
- Turn off any inhalational anesthetic gases or IV anesthetic medications.
- If the patient is already intubated, ensure delivered FiO$_2$ is 100%.
- If the patient is not intubated, start bag-mask ventilation with 100% oxygen if not breathing, or 100% oxygen by facemask if respirations are adequate.

Call for the defibrillator and perform synchronized cardioversion ASAP with an initial dose of 100 J in adults. For neonates, infants, and children, deliver 1 J/kg synchronized and increase to 2 J/kg if unsuccessful (Figures 12.6A–D).

Sequence to follow for synchronized cardioversion:

- Apply defibrillator pads or paddles to the patient and turn on the defibrillator.
- **MAKE SURE TO ACTIVATE THE SYNCHRONIZATION FUNCTION ON THE DEFIBRILLATOR.**
- When synchronization is activated you should see marks on the ECG display on the defibrillator and/or hear beeps with each QRS.
- Charge the defibrillator to 100 J.
- Ensure no one is in contact with the patient and clearly state "all clear."
- Press and hold the defibrillate button until a shock is delivered.
- If the initial cardioversion is unsuccessful, repeat at 200 J.

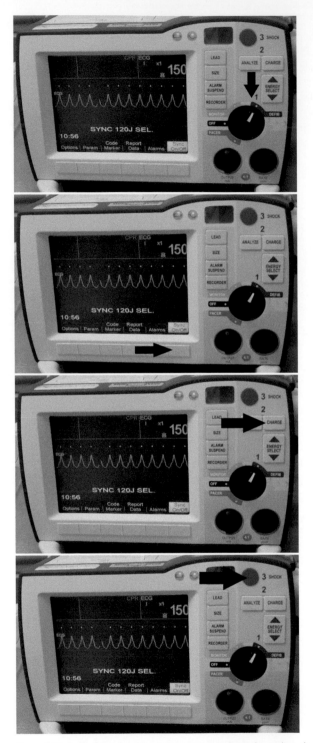

Figure 12.6 A–D. Sequence to cardiovert ventricular tachycardia—A: synchronized cardioversion step 1: activate defibrillation mode. B: synchronized cardioversion step 2: synchronize. C: synchronized cardioversion step 3: charge. D. synchronized cardioversion step 4: shock.

> **Caution!** A narrow-complex ECG is not a ventricular rhythm and is not covered in this chapter. A loose ECG lead may produce artifact that resembles VT or VF. Corroborate the ECG findings with the palpable pulse or pulse oximeter data.

7. Post-ROSC care.

Signs of ROSC include a return of pulse and blood pressure as well as a sustained increase in $EtCO_2$ (>40 mmHg). Discuss disposition of the patient and whether to continue the procedure, if applicable, with the surgeon and code team. Check electrolytes and troponin levels to rule out potential causes. Avoid hyperoxia by delivering the lowest FiO_2 necessary with a target SpO_2 ≥94%. Avoid hyperventilation by starting ventilation at 10 breaths per minute and titrate to an $EtCO_2$ of 35–40 mmHg.

Treat hypotension, if present. Consider giving a bolus of isotonic IV fluids (1–2 L) or vasoactive infusions:

- Epinephrine 0.1–0.5 mcg/kg/min IV
- Dopamine 5–10 mcg/min IV
- Norepinephrine 0.1–0.5 mcg/kg/min IV

Evaluate for ischemia by checking a 12-lead ECG and sending troponin levels. Consider coronary reperfusion with percutaneous coronary intervention (PCI) by cardiologist if ST-elevation myocardial infarction (STEMI) is present on ECG. Institute targeted temperature management in patients who remain comatose. Select and maintain a constant temperature between 32 and 36°C for at least 24 hours.

B. Treatment of Stable Ventricular Tachycardia

If a pulse is present and the patient is in stable VT (SBP >90 mmHg) and awake and oriented (if not under anesthesia), management is urgent but not emergent (Figure 12.7).

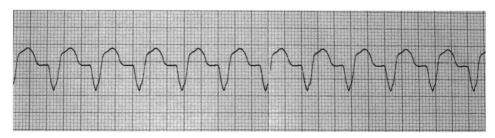

Figure 12.7 Stable ventricular tachycardia—regular rhythm with a wide QRS.

Step by Step

1. If the patient is in the operating room with an ongoing surgery, notify the surgeon and halt the procedure.

If surgery is nonemergent, consider cancelling the procedure.

2. Administer 100% oxygen.

If the patient is awake and oriented, administer 100% oxygen by facemask. If the patient is in the operating room under general anesthesia, administer 100% oxygen via the endotracheal tube.

3. **Check electrolytes and obtain a 12-lead ECG.**

Send electrolytes to check for any abnormalities and obtain a 12-lead ECG to look for ischemia. Consult cardiology to assist with management.

4. **Administer antiarrhythmic medications.**

If the pulse is regular and monomorphic, administer adenosine 6 mg IV rapid bolus, followed by a 10-ml saline flush to ensure rapid delivery. If there is no response after the first dose, administer a second dose of 12 mg IV followed by a 10-ml saline flush.

If the ECG exhibits a QRS >0.12 seconds (wide complex), administer amiodarone 150 mg IV bolus over 10 minutes followed by an infusion of 1 mg/min IV for 6 hours, and then 0.5 mg/min IV for 18 hours to achieve a full loading dose. Additional boluses can be given as needed if VT recurs. If amiodarone is not effective, other second-line agents to consider include procainamide 20–50 mg/min IV until arrhythmia suppressed, then decreasing to a maintenance rate of 1–4 mg/min IV, or sotalol 100 mg IV over 5 minutes.

5. **Consider overdrive pacing if not responsive to medications.**

Overdrive pacing can be considered in sustained VT refractory to antiarrhythmic medications. Consult cardiology as the patient may require workup for a permanent pacemaker and will require a monitored setting to manage external pacing.

> **Caution!** Overdrive pacing can precipitate VF.

Other Management Considerations

A patient may appear to have VT if they are paced with a ventricular lead and the ECG display does not show the pacemaker spikes. A patient may also appear to have VT if they have a wide QRS from an aberrant conduction pathway or a bundle branch block and small and absent p-waves such as in atrial fibrillation.

If this is a new onset of VT as confirmed by the patient's medical history, delay nonemergent surgery for a cardiac workup.

References

1. Donnino M, Navarro K, Berg K, et al. *Advanced Cardiovascular Life Support Provider Manual.* Dallas, Texas: American Heart Association; 2016:92–109, 145–155.
2. Henry M, Deegan R. Cardiac Dysrhythmias. In: Matthew M, Furse C, eds. *Advanced Perioperative Crisis Management.* New York: Oxford University Press; 2017:35–51.
3. Neumar R, Shuster M, Callaway C, et al. Part 1: Executive Summary. *Circulation.* 2015;132(18 suppl 2):S315–S367. doi:10.1161/cir.0000000000000252
4. Miller R, Cohen N, Eriksson L, Fleisher L, Wiener-Kronish J, Young W. *Miller's Anesthesia.* 7th ed. Philadelphia: Elsevier; 2010:2970–3001.
5. Oropello J, Pastores S, Kvetan V. *Critical Care.* New York: McGraw-Hill Education; 2017:289–302.
6. Pettit SJ, Petrie MC, Connelly DT, et al. Use of Implantable Cardioverter Defibrillators in Patients with Left Ventricular Assist Devices. *Eur J Heart Fail.* 2012 Jul;14(7):696–702.
7. Vincent J, Abraham E, Moore F, Kochanek P, Fink M. *Textbook of Critical Care.* 7th ed. Philadelphia: Elsevier; 2017:541–549.
8. Watson K. Abnormalities of Cardiac Conduction and Cardiac Rhythm. In: Hines R, Marschall K, eds. *Handbook for Stoelting's Anesthesia and Co-Existing Disease.* 3rd ed. Philadelphia: Saunders Elsevier; 2018:52–53.

Chapter 13

Tension Pneumothorax

Matthew Desmond and Yury Zasimovich

Summary Page

Symptoms:

- Cough, chest pain, and respiratory distress if awake
- Increasing airway pressure/decreasing lung compliance with mechanical ventilation
- Decreased breath sounds
- Asymmetric chest expansion
- Hypoxemia and hypercapnea
- Tachycardia
- Jugular venous engorgement/increased central venous pressure
- Subcutaneous emphysema
- Tracheal deviation
- Systemic arterial hypotension
- Cardiopulmonary compromise

Differential Diagnosis:

- Myocardial ischemia
- Cardiac tamponade
- Bronchospasm/laryngospasm
- Obstruction of mainstem bronchus or endotracheal tube
- Anaphylaxis
- Bronchial intubation
- Hemothorax/capnothorax/hydrothorax
- Congenital diaphragmatic hernia
- Tension viscerothorax

Introduction

Tension pneumothorax is an emergency that requires timely diagnosis and management to prevent mortality. Any procedure that may violate the pleura can cause a pneumothorax, such as nerve blocks and surgical procedures in that area. Others are prone to pneumothorax simply due to their anatomy and physiology, including neonates undergoing mechanical ventilation, tall adolescents, and older patients with chronic obstructive pulmonary disease (COPD). Every anesthesiologist should be familiar with tension pneumothorax, which may present after the initiation of artificial, positive pressure ventilation. Here the approach is presented, including step-by-step guidance for needle decompression and definitive drain placement. The use of ultrasound is emphasized. Ultrasound is extremely useful for both diagnostic and therapeutic purposes.

Treatment

Tension pneumothorax is a true emergency, which, if not diagnosed and treated in a timely manner, can lead to cardiac arrest. Maintain a high index of suspicion at all times.

One should have a heightened suspicion in a number of settings: premature infants under positive pressure ventilation; transtracheal or translaryngeal jet ventilation; use of an airway exchange catheter;[1-3] subclavian or internal jugular venous cannulation (especially without ultrasound guidance); supraclavicular, infraclavicular, thoracic paravertebral,[4] or intercostal nerve block (again, especially without ultrasound guidance); COPD; Marfan's syndrome;[5] thoracic or scoliosis[6] surgery; polytrauma (especially rib fracture); high airway pressure; previous pneumothorax; and nitrous oxide anesthesia. Nitrous oxide does not cause a pneumothorax in general but may lead to it in the setting of communicating pulmonary bullae.[7] Tension capnothorax risk is increased with laparoscopic esophageal[8] and thoracoscopic mediastinal[9] surgery.

> **WARNING!!** If a patient has a cardiac arrest due to tension pneumothorax, proceed according to advanced cardiac life support (ACLS) guidelines but do not stop decompression maneuvers, since without pneumothorax treatment, successful resuscitation is unlikely.

Step by Step

1. Suspect diagnosis of tension pneumothorax.

Signs and symptoms include cough, chest pain, and respiratory distress if awake; decreased breath sounds and asymmetric chest expansion; increasing airway pressure/decreasing lung compliance with mechanical ventilation; hypoxemia; hypercapnia and tachycardia; jugular venous engorgement/increased central venous pressure; and subcutaneous emphysema. The presence of tracheal deviation is highly diagnostic.

> **Caution!** Symptoms can progress to systemic arterial hypotension and cardiopulmonary compromise if not treated quickly.

> **WARNING!!** In the setting of cardiopulmonary compromise, begin ACLS and go **DIRECTLY to step 5** and perform emergent decompression.

2. **Administer 100% oxygen.**

Administer 100% oxygen. Turn off nitrous oxide, if using. If the patient is not intubated, place a nonrebreathing oxygen mask.

>> **Tip on Technique:** If one-lung ventilation is being performed, immediately convert to two-lung ventilation.

3. **Rule out mainstem intubation.**

Check the endotracheal tube (ETT) position/depth at the mouth. Extend the neck and recheck breath sounds and airway pressure. Perform laryngoscopy to check ETT placement or place a flexible bronchoscope through the ETT to rule out mainstem intubation.

> **WARNING!!** Mainstem intubation may lead one to both suspect tension pneumothorax and falsely diagnose it due to high airway pressure, a lack of breath sounds, and (on ultrasound) a lack of lung sliding on the side of the nonventilated lung.

4. **Verify the diagnosis with chest x-ray and/or ultrasound.**

Verify pneumothorax by clinical examination, chest x-ray, and ultrasound, if available.

Clinical diagnosis can be made via auscultation and a high index of suspicion after an airway or breathing circuit problem has been ruled out. Asymmetric chest rise is a particularly noticeable and helpful sign in small children.

Perform transthoracic ultrasound (preferred), transesophageal ultrasound, or chest x-ray if immediately available in the room. Place the transthoracic ultrasound probe longitudinally at multiple intercostal spaces along the anterolateral chest wall. Note the distance for decompression. The absence of lung sliding strongly suggests but is not diagnostic of pneumothorax.

The "lung point" sign, where an area intermittently has lung sliding or B lines, has a specificity of 100% for pneumothorax.[10] Time-motion display (M mode) on ultrasound can be used, with the "seashore sign" equivalent to lung sliding and the "barcode sign" consistent with pneumothorax (Figure 13.1).

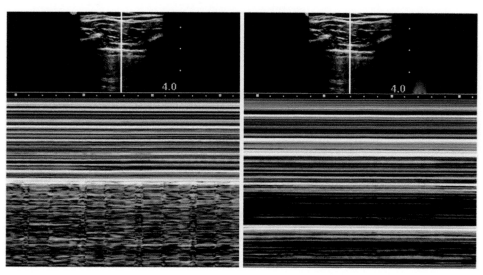

Figure 13.1 Time-motion display (M mode) on ultrasound can be used, with the "seashore sign" equivalent to lung sliding (on the left) and the "barcode sign" consistent with pneumothorax (on the right).

>> **Tip on Technique:** X-ray is often already in the room; otherwise, this modality is too time consuming. The absence of lung sliding strongly suggests but is not diagnostic of pneumothorax, as any entity that prevents the pleura from moving (e.g., pleural adhesions) can lead to this. The absence of ultrasound comet-tail artifact (B lines) increases diagnostic accuracy.[11]

If thoracoscopy is being performed, alert the surgeon to look for mediastinal herniation toward the operative side.

>> **Tip on Technique:** If a transesophageal echo (TEE) probe is already in place, it can be useful for ruling out a cardiac cause of hypoxemia (e.g., pulmonary embolism).[12,13] It is invaluable if the chest wall cannot be adequately imaged externally (e.g., subcutaneous emphysema, obesity). Tension pneumothorax is obvious on both lung and cardiovascular analysis (the latter showing right heart compression and venae cavae engorgement).

Note: If cardiopulmonary compromise is present, complete steps 5–7 immediately! If the patient is stable, go to step 8.

5. **If cardiopulmonary compromise is present, start ACLS immediately.**

   Start ACLS and chest compressions, if indicated. Call for help. Step 6 can be performed during resuscitation, as hemodynamics are more likely to improve if the tension pneumothorax is decompressed. Additional personnel will be needed to perform steps 5 and 6 simultaneously.

6. **Perform needle decompression (Figure 13.2).**

   Sterilize the skin and identify the mid- to anterior axillary line of the fifth intercostal space (AL5ICS).[14,15] Insert an 8-cm, 10- to 14-gauge angiocatheter perpendicular to the skin just above the rib while the other hand continues to palpate the bony landmarks. If bone is encountered, angle cephalad and advance again. Air should be released via the needle/angiocatheter.

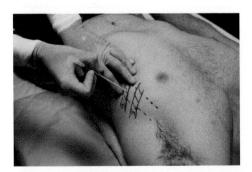

Figure 13.2 Needle decompression at AL5ICS.

WARNING!!   Failed needle decompression is common. If no air is released, attempt again in a slightly different location with a larger, longer needle. If the patient continues to deteriorate, move rapidly to open thoracostomy (step 11).

!! **Potential Complication:** Pulmonary laceration may occur. Hemothorax (from severing an intercostal vessel) or intercostal nerve injury can result from inserting the needle along the inferior rib edge.

>> **Tip on Technique:** The decompression site is found most quickly by moving directly lateral to the nipple in patients with no or small breasts, but with larger breasts this relationship is not reliable. The site is identified by moving caudally from the manubrium 80% of the distance between the sternal notch and xiphoid process.[16] Ultrasound can be used by finding the second rib as it joins the sternomanubrial joint and following it laterally and then inferiorly, counting ribs.[17]

>> **Tip on Technique:** Advanced Trauma Life Support still recommends the second intercostal space, midclavicular line in children due to a dearth of pediatric studies.[18] Palpate the sternomanubrial joint, where the second rib articulates, and lateral to this lies the second intercostal space. If decompression fails, attempt again at the AL5ICS. A shorter angiocatheter may suffice. Needle placement is commonly too medial, and if so injury to the internal mammary artery can occur.[19]

7. **Remove the needle and leave the angiocatheter in place.**

Leave the needle in place for 5–10 seconds, or until air is no longer heard evacuating, as the catheter could collapse or kink.[20] Needle removal prevents pulmonary laceration.

!! **Potential Complication:** Angiocatheters are prone to dislodgement or obstruction by external compression, clots, or kinking. Dislodgement may be more likely at the second intercostal, midclavicular site.[21]

8. **If laparoscopy is being performed, look for a diaphragm breach and deflate the pneumoperitoneum.**

This identifies a tension capnothorax and improves cardiac preload in any situation.

> **Caution!** Tension capnothorax is found in 22% of laparoscopic repairs of massive hiatal hernia.[8] These can almost always be managed without external decompression. The surgeon should suction through the defect and decrease insufflation pressure. After hypotension has resolved, increased airway pressure and positive end-expiratory pressure (PEEP) may be applied to prevent recurrence.[8]

9. **Stabilize the patient.**

Give IV fluids rapidly to increase cardiac preload and quickly deliver needed medications.

To improve hemodynamics, turn off volatile anesthetics and consider administering midazolam 0.1 mg/kg IV for amnesia. If the patient is hypotensive, administer phenylephrine 1–4 mcg/kg IV to increase preload and blood pressure.[22] If the patient is both hypotensive and bradycardic, administer epinephrine 0.1–0.5 mcg/kg IV.

If the patient is breathing spontaneously, do not initiate mechanical support, and ensure there is no PEEP or pressure support to prevent/slow enlargement of the pneumothorax. If the patient is intubated and receiving positive pressure ventilation, advance the endotracheal tube under bronchoscopic guidance (if possible) into the opposite mainstem bronchus to prevent enlargement of the pneumothorax.

10. Place a small-bore (8 to 14 French) drain.

Often this is performed by the surgeon if he or she has more experience. If there is insufficient time or as an alternate next step, a thoracostomy tube can be placed (step 11).

Position the patient (Figure 13.3). The ipsilateral arm should be abducted, securing the hand on top of or under the head. A bump is placed under the ipsilateral flank. Decompression may also be performed in the lateral decubitus position, moving the arm anteriorly.

Sterilize the skin and, if time allows, numb the insertion site (just inferior to AL5ICS) with 0.25% bupivacaine 0.25–0.5 ml/kg or 1% lidocaine with epinephrine 1:200,000 (up to 30 ml) SC and IM. Attach the finder needle to a syringe and aspirate while advancing cephalad with ultrasound guidance (Figure 13.4).

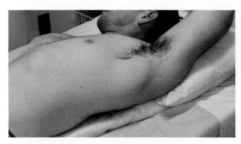

Figure 13.3 Ideal positioning for tube thoracostomy (often not possible during surgery), with the arm abducted, the hand secured under or on top of the head, and a bump under the ipsilateral flank.

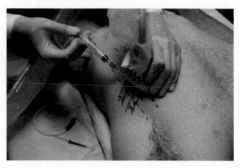

Figure 13.4 Using ultrasound guidance, angle cephalad while inserting the needle for percutaneous drain placement.

>> **Tip on Technique:** The needle should pass just superior to the edge of the rib to avoid neurovascular injury. Keep the angle between the skin and angiocatheter <45 degrees. This is associated with decreased complications.[23]

After reaching air or liquid, remove the syringe and pass the wire. Remove the needle, marking the depth to the pleural space with fingertips. Make a skin incision and pass the dilator not more than a centimeter beyond the distance to the pleural cavity.[24] Exchange the dilator for the drain, then advance until the last drainage hole is intrapleural, and remove the wire. Attach a large-bore stopcock and secure the drain as one would a central venous catheter. Attach a Heimlich flutter valve if there is no significant liquid draining; otherwise, use a standard suction device (Figure 13.5).

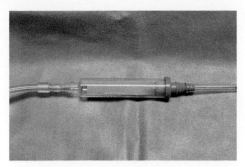

Figure 13.5 The Heimlich flutter valve is an easily portable, one-way check valve used for pneumothorax.

WARNING!! Reversing the Heimlich valve can lead to tension pneumothorax.

>> **Tip on Technique:** A larger drain should be placed with an open technique if there is a suspected or proven hemothorax, bronchial dehiscence (as after lung surgery), or penetrating chest injury ipsilaterally. In severe trauma, where the possibilities of massive pleural hemorrhage or bronchopleural disruption are significant, use a large-bore drain. Specialized kits are available but single-lumen central venous kits or individual percutaneous drainage catheters can be used.

>> **Tip on Technique:** Avoid standard stopcocks as they are the flow-limiting point in drains as small as 8F.[25]

11. If needle decompression or drain placement fails, perform an open thoracostomy at AL5ICS.

Position the patient (see Figure 13.3), sterilize, and numb the site if time allows. Make a 3- to 4-cm horizontal incision at the sixth rib's inferior edge. With a curved Kelly clamp, dissect a subcutaneous tunnel superiorly over the sixth rib, entering the pleural cavity. Spread the clamp, ensuring decompression. Remove the clamp and sweep a finger in the pleural space, confirming the correct location.

Load the drain on the clamp such that the drain ends 1 cm beyond the clamp (Figure 13.6). Reinsert the clamp with the drain attached, digitally palpating to confirm that the drain is intrapleural and not subcutaneous. Advance the drain anterosuperiorly (posterosuperiorly if a hemopneumothorax is present). Remove the clamp while advancing the drain, ensuring the last side hole is intrapleural.

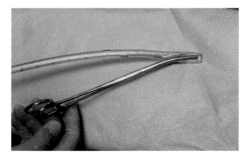

Figure 13.6 A curved Kelly clamp properly loaded, with the chest drain extending just past the clamp.

If the patient had lung isolation initiated to treat the pneumothorax, return to two-lung ventilation and assess drain adequacy. Suture the drain in place using 0 silk, forming an airtight seal, and place an occlusive petrolatum dressing, gauze, and tape. Place an "omental" tape further down the drain to keep tension off sutures. Connect a chest drainage system with suction set to −20 cm of water.

>> **Tip on Technique:** Historically a 16–22 French chest tube has been placed with the open technique; however, often a small-bore drain suffices.[26] If there is concern for hemothorax, a large air leak (e.g., bronchial disruption), or penetrating chest wound ipsilaterally, use a 28–32 French chest tube.[18]

!! **Potential Complication:** Horner's syndrome occurs in almost 1% of cases, likely from a drain placed at the apex that compresses the stellate ganglion.[27] This neurapraxia should resolve with tube retraction by several centimeters. Subcutaneous drain placement occurs in 0.8% and is catastrophic if placed for tension pneumothorax.[23] This tends to occur due to an inadequate incision and/or lack of palpating the drain entering the intercostal space.

> **Caution!** Continuous air bubbling in the chest drainage system is a clue that the skin suture may not be airtight or the last side hole is not intrapleural. Chest x-ray rules out the latter. The other possibility is a pulmonary air leak.

12. Confirm decompression and drain placement.

Perform a chest x-ray. If the pneumothorax remains and the drain is in good position, confirm suction is functioning and manually inject and aspirate sterile saline. If the drain fails and the patient is unstable, have a proceduralist place a second drain. If the drain fails and the patient is stable, obtain a chest computed tomography scan to determine the cause of failure.

Other Management Considerations

Decompression is emergent, whereas drain placement is not. Thus, drains are omitted in many places in the world as air simply escapes through the thoracostomy. Drains are only placed if there is repeated air accumulation, excessive adipose tissue likely to impede air egress, a prolonged medical evacuation with difficult patient access, etc.

Needle decompression can also be done at the second intercostal space along the midclavicular line (Monaldi position). However, depth is greater and placement less accurate.[28,29]

Small-bore chest drains have markedly decreased complications, including infections,[30] injury,[14] malposition, and pain,[31] but have a somewhat higher occlusion rate (8.1 versus 5.2%).[24] The British Thoracic Society, which publishes the most comprehensive guidelines, recommends a small drain as first-line treatment for pneumothoraces.[24]

References

1. Hulst AH, Avis HJ, Hollmann MW, Stevens MF. Massive subcutaneous emphysema and bilateral tension pneumothoraces after supplemental oxygen delivery via an airway exchange catheter: a case report. A A Case Rep. 2017 Jan 15;8(2):26–28.
2. Duggan LV, Law JA, Murphy MF. Brief review: supplementing oxygen through an airway exchange catheter: efficacy, complications, and recommendations. Can J Anaesth. 2011;58:560–568.

3. McLean S, Lanam CR, Benedict W, Kirkpatrick N, Kheterpal S, Ramachandran SK. Airway exchange failure and complications with the use of the Cook Airway Exchange Catheter®: a single center cohort study of 1177 patients. Anesth Analg. 2013 Dec;117(6):1325–1327.

4. Naja Z, Lönnqvist PA. Somatic paravertebral nerve blockade. Incidence of failed block and complications. Anaesthesia. 2001;56:1184–1188

5. Hao W, Fang Y, Lai H, Shen Y, Wang H, Lin M, Tan L. Marfan syndrome with pneumothorax: case report and review of literatures. J Thorac Dis. 2017 Dec;9(12):E1100–E1103.

6. Soroceanu A, Burton DC, Oren JH, Smith JS, Hostin R, Shaffrey CI, Akbarnia BA, Ames CP, Errico TJ, Bess S, Gupta MC, Deviren V, Schwab FJ, Lafage V, International Spine Study Group. Medical complications after adult spinal deformity surgery: incidence, risk factors, and clinical impact. Spine (Phila Pa 1976). 2016 Nov 15;41(22):1718–1723.

7. Sahoo RK, Nair AS, Kulkarni V, Mudunuri R. Anesthetic consideration in a patient with giant bilateral lung bullae with severe respiratory compromise. Saudi J Anaesth. 2015 Oct–Dec;9(4):493–495.

8. Phillips S, Falk GL. Surgical tension pneumothorax during laparoscopic repair of massive hiatus hernia: a different situation requiring different management. Anaesth Intensive Care. 2011 Nov;39(6):1120–1123.

9. Pandey R, Garg R, Chandralekha, Darlong V, Punj J, Sinha R, Jyoti B, Mukundan C, Elakkumanan LB. Robot-assisted thoracoscopic thymectomy: perianaesthetic concerns. Eur J Anaesthesiol. 2010 May;27(5):473–477.

10. Lichtenstein D, Mezière G, Biderman P, Gepner A. The "lung point": an ultrasound sign specific to pneumothorax. Intensive Care Med. 2000 Oct;26(10):1434–1440.

11. Lichtenstein D, Mezière G, Biderman P, Gepner A. The comet-tail artifact: an ultrasound sign ruling out pneumothorax. Intensive Care Med. 1999 Apr;25(4):383–388.

12. Cavayas YA, Girard M, Desjardins G, Denault AY. Transesophageal lung ultrasonography: a novel technique for investigating hypoxemia. Can J Anaesth. 2016 Nov;63(11):1266–1276.

13. Vetrugno L, Bignami E, Bove T. Transesophageal lung ultrasound should be the first-line tool to evaluate intraoperative hypoxia. Anesth Analg. 2018 Jun;126(6):2145–2146.

14. Inaba K, Branco BC, Eckstein M, Shatz DV, Martin MJ, Green DJ, Noguchi TT, Demetriades D. Optimal positioning for emergent needle thoracostomy: a cadaver-based study. J Trauma. 2011 Nov;71(5):1099–1103; discussion 1103.

15. Inaba K, Ives C, McClure K, Branco BC, Eckstein M, Shatz D, Martin MJ, Reddy S, Demetriades D. Radiologic evaluation of alternative sites for needle decompression of tension pneumothorax. Arch Surg. 2012;147(9):813–818.

16. Marcus F, Hughes T, Barrios P, Borgstrom M. Clinical location of the fourth and fifth intercostal spaces as a percent of the length of the sternum. J Electrocardiol. 2018 Jan–Feb;51(1):55–59.

17. Bowness JS, Nicholls K, Kilgour PM, Ferris J, Whiten S, Parkin I, Mooney J, Driscoll P. Finding the fifth intercostal space for chest drain insertion: guidelines and ultrasound. Emerg Med J. 2015 Dec;32(12):951–954.

18. American College of Surgeons. Advanced Trauma Life Support Student Course Manual, 10th Edition. 2018.

19. Ferrie EP, Collum N, McGovern S. The right place in the right space? Awareness of site for needle thoracocentesis. Emerg Med J. 2005 Nov;22(11):788–789.

20. Butler FK Jr, Holcomb JB, Shackelford S, Montgomery HR, Anderson S, Cain JS, Champion HR, Cunningham CW, Dorlac WC, Drew B, Edwards K, Gandy JV, Glassberg E, Gurney J, Harcke T, Jenkins DA, Johannigman J, Kheirabadi BS, Kotwal RS, Littlejohn LF, Martin M, Mazuchowski EL, Otten EJ, Polk T, Rhee P, Seery JM, Stockinger Z, Torrisi J, Yitzak A, Zafren K, Zietlow SP. Management of suspected tension pneumothorax in tactical combat casualty care: TCCC guidelines change 17-02. J Spec Oper Med. 2018 Summer;18(2):19–35.

21. Leatherman ML, Held JM, Fluke LM, McEvoy CS, Inaba K, Grabo D, Martin MJ, Earley AS, Ricca RL, Polk TM. Relative device stability of anterior versus axillary needle decompression for tension pneumothorax during casualty movement: preliminary analysis of a human cadaver model. J Trauma Acute Care Surg. 2017 Jul;83(1 Suppl 1):S136–S141.

22. Cannesson M, Zhongping J, Chen G, Vu TQ, Hatib F. Effects of phenylephrine on cardiac output and venous return depend on the position of the heart on the Frank–Starling relationship. J Appl Physiol. 2012;113:281–289.

23. Hernandez MC, Laan DV, Zimmerman SL, Naik ND, Schiller HJ, Aho JM. Tube thoracostomy: increased angle of insertion is associated with complications. J Trauma Acute Care Surg. 2016 Aug;81(2):366–370.

24. Havelock T, et al. Pleural procedures and thoracic ultrasound: British Thoracic Society pleural disease guideline 2010. Thorax 2010;65(Suppl 2):ii61–ii76.

25. Macha DB, Thomas J, Nelson RC. Pigtail catheters used for percutaneous fluid drainage: comparison of performance characteristics. Radiology. 2006 Mar;238(3):1057–1063.

26. Kaya SO, Liman ST, Bir LS, Yuncu G, Erbay HR, Unsal S. Horner's syndrome as a complication in thoracic surgical practice. Eur J Cardiothorac Surg. 2003 Dec;24(6):1025–1028.

27. Porcel JM. Chest tube drainage of the pleural space: a concise review for pulmonologists. Tuberc Respir Dis (Seoul). 2018 Apr;81(2):106–115.

28. Benton IJ, Benfield GF. Comparison of a large and small-calibre tube drain for managing spontaneous pneumothoraces. Respir Med. 2009 Oct;103(10):1436–1440.

29. Inaba K, Karamanos E, Skiada D, Grabo D, Hammer P, Martin M, Sullivan M, Eckstein M, Demetriades D. Cadaveric comparison of the optimal site for needle decompression of tension pneumothorax by prehospital care providers J Trauma Acute Care Surg. 2015 Dec;79(6):1044–1048.

30. Kulvatunyou N, Erickson L, Vijayasekaran A, Gries L, Joseph B, Friese RF, O'Keeffe T, Tang AL, Wynne JL, Rhee P. Randomized clinical trial of pigtail catheter versus chest tube in injured patients with uncomplicated traumatic pneumothorax. Br J Surg. 2014 Jan;101(2):17–22.

31. Wax DB, Leibowitz AB. Radiologic assessment of potential sites for needle decompression of a tension pneumothorax. Anesth Analg. 2007;105(5):1385–1388.

Chapter 14

Vascular Access
Peripheral Venous, Central Venous, and Intraosseous Access

Linda Le-Wendling, Jayme N. Looper, and Lisa Gu

Introduction

Access to the venous system can be used for both drug delivery and volume resuscitation. Peripheral intravenous (PIV) access is the main route of drug delivery. Central venous line (CVL) access is indicated for delivery of vasoactive or caustic medications, large and rapid volume infusions, total parenteral nutrition, invasive monitoring (central venous pressures, pulmonary artery pressures), and certain procedures (extracorporeal membrane oxygenation, transvenous pacing, dialysis). Intraosseous (IO) access can be used when PIV access is difficult, especially in emergency situations such as cardiac arrest due to more rapid and successful access, though it is usually a temporary (usually <24 hour) modality. For PIV and CVL access, ultrasound can be used to visualize the target vein in real time as well as neighboring neurovascular structures to determine the optimal entry point and needle trajectory. Maintaining sterility is important. Visualizing the vessel in cross-section and advancing the needle in an out-of-plane approach is the simplest technique when using ultrasound. Local lidocaine infiltration can be used to increase patient comfort. Confirming venous, and not arterial or extravascular, placement is key in minimizing complications. Other complications include hematoma, vascular or nerve damage, fluid extravasation, compartment syndrome, air embolism, hemo-/pneumothorax (with CVL), and infection.

In an emergent situation (e.g., cardiac arrest), central lines may take too long to obtain. IO access is much quicker and preferred. Femoral CVL access is usually the easiest to obtain in an emergency and does not interrupt airway manipulation and chest compressions.

The three sections below will provide step-by-step guidance for PIV access placement, IO access placement, and CVL placement both with and without the use of ultrasound.

Peripheral Intravenous Access Placement

Step by Step

1. Prepare your materials.

To place a peripheral IV, you will need a tourniquet, antiseptic (alcohol or ChloraPrep), IV catheters of various sizes, tape, gauze and dressings, a saline-filled syringe, and IV connector tubing. Optional materials include an ultrasound machine with sterile gel and a probe cover, and local anesthetic to topicalize the area.

>> **Tip on Technique**: Remove jewelry, wash hands, and wear clean gloves to prevent infection.

2. Select the vein.

Choose the most distal, superficial, straight, and large vein.

>> **Tip on Technique**: Start distally. If you rupture a vein more proximally, then placing an IV in the same vein distally will cause fluid extravasation. Consider the use of ultrasound to identify and select a vein if IV access is difficult and veins are not easily seen or palpated (see step 6).

WARNING!!   IVs should NOT be placed distal to an arteriovenous fistula or lymph node dissection (e.g., history of mastectomy).

---

3. Choose the appropriate gauge catheter.

Consider placement of smaller gauge IVs (24–20 gauge) for drug delivery. Larger gauge IV catheters (18–14 gauge) are recommended for volume resuscitation.

>> **Tip on Technique**: Ultrasound allows access to deeper, more proximal veins but requires longer catheters to reach the vessel and minimize catheter dislodgement.

WARNING!!	Large diameter catheters (16 gauge and larger) increase risk of rupturing the vessel (aka a "blown vein") and rarely last as long as smaller ones.

4. Apply tourniquet to increase vein size.

Apply the tourniquet proximal to the selected vein and position the arm below the level of the heart. Stroking the vein proximal to distal and keeping the patient's limb warm can assist in increasing vein size.

WARNING!!	Remember to undo the tourniquet at the end of procedure. Failure to release the tourniquet can lead to limb ischemia or local tissue injury.

5. Disinfect the skin with antiseptic and administer local anesthesia if needed.

Options for disinfection include alcohol prep pads, iodine/betadine prep, and chlorhexidine prep.

!! **Potential Complications:** Patients may have allergic and skin reactions to antiseptic solution.

Consider administration of local anesthetic if the patient is awake (optional). Options for local anesthetic include lidocaine injection with small needle (27 gauge), eutectic mixture local (EMLA) cream, or vapocoolant spray.

6. Place IV with or without ultrasound.

IV placement without ultrasound: Retract the skin near the insertion site. Insert the needle of the IV catheter at a 10- to 20-degree angle with the bevel facing up toward the selected vein until a flash of blood can be seen in the flashback chamber. Advance the catheter another ½ cm before sliding the catheter off the needle and into the vein to ensure that the catheter tip and not just the needle tip is inside the vessel.

If unsuccessful the first time, try more proximally. If not successful the second time, proceed with an ultrasound-guided technique. Release the tourniquet after successful IV placement.

>> **Tip on Technique**: Avoid touching the IV catheter shaft with your gloved hand (especially if using nonsterile gloves) to reduce the risk of infection.

IV placement using ultrasound: Apply sterile gel to the skin and cover the ultrasound probe with a sterile sleeve or Tegaderm dressing. Hold the probe so that your left = left on the ultrasound screen. Manipulate the ultrasound probe so that the vein appears in cross-section (as a dark circle on the screen) and centered. Fluid (and blood) will appear anechoic (black) on ultrasound.

Determine whether the vascular structure seen on ultrasound is arterial or venous. An artery will appear pulsatile. Tilt the probe and use the doppler feature to help determine whether the flow is pulsatile. Apply downward pressure on the ultrasound probe to check compressibility. Veins should easily collapse compared to arteries.

Place the IV needle through the skin and advance at a 10- to 20-degree angle. The needle tip will be seen as a bright dot within the vein (Figure 14.1). Advance the needle under ultrasound until another 1 cm of needle catheter is within the vein before sliding the catheter off the needle.

Release the tourniquet after successful IV placement.

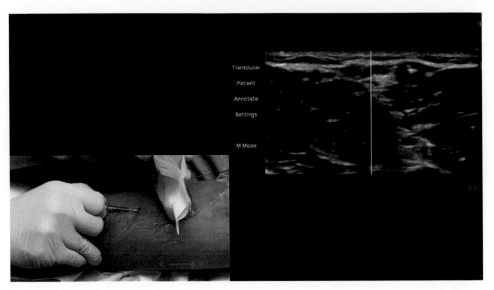

Figure 14.1 Needle visualized as a dot within the vein as it is advanced out of plane under ultrasound guidance.

>> **Tip on Technique**: Keep the ultrasound machine in front of you so you do not have to turn your head. Use a high-frequency linear probe for better resolution. Transparent dressings (Tegaderm) provide a tighter seal over the probe and will limit image distortion. A needle entry point too close to the probe will risk probe damage and needle contamination. Avoid applying too much pressure with the ultrasound probe as this will compress the vessel. If you see swelling with saline injection, the catheter is likely extravascular. Remove the catheter and apply pressure with gauze to the cannulation site to avoid hematoma formation.

!! **Potential Complication**: Failure to recognize an extravascular catheter may lead to fluid extravasation in the limb and compartment syndrome. Arterial cannulation instead of venous cannulation can occur. Pulsatile blood implies cannulation into an artery. Remove the catheter and apply pressure for 10 minutes if arterial cannulation is suspected.

7. **Secure the IV and connect to IV tubing.**

Place some gauze underneath the catheter hub to absorb any blood that bleeds back through the cannula after removal of the stylet. Remove the stylet and connect IV tubing or a saline syringe to the catheter. Aspirate via the syringe or tubing to confirm blood return (this may be difficult or impossible with smaller gauge IV catheters).

If ultrasound was used for placement, wipe the sterile ultrasound gel off the skin. Reapply skin antiseptic. Apply skin adhesive if desired, and secure the IV with a transparent sterile occlusive dressing and tape.

Intraosseous Access Placement

Consider IO access in emergent/urgent situations in which IV access is difficult (trauma, cardiac arrest, status epilepticus, burn, shock). Absolute contraindications include fracture at the intended IO access site, compartment syndrome/vascular injury in the target extremity, infection at the site, previous hardware (orthopedic surgery) at the site, or a recent failed IO attempt (within 24 hours).

Step by Step

1. Select the site for IO access.

Options for IO access include the proximal tibia, distal tibia, and proximal humerus. The proximal tibia is the easiest site to palpate, but the proximal humerus allows for the highest flow rates.

> **WARNING!!** Avoid any site of previous fracture, failed attempt at IO access, or infection.

!! **Potential Complication:** Osteomyelitis or bone fracture can occur.

> **Caution!** Consider avoiding IO access if there is a history of osteopenia. The sternum is not recommended due to interference with chest compressions and risk of injury to the heart and great vessels.

2. Prepare materials.

You will need the appropriate length needle and a drill if using machine-driven IO access (EZ-IO, FAST 1), as well as sterile prep solution, 3 to 5 ml of lidocaine in a syringe with a needle for injection, a needle/IV tubing adapter, a half-filled syringe of saline for aspiration, and a pressure bag.

>> **Tip on Technique**: For proximal tibia IO access, use a 2.5-cm needle length if the tibia is palpable, 4.5 cm if it is not palpable. For proximal humerus IO access, use a 4.5-cm length if body mass index (BMI) is >40, 2.5 cm if BMI is <40. For a 3–39-kg patient, use 1.5-cm needle length. Ultrasound can be used to determine needle length. Bone must be at most 2 cm deep to use a 2.5-cm needle and 4.0 cm deep to use a 4.5-cm needle.

!! **Potential Complication**: Selection of a too-short needle increases the risk of fluid/ drug extravasation from inadequate needle depth or future needle displacement, which may result in compartment syndrome or an ischemic limb. Selection of a too-long needle (needle will protrude above the skin) increases the risk of needle dislodgement.

3. Prepare the selected site and position the patient.

Externally rotate the lower extremity if tibial access is selected. Place the patient's hand over the abdomen (adduct and internally rotate arm) for humerus IO access. Prep the site with antiseptic. Use lidocaine (optional) if the patient is conscious.

4. Place IO access.

For the proximal tibia (Figure 14.2):

- In adults, access at the flat part of the tibia 2 fingerbreadths below the tibial tuberosity.
- In newborns, access at 10-mm distal to the tibial tuberosity with needle aimed slightly caudad to avoid the growth plate.

For the proximal humerus (Figure 14.3):

- It may require longer needles, but it allows for higher flow rates.
- Stay lateral to the biceps tendon.

For the distal tibia (Figure 14.4):

- Access at the flat part of the tibia 1–2 cm above the medial malleolus (2 cm for adults, 1 cm for children).

Place the needle at 90 degrees (perpendicular) to the bone plane and advance the needle. Drive the needle in. Remove the drill and trocar/stylet once loss of resistance is felt. Connect to the adaptor and syringe and place dressing. Aspirate bone marrow to confirm correct placement. Once confirmed, inject saline. Look and feel for evidence of extravasation. Inject lidocaine 2 ml for patient comfort. Use a transparent dressing to allow visualization of the needle and adaptor. Secure well to avoid needle dislocation.

>> **Tip on Technique**: If placing the needle manually, twist as you advance until a loss of resistance is felt. Avoid a rocking motion. If using a spring-loaded (impact-driven) or battery-powered device, hold both the device and the target limb firmly in place to allow enough driving pressure for needle penetration of the cortex.

>> **Tip on Technique**: An initial saline flush can break the trabecular meshwork and improve flow rates.

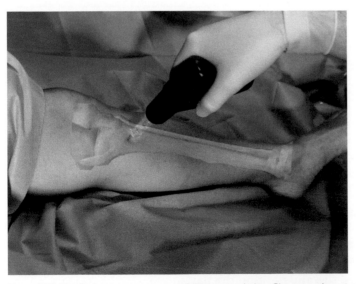

Figure 14.2 Site for intraosseous access of the proximal tibia. Chapter author pictured in the figure.

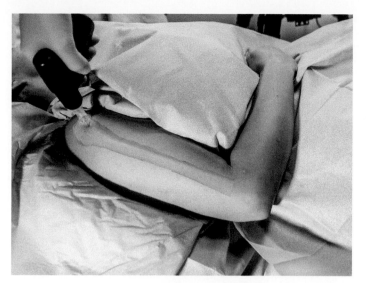

Figure 14.3 Site for intraosseous access for proximal humerus. Chapter author pictured in the figure.

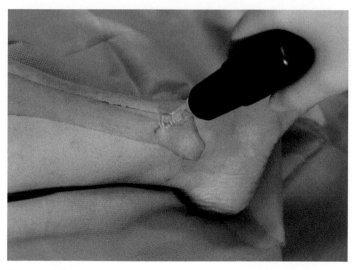

Figure 14.4 Site for intraosseous access for distal tibia. Chapter author pictured in the figure.

!! **Potential Complication**: Rocking the needle during manual placement increases bone opening and extravasation.

Caution! Manual needle placements have a greater risk of needle bending or breaking.

7. Connect drugs or IV fluids to the IO access.

Apply a pressure bag to fluids for higher infusion rates. Watch for fluid/drug extravasation. IO access should be discontinued once reliable IV access has been obtained or if there is concern for displacement or infection. Recommend removing IO lines within 24 hours of placement. Extravasation occurs 1–2% of the time, and risk factors include incorrect needle placement, multiple punctures in the same bone, and incorrect needle length.

>> **Tip on Technique**: All medications, IV fluids, and blood products can be given IO.

Central Venous Access Placement

Step by Step

1. Select the site.

Options for CVL placement include:
- Internal jugular (IJ) vein: straightest trajectory to right atrium
- Subclavian (SC) vein: lowest infection risk
- Femoral (FEM) vein: highest infection risk

> **WARNING!!**   Reconsider target vein if there is a clot in the target vessel, significant coagulopathy or current anticoagulation (SC or IJ), trauma or infection at the target site, or respiratory compromise (avoid SC).

2. Select catheter size and length.

Consider a smaller size (7 or 7.5 French) for delivery of medications. Consider a larger size (9 or 12 French) for volume resuscitation or pulmonary artery catheter placement.

A 15-cm length catheter is recommended for right-sided IJ/SC placement, while a 20-cm length is recommended for left-sided IJ/SC placement or FEM placement.

3. Place patient in Trendelenburg for IJ/ SC placement.

Trendelenburg position is preferred for central venous access if tolerated by the patent.

For IJ placement, turn the head up to 30 degrees away from the target site to improve access to the neck.

> **Caution!**   Excessive head turn increases carotid artery and IJ overlap and risks arterial puncture, especially on the left side.

> **WARNING!!**   Without Trendelenburg positioning for IJ/SC, air embolism may occur, especially in patients with low central venous pressure.

4. Prepare the CVL kit and patient.

Apply antiseptic solution to the chosen site. Remove any jewelry, wash hands, and don a mask, hat, sterile gown, and gloves. Open the CVL kit sterilely and confirm all contents are present in the kit. Flush central line ports to remove air. Clamp all ports (except the end port) after flushing.

Place a drape over the patient. In awake patients, consider local anesthetic. Aspirate before injecting local anesthetic to confirm no vascular injection. Apply sterile probe cover over ultrasound probe, if using.

>> **Tip on Technique**: Chlorhexidine is preferred for the best microbial coverage, longer duration, and quicker onset of action. Use of colored antiseptic allows you to visualize your sterile field.

WARNING!!   Central line associated bloodstream infections (CLABSIs) can occur with improper sterile technique.

---

5. Find the landmarks using both surface anatomy and ultrasound.

Use of ultrasound is STRONGLY encouraged to help determine safer trajectories and minimize the number of passes with the needle.

Landmarks for CVL placement include:

- IJ: Apex of the triangle created by the clavicle and the sternal and clavicular heads of the sternocleidomastoid, lateral to the carotid pulse. Aim the needle toward the ipsilateral nipple.
- FEM: 1–2 cm below inguinal ligament, 1 cm medial to the femoral pulse. Aim the needle cephalad.
- SC: 1 cm below the lateral edge of the proximal one-third of the clavicle. Aim the needle toward the sternal notch.

If using, place the ultrasound over the above landmarks with the vessels in cross-section (Figure 14.5). Suitable access includes a lack of a thrombus, minimal tortuosity, large size, and no overlapping artery. Position the ultrasound machine in front of you to minimize head movements during CVL placement. Confirm correct probe orientation (your left = left on the screen). Adjust depth and gain to maximize view. Locate and identify nearby arteries to avoid arterial puncture. Arteries are pulsatile, while veins are nonpulsatile and collapsible. Color doppler can help differentiate between vein and artery.

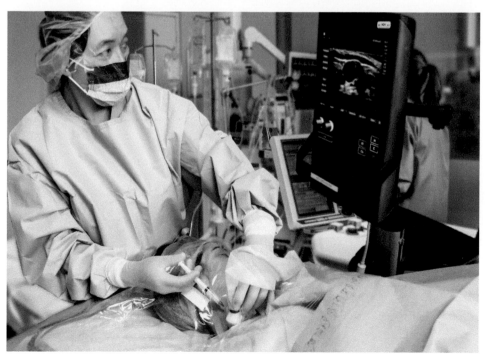

Figure 14.5 Place the target vein in cross-section. Place ultrasound monitor in front of you to minimize head movements. Chapter author pictured in the figure.

!! Potential Complications: Arterial puncture or pneumothorax can occur. Risks are higher with landmark-based approaches as compared to ultrasound-guided approaches.

WARNING!!   Too caudad a needle entry point with IJ access increases the risk of lung and SC injury.

---

6. Obtain venous access.

Obtain an image of the target vessel in cross-section with ultrasound (previous step). Center the vein on the ultrasound screen. Note vein depth using markers on the side of the ultrasound screen.

Enter the skin 1 cm from the probe with a needle or catheter attached to a syringe (to avoid penetrating the ultrasound probe sleeve and contaminating the needle). Advance the needle at about a 30-degree angle under ultrasound visualization into the target vein. Confirm blood return via syringe.

>> **Tip on Technique**: Avoid excessive downward pressure on the ultrasound probe to avoid collapsing the target vein.

In hypovolemic patients, veins collapse with needle advancement and can result in no blood return. Blood return will occur with needle retraction in this case, so constantly aspirate as you pull the needle back.

WARNING!!   Arterial access can occur, even with ultrasound guidance. Pneumothorax/hemothorax/chylothorax can occur with IJ or SC placement (risk is higher on the left side).

---

7. Confirm venous (and lack of arterial) access.

Disconnect the syringe from the needle, or remove the introducer needle from the catheter and attach manometry tubing to the catheter or the needle. Hold the unattached end toward the ceiling, and visualize a nonpulsatile column of blood that should not continue to rise above the expected central venous pressure (Figure 14.6).

>> **Tip on Technique**: A catheter is less likely to migrate out of the blood vessel when the operator removes the syringe and attaches the manometry tubing.

WARNING!!   If arterial access is accidentally obtained, it is important to abort the procedure IMMEDIATELY. Dilating an artery can lead to serious damage. Remove the needle and apply pressure.

Caution!   Blood color is not an accurate predictor of venous or arterial blood. Manometry and ultrasound visualization of the entire guidewire within the vein are more accurate predictors.

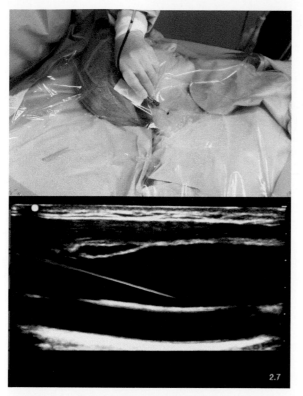

Figure 14.6 Top: Manometry used to confirm venous, and not arterial, access. Connect manometry tube to the needle/catheter and allow blood to fill tubing. Then raise tubing upward, watching for a lowering of the column of blood, confirming the low pressure associated with venous access. Bottom: Confirmation of guidewire placement with ultrasound using longitudinal view of the internal jugular vein. The hypoechoic structure underneath is the carotid artery.

8. Place the guidewire through the needle or catheter.

Place the guidewire through the needle/catheter to about 5–10 cm beyond the needle/catheter tip. It should advance easily. If there is resistance to guidewire advancement, STOP. Withdraw the guidewire and reposition the needle, using ultrasound if necessary. Observe the electrocardiogram for ectopy, which often occurs when the guidewire enters the right ventricle. If this occurs, pull back the guidewire. Remove the needle over the guidewire once it is advanced while maintaining a constant grip on the guidewire.

!! Potential Complication: The guidewire can be lost during the procedure. The wire can also trigger ventricular ectopy during advancement.

> **WARNING!!** DO NOT lose hold of the guidewire. A lost guidewire requires surgical retrieval.

9. Place the catheter over the guidewire.

Use a scalpel to make a skin nick where the guidewire enters the skin. Advance the dilator if needed over the guidewire to enlarge the vessel entry point. A dilator may not be needed for smaller CVL (e.g., 5 French) sizes. Withdraw the dilator over the guidewire, holding pressure at the skin to reduce bleeding.

>> **Tip on Technique**: Advance the dilator enough to dilate the vessel entry point and do not advance too much further. If resistance is met, gently retract and advance a few times instead of forcing it. If it still does not advance, make a bigger and deeper skin nick with the scalpel. Maintain a grip on the guidewire at all times.

Caution! Too small a skin nick with the scalpel can result in a blunt trauma to the vessel when attempting to advance the dilator into the vessel.

!! **Potential Complication**: In the case of SC and IJ placement, dilator injury to neighboring major vessels (such as the SC or carotid artery) can result in life-threatening bleeding (hemothorax, neck hematoma). Thus, avoid too caudad of a skin entry point for placement, as this complication requires a vascular or cardiothoracic surgery consult for management.

Advance the central venous catheter over the guidewire. Firmly grasp the guidewire when inserting the catheter. When the catheter is fully inserted, remove the guidewire. Sequentially unclamp each port, ensure blood flows back via syringe, flush the port with saline, and cap the port to avoid air entry. Place an antibiotic-coated disk around the skin entry site (if using) and secure the catheter with staples or suture. Cover with a transparent occlusive dressing.

WARNING!! Make sure all the air in the central line catheter ports is aspirated before flushing with saline to avoid air embolism.

>> **Tip on Technique**: If the guidewire is not visualized coming out of the proximal end of the catheter, feed more wire back through the central venous catheter until the guidewire is seen. Then, grasp the proximal end of the guidewire and slide the catheter until its hub is against the skin.

Other Management Considerations

Consider ordering a chest x-ray after the procedure to verify CVL placement. The tip of the catheter should be at the cavo-atrial junction. If it is too shallow, there is a risk of vessel damage with vasoactive and caustic medications. If it is too deep, there is a risk of myocardial perforation.

To minimize risk of infection, assess the CVL site daily for infection. To minimize risk of infection and vein damage, remove the central line as early as clinically possible and keep the ports capped when not in use.

Potential complications of IV catheter placement include thrombus formation and thrombophlebitis, peripheral nerve injury (e.g., radial nerve with cephalic vein at wrist, median nerve with basilic vein at antecubital fossa), and inadvertent arterial placement of the catheter (e.g., carotid artery instead of the internal jugular vein, subclavian artery instead of the subclavian vein, femoral artery instead of femoral vein).

Further Reading

Dev SP, Stefan RA, Saun T, Lee S. Insertion of an intraosseous needle in adults. *N Engl J Med* 2014;370:e35.

Anson JA. Vascular access in resuscitation: is there a role for the intraosseous route? *Anesthesiology* 2014;120:1015–31.

American Society of Anesthesiologists Task Force on Central Venous Access, Rupp SM, Apfelbaum JL, Blitt C, Caplan RA, Connis RT, Domino KB, Fleisher LA, Grant S, Mark JB, Morray JP, Nickinovich DG, Tung A. Practice guidelines for central venous access. *Anesthesiology* 2012;116(3):539–73.

References

Kehrl T, Becker BA, Simmons DE, Broderick EK, Jones RA. Intraosseous access in the obese patient: assessing the need for extended needle length. *Am J Emergency Med* 2016;34:1831–34.

Luck RP, Haines C, Mull CC. Technical tips: intraosseous access. *J Emergency Med* 2010;39(4): 468–75.

McGee DC, Gould MK. Preventing complications of central venous catheterization. *N Engl J Med* 2003;348(12):1123–33.

Chapter 15

Venous Air Embolism

Sindhu Reddy Nimma and Christoph Nikolaus Seubert

Summary Page

Symptoms:

- Persistent coughing and dyspnea in an awake patient
- Stepwise decrease in $EtCO_2$
- Hypotension
- Sound changes associated with air bubble test on precordial Doppler
- Air bubbles on transesophageal echocardiography
- Cardiovascular collapse

Differential Diagnosis:

- Pulmonary embolus
- Acute myocardial infarction
- Anaphylaxis

Introduction

Venous air embolism (VAE) is a gas embolism that may quickly lead to cardiovascular collapse if unrecognized or insufficiently treated. VAE is a well-known complication of neurosurgical procedures performed in the sitting position but has also occurred during central venous access, spine surgery, liver resections, penetrating and blunt chest trauma, and procedures using pressurized gas sources.[1,2] VAE is typically an iatrogenic complication that occurs when gas enters the venous system. Two factors that determine morbidity and mortality are the total volume of gas entrained and the rate of gas entrainment. The higher the pressure gradient between the site of air entry and right atrium, the greater the risk for VAE. The clinical presentation of a VAE may range from mild hypotension and respiratory changes to complete cardiovascular collapse. If VAE is diagnosed or suspected, prompt treatment should encompass three steps: preventing further air entry, providing hemodynamic support, and decreasing the volume of air already entrained.

Treatment

It is important to know the baseline risk of VAE for a procedure and assess patients for heightened risk for complications. Certain procedures carry a higher risk of VAE than others (Table 15.1), and certain patients also carry a higher risk. Patients with a patent foramen ovale (PFO) are at increased risk of paradoxical air embolism (i.e., air entry into the systemic circulation). Since air rises, two structures at particular risk from paradoxical embolism are the right heart, because the right coronary ostium is on the ventral side of the aorta, and the brain in a sitting position. Significant right heart failure reduces the tolerance for entrained air.

Table 15.1 Risk of Venous Air Embolism by Type of Surgical Procedure

High Risk	Medium Risk	Low Risk
Craniotomy in sitting position Craniosynostosis repair	Spinal fusion	Peripheral nerve procedures
Posterior fossa surgery	Cervical laminectomy	Anterior neck surgery
Laparoscopic procedures	Prostatectomy	Burr hole procedure
Total hip arthroplasty	GI Endoscopy	Vaginal procedures
Cesarean section	Coronary surgery	Hepatic surgery
Placement/removal of central venous access	Blood transfusion	Surgery on extremity

Adapted from Cottrell, James E., and William L. Young. Cottrell and Young's Neuroanesthesia. 5e ed., Elsevier Health Sciences, 2010, chapter 12.)

Consider a preoperative echocardiogram to determine patients at risk. If the surgical procedure poses a high risk of VAE, a preoperative echocardiogram is indicated to evaluate right heart function and the presence of a PFO (Figure 15.1). If the patient has a PFO, putting them at risk for stroke from paradoxical embolism, consideration should be given to altering the surgical position to minimize this risk. If altering the position is not an option, consider using intraoperative transesophageal echocardiography (TEE), because it is the only monitor able to detect paradoxical embolism.

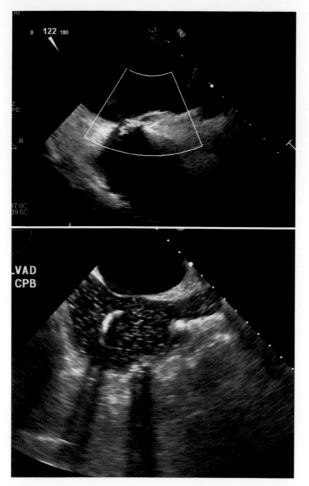

Figure 15.1 Assessment for patient foramen ovale. **Upper panel:** Patent foramen ovale with flow across the intraatrial septum. The right atrium is at the top of the screen near the probe in this mid-esophageal view. The left atrium is towards the bottom of the screen. **Lower panel:** Bi-caval view of the atria during a bubble study to evaluate for a patent foramen ovale. Air can be seen as white speckles filling the right atrium located towards the bottom of the screen. No bubbles pass to the left atrium seen at the top of the screen.

Diagnostic Monitors

Consider specific monitoring for cases and patients at risk of VAE: TEE, precordial doppler, a multiorifice central venous catheter, and/or an esophageal stethoscope to detect entrained air. TEE is the most invasive but has the highest sensitivity for detecting VAE and is the only monitor that can detect paradoxical embolism. Precordial doppler (Figure 15.2) is noninvasive and highly sensitive for detecting VAE but may be difficult to secure in place.

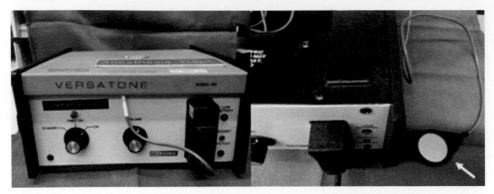

Figure 15.2 Precordial Doppler. Left panel: Precordial Doppler box with volume adjustment. Right panel: The circular probe that is placed over the precordium.

>> **Tip on Technique:** Place the doppler probe at the right sternal border near the superior vena cava–right atrial junction (third to fourth intercostal space). Adjust the volume to make the venous flow pattern audible. Verify proper position by injecting agitated saline and listening for a change in pitch as the bubbles pass beneath the probe.

End-tidal capnography ($EtCO_2$) is noninvasive and has moderate sensitivity for early detection but good correlation with the effect of VAE on cardiac output. It can be used in awake and anesthetized patients and is part of standard monitoring during anesthesia. A multiorifice central venous catheter (Figure 15.3) is an invasive catheter that can be placed for procedures performed in the sitting position. The intent is to place the distal tip of the catheter at the superior vena cava–right atrial junction, which is the most effective position for air aspiration.[2,3] Use of an esophageal stethoscope is relatively noninvasive but has low sensitivity.

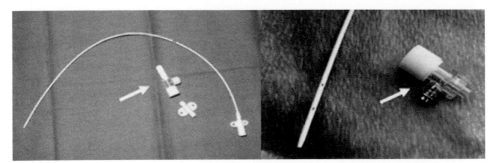

Figure 15.3 Right atrial multiorifice catheter. Left panel: Multiorifice catheter specialized with multiple distal side holes. Johans connector (arrow) for recording of intraatrial ECG. The yellow clamp is used to secure the catheter at the skin entry site at the correct depth. Right panel: Zoomed-in view of the multiple side holes. The metal piece is the connection for ECG recording.

>> **Tip on Technique:** This central line can be placed via the internal jugular or subclavian route either by itself or through an introducer. Upon initial placement, insert the catheter to its full length, which typically places its distal tip in the inferior vena cava. Hand off the

Johans connector to an assistant. Connect the Johans connector through a piece of sterile extension tubing to the multiorifice catheter. Prime the Johans connector, extension tubing, and central line with electrolyte solution (8.4% sodium bicarbonate solution preferred). Connect lead II or V to the Johans connector. Withdraw the catheter until the P wave approximates the height of the QRS complex. Withdraw an additional 1 cm and secure the catheter in place.[4,5]

> **WARNING!!** Once the catheter is positioned, remove the Johans connector because it is a potential source of microshock.

Step by Step

1. **Recognize and alert the team to the VAE.**
   The clinical presentation of a VAE may range from mild hypotension and respiratory changes to complete cardiovascular collapse.[6] Signs and symptoms of VAE include stepwise decrease in EtCO$_2$, hypotension, sound changes associated with air bubble test on precordial doppler, air bubbles on TEE, cardiovascular collapse, nonspecific electrocardiogram (ECG) changes (ST changes, T-wave inversion, peaked P waves), and/or "mill-wheel" murmur heard via esophageal stethoscope. Detection of VAE by ECG has low sensitivity and specificity. Look for right heart strain such as ST-segment changes, T-wave inversions in anterior leads (V1–4, lead III), and peaked P waves.
   Inform the surgeon and the operating room (OR) team immediately. A coordinated response of the entire team is essential to a good patient outcome.

2. **Prevent further air entry from the surgical field.**
   Have the surgeons flood the surgical field with saline irrigation or saline-soaked dressings and place bone wax on cut bony surfaces. Turn off pressurized gas sources in laparoscopic or endoscopic procedures. Lower the site of air entry below the level of the heart to decrease the pressure gradient for air entry (e.g., head down or Trendelenburg position for sitting cranio-cervical procedures). Consider placing the patient in left lateral decubitus position (Durant maneuver) to relieve the airlock that is causing outflow obstruction of the right heart. Transient jugular venous compression (Queckenstedt maneuver) can help the surgeon visualize actual or potential sites of air entry in cranial surgeries. This raises venous pressures in the surgical field, indicating missed opportunities for hemostasis.

> **Caution!** If the Mayfield pin attachment is not fixed to the top segment of the OR table, lowering just the head will tear the patient's head out of the pins.
>
> **Caution!** The left lateral decubitus position minimizes the effectiveness of chest compressions during cardiopulmonary resuscitation (CPR).

3. **Provide hemodynamic support as needed to maintain hemodynamics.**
   Initiate chest compressions for profound hypotension or cardiac arrest. Turn off anesthetic agents and increase FiO$_2$ to 100%. Deliver inotropic agents to decrease right

ventricular size and improve forward flow to prevent right heart failure. Recommended initial doses (titrate to effect) include ephedrine 10–15 mg IV bolus, epinephrine 8–100 mcg IV bolus, or norepinephrine 8–16 mcg IV bolus. Direct-acting agents are preferred in a crisis.

Other medications that may be used include dobutamine 5 mcg/kg/min, phenylephrine 150–200 mcg IV, or vasopressin 5–10 units IV.

>> **Tip on Technique:** Use inotropic agents before vasoconstrictors to increase contractility, stroke volume, and cardiac index as well as decrease pulmonary vascular resistance. Give IV fluids to raise central venous pressure and improve right ventricular filling.

Pearl: Start with 1–2 liters of normal saline/Plasma-Lyte and continue for continuous hemodynamic support.

4. **Reduce the volume of gas in the vascular system.**

Discontinue nitrous oxide and any other pressurized sources of gas. In surgeries at high risk for VAE, nitrous oxide should not be used because nitrous oxide exchanges at a ratio of 20:1 for the nitrogen in the entrained air, massively expanding the size of the bubbles.

5. **Aspirate air from a multiorifice catheter (if already in place).**

Aspiration of air unequivocally confirms the diagnosis of VAE. If a multiorifice catheter is NOT already in place, do not attempt placement during the acute treatment of VAE. Maintaining hemodynamics and stopping further entrainment of air is the priority. Aspiration is most effective for VAE in a patient in the sitting position, because entrained air flows past the superior vena cava–right atrium junction, where the catheter tip sits.

6. **Follow-up after VAE event.**

After the patient is hemodynamically stable, discuss continuing or aborting the surgical procedure with the surgeon and the operative team. Weigh the importance of the procedure versus the current physiologic state of the patient. Consider hyperbaric treatment of paradoxical embolism. After a clinically significant VAE intraoperatively, postoperative care will be dictated by the patient's ongoing symptoms. Consider hyperbaric oxygen therapy for a stroke due to paradoxical embolism.

Other Management Considerations

Sitting position craniotomy (Figure 15.4) is sometimes considered for posterior fossa and upper cervical surgeries because it offers the surgeon easy orientation and low local venous pressures (a dry field) because blood and cerebrospinal fluid drain away from the surgical site.[7] Although from the anesthesiologist's perspective a sitting position may facilitate ventilation, major risks include VAE, inadequate cerebral perfusion pressure, quadriplegia due to stretch/compression of the cervical spinal cord, mid-cervical tetraplegia, tongue swelling, and postoperative pneumocephalus. All of the surgeries that are appropriate for the sitting position can also be done in a three-quarter prone or full prone position, which has a lower VAE risk.

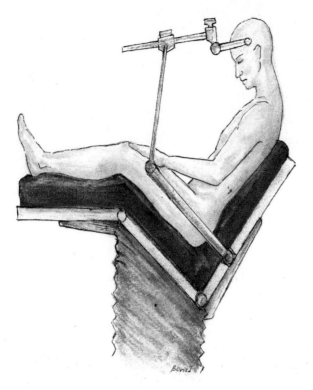

Figure 15.4 Positioning for sitting craniotomy. Note that the Mayfield pin attachment is properly fixed to the top part of the OR table allowing lowering of the head relative to the heart via either head-down or reverse Trendelenburg positioning.

The lethal volume of gas ranges from 200 to 300 ml or 3 to 5 ml/kg of air.[8] A pressure gradient of 5 cmH$_2$O across a 14-gauge needle (internal diameter of 1.8 mm) allows entrainment of 100 ml of air/sec. This illustrates why rapid intervention is required and why the first step in preventing cardiovascular collapse is immediate termination of air entrainment.

There are diseases and settings that put the patient at risk for entraining a large volume of gas over a short period of time, risking cardiac arrest from VAE without much warning. Examples include:

- A parasagittal brain tumor, because of its proximity to a dural sinus, that is, a large noncollapsible venous structure
- A surgery that uses pressurized gas near large veins, for example, the initial insufflation of the abdominal cavity, if the insufflating needle was misplaced into the inferior vena cava
- The use of rapid infusion devices in the setting of inadequate air traps or a failure to eliminate air from bags of IV fluid

Extensive exposure of venous channels within bone (i.e., cancellous bone), as occurs during extensive spine surgery or craniosynostosis repair, allows air to access venous channels. The extent of air entrainment can be increased by low central venous pressure in the setting of underresuscitation and significant blood loss.

References

1. Bebawy JF, Pasternak JJ. Anesthesia for neurosurgery. In Barash PG. *Clinical Anesthesia*. Wolters Kluwer; 2017:1003–28.
2. Smith DS. Anesthetic management for posterior fossa surgery. In Cottrell JE, Young WL. *Cottrell and Young's Neuroanesthesia*. 5th ed. Elsevier Health Sciences; 2010:Chapter 12; 203–17.
3. Colley PS, Artru AA. ECG-guided placement of Sorenson CVP catheters via arm veins. Anesthesia & Analgesia. 1984;63(10):953–6.
4. Johans TG, et al. Multiorificed catheter placement with an intravascular electrocardiographic technique. Anesthesiology. 1986 Mar;64(3):411–13.
5. Warner DO, Cucchiara RF. Position of proximal orifice determines electrocardiogram recorded from multiorificed catheter. Anesthesiology. 1986 Aug;65(2):235–36.
6. Mirski MA, et al. Diagnosis and treatment of vascular air embolism. Anesthesiology. 2007;106(1):164–77.
7. Papadopoulos G, Kuhly P, Brock M, Rudolph KH, Link J, Eyrich K. Venous and paradoxical air embolism in the sitting position: a prospective study with transesophageal echocardiography. Acta Neurochir (Wien). 1994;126:140–43.
8. Toung TJ, Rossberg MI, Hutchins GM. Volume of air in a lethal venous air embolism. Anesthesiology. 2001;94:360–61.

PART 3

BLEEDING, BLOOD, TRANSFUSIONS

Chapter 16

Hemorrhage and Massive Transfusion Protocols

Christopher Heine and Tod Brown

Summary Page

Symptoms:

- Tachycardia
- Hypotension
- Anemia

Differential Diagnosis:

- Traumatic hemorrhage
- Dilutional coagulopathy
- Disseminated intravascular coagulation
- Pharmacologic (aspirin, heparin, warfarin, and many other oral anticoagulants)
- von Willebrand disease
- Thrombocytopenia
- Hemophilia A or B
- Specific factor deficiencies

Introduction

Acute, major hemorrhage, like that seen in the setting of a traumatic injury, carries a high risk of morbidity and mortality. This is the result of the inciting injury, the treatment with intravenous infusions and transfusions, and the body's subsequent response to both. While the ultimate treatment of the insult is either surgery or conservative critical care, the resuscitation is often managed by paramedics and other first responders, emergency room physicians, and potentially anesthesiologists if the patient is brought to the operating room (OR). Proper use of blood products, protocols, pharmacologic and nonpharmacologic therapy, and testing can help mitigate the damage caused by the trauma and the therapy. The principles of damage control surgery and resuscitation allow for the care team to initially stabilize the patient in the OR and then the critical care team to further resuscitate and treat coagulopathies before returning for the definitive repair hours or days later.

Treatment

The steps below apply to acute hemorrhage that is managed in the emergency room as well as in the intensive care unit (ICU) or OR, depending on the clinical scenario.

Step by Step

1. Perform initial trauma survey.

This step will likely be performed in the emergency room where the anesthesia team may or may not be present. A brief clinical history should be obtained, including the mechanism of injury. For trauma to the chest or abdomen, major vascular injury, or pelvic or femur fracture, have a high index of suspicion for major blood loss.

Perform the *primary* survey:

- *Airway*—with cervical spine stabilization
- *Breathing*—oxygenation and ventilation
- *Circulation*—hemorrhage control and volume restoration
- *Disability*—neurological status
- *Exposure*—environmental control

Perform the *secondary* survey:

- Head-to-toe examination
- Diagnostic studies and imaging
- Focused Assessment with Sonography for Trauma (FAST)
- X-ray, computed tomography, or magnetic resonance imaging if stable
- Angiography may occasionally be needed

Send blood for baseline labwork:

- Complete blood count (CBC), complete metabolic panel (CMP), arterial blood gas (ABG), lactate, prothrombin and partial thromboplastin Time (PT/PTT), and fibrinogen[1]
- Type and cross for patient-specific blood products
- Preoperative lactate and base deficit[1]
- Monitor hypotension and heart rate, shock index (heart rate/systolic blood pressure[2])

Assess the adequacy of IV access (should have a minimum of two large-bore IVs (14–18 gauge)) and obtain history of what patient has received for resuscitation.

> **WARNING!!** Repeat the initial survey in the event of instability and consider other unknown/not yet identified injuries that may be the cause such as pelvic or long bone fractures, solid organ injury, or cardiac tamponade.

> **Caution!** Patients may arrive from the emergency room having undergone resuscitative endovascular ballooning of the aorta (REBOA).[3] This catheter is placed into a femoral artery and a balloon is inflated to control bleeding temporarily below the diaphragm and will look similar to a femoral central venous line (Figure 16.1).

>> **Tip on Technique:** Also consider nontraumatic causes of bleeding that may have specific treatments: disorders such as hemophilia A or B or von Willebrand disease, factor deficiencies, thrombocytopenia due to malignancy, or anticoagulants such as warfarin, dabigatran, and apixaban.

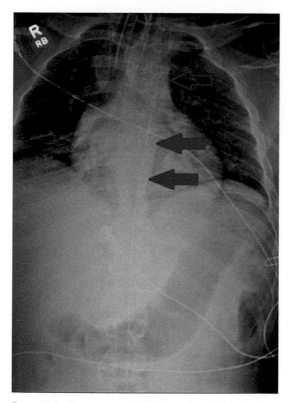

Figure 16.1 Chest x-ray with REBOA in place. The hollow arrow indicates the tip of the catheter in the distal aortic arch and the solid arrows indicate the markings on the catheter for the proximal and distal ends of the balloon.

2. **Support hemodynamics.**

   Resuscitate the patient with volume using balanced crystalloid solutions in 10–20 ml/kg boluses until blood is available (ideally 1–2 liters total).

   Judiciously use vasopressors to maintain goal blood pressure:

   - Epinephrine: 1–10 mcg/kg IV, 0.1–1 mcg/kg/min infusion
   - Phenylephrine: 0.5–1 mcg/kg IV, 0.2–1 mcg/kg/min infusion
   - Vasopressin: 0.01–0.06 U/min infusion
   - Norepinephrine: 0.1–0.5 mcg/kg/min infusion, bolus not recommended

   Give blood products. Until cross-matched blood is available, minimize crystalloid administration by transfusing un-cross-matched, universal donor, packed red blood cells (PRBCs) and fresh frozen plasma (FFP) in a 1:1 ratio if blood is needed. Place a tourniquet temporarily if there is bleeding from an extremity. Utilize cell saver if available.

   >> **Tip on Technique:** Permissive hypotension (goal SBP 90–100 mmHg) helps minimize blood loss. Excessive crystalloid infusion can dilute clotting factors and worsen coagulopathy. Higher blood pressure goals to maintain perfusion may be needed if concurrent traumatic spine or brain injury is present or in elderly or chronically hypertensive patients.

3. **Rapidly transfer patient to the OR if surgery is indicated.**

   Quickly transport the patient to the OR, place monitors, and reconfirm identity (procedural timeout). Call for help if not already done.

   Reconfirm adequacy of IV access:

   - Central venous or multiple large-bore peripheral access, preferably above the diaphragm
   - Place an arterial line if not already in place
   - Set up rapid infusion equipment (Belmont or Level 1)

   >> **Tip on Technique:** These steps will be performed as resuscitation is continued by team members.

   > **WARNING!!** Do not delay resuscitation to establish arterial or central venous access if peripheral access is adequate.

4. **Initiate massive transfusion protocol (MTP).**

   Place an order or call the blood bank to initiate the institution's MTP. Obtain type and cross if not already sent. Transfuse un-cross-matched PRBCs and FFP in a ratio of 1:1. Transfuse platelets and cryoprecipitate as they arrive per the MTP. Switch to cross-matched blood once it becomes available.

   Once bleeding is controlled, deactivate the MTP after discussion with the surgical team.

   >> **Tip on Technique:** The MTP may be initiated anytime between arrival to the hospital and the end of the case. If it was initiated prior to the OR, the anesthesia team should continue the protocol.

   >> **Tip on Technique:** If you have a patient with a massive hemorrhage in an institution that does not have an MTP in place, then the goals are still the same: transfuse PRBCs

and FFP in a 1:1 ratio. Platelets can be transfused to make the ratio 1:1:1. Cryoprecipitate can be given as needed if fibrinogen levels are low via lab testing or if there is concern that resuscitation has led to a low fibrinogen state.

> **Caution!** If unable to obtain a cross-match for the patient, continue transfusion with un-cross-matched blood while the blood bank continues to work on cross-match.

5. Administer antifibrinolytics.

Give tranexamic acid (TXA) as a 1-gram bolus followed by 1-gram infusion over 8 hours to prevent hyperfibrinolysis.

> **WARNING!!** Late administration of TXA (>3 hours) is associated with increased mortality.[4] High-dose TXA has been associated with new-onset seizures in some case reports.

> **Caution!** ε-Aminocaproic acid (Amicar), another lysine analogue antifibrinolytic, is not recommended in trauma.

6. Send labwork for testing.

Send CBC, CMP, and coagulation studies if not already sent. Send thromboelastogram (TEG) or rotational thromboelastogram (ROTEM) to assess for reversal of coagulopathy and to guide further transfusion (Figures 16.2 and 16.3).

>> **Tip on Technique:** ROTEM can provide earlier guidance (within 15 minutes) of coagulation resuscitation compared to traditional coagulation studies like PT/PTT/international normalized ratio (INR).

>> **Tip on Technique:** Measurement of fibrinogen is important because deficiency develops early in hemorrhage. Levels below 100 mg/dl should be treated with cryofibrinogen.[1]

> **Caution!** Watch closely for hypocalcemia due to citrate present in blood products that binds calcium. The goal is an ionized calcium level above 0.9 mmol. If low, treat with calcium chloride 10–20 mg/kg IV *or* calcium gluconate 30–50 mg/kg IV (up to 1000 mg).

The use of lab testing to assess the causes of coagulopathy is important to ensure the patient is receiving the appropriate treatment. Historically, this was done with coagulation studies like platelets, fibrinogen, and PT/PTT/INR. In the event of active bleeding and transfusion, the 30–45 minutes these labs require offer little utility. TEG or ROTEM technology allows for earlier data (within 15 minutes) and more specific pathology identification. Figure 16.3 shows several possible pathologies.

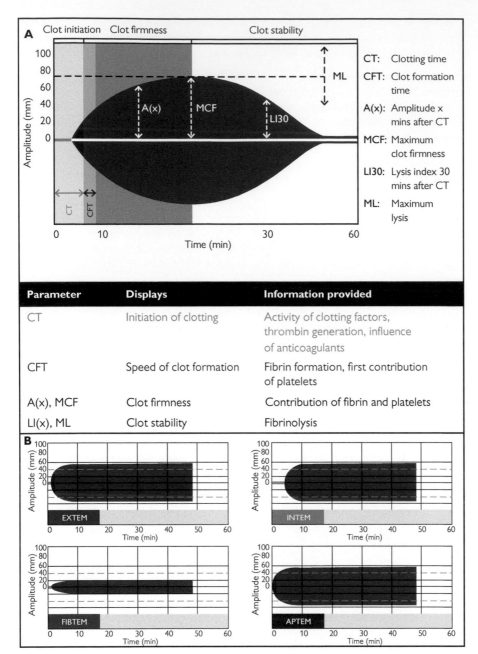

A Clot initiation Clot firmness Clot stability

CT: Clotting time
CFT: Clot formation time
A(x): Amplitude x mins after CT
MCF: Maximum clot firmness
LI30: Lysis index 30 mins after CT
ML: Maximum lysis

Parameter	Displays	Information provided
CT	Initiation of clotting	Activity of clotting factors, thrombin generation, influence of anticoagulants
CFT	Speed of clot formation	Fibrin formation, first contribution of platelets
A(x), MCF	Clot firmness	Contribution of fibrin and platelets
LI(x), ML	Clot stability	Fibrinolysis

B

EXTEM

INTEM

FIBTEM

APTEM

Figure 16.2 Example of a normal ROTEM, a type of thromboelastogram (TEG). EXTEM, INTEM, FIBTEM, and APTEM are different versions of the original curve and help differentiate between pathologies. Images used with the permission of Instrumentation Laboratory.

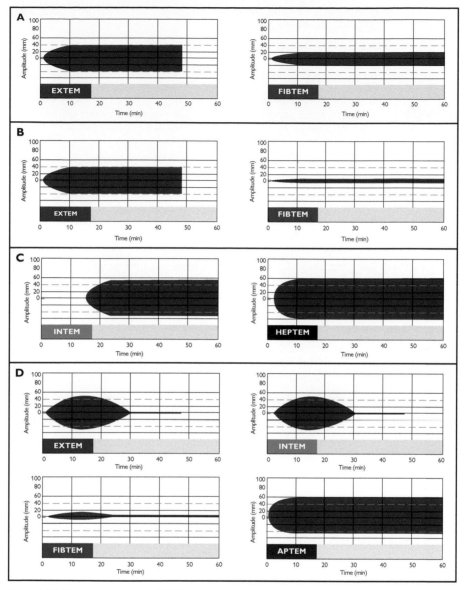

Figure 16.3 Common abnormal ROTEM curves seen during traumatic hemorrhage. A: Decreased clot firmness in EXTEM and normal clot firmness in FIBTEM may suggest decreased platelet contribution. B: Decreased clot firmness in EXTEM and FIBTEM may suggest fibrinogen deficiency. C: Prolonged INTEM CT versus normal HEPTEM CT may suggest presence of heparin. D Increased EXTEM ML versus normal APTEM ML may confirm fibrinolysis. Images used with the permission of Instrumentation Laboratory.

7. Treat coagulopathy.

Transfuse blood products using TEG or ROTEM results if no longer following the MTP.
If bleeding continues despite adequate transfusion, or if specific pathology is noted on testing, consider the following:

- Prothrombin complex concentrates (PCCs) for the reversal of vitamin K antagonists (warfarin). **Note:** The use of PCC or recombinant factor VIIa (rFVIIa) for refractory traumatic coagulopathy is off-label, but clinical trials have shown benefit, particularly with rFVIIa use for blunt-force trauma.[5]

- Cryofibrinogen or human fibrinogen concentrate (RiaSTAP) 70 mg/kg bolus if patient has low fibrinogen levels
- rFVIIa (NovoSeven) 90 mcg/kg bolus

> **WARNING!!** PCCs are not recommended for reversal of thrombin inhibitors like dabigatran, which has a specific reversal agent: idarucizumab 5g IV bolus.

8. Consider and manage risks of transfusion.

- Hyperkalemia:

Monitor for electrocardiogram changes (Figure 16.4).

Treatment includes hyperventilation, calcium chloride 10–20 mg/kg (up to 500 mg) or calcium gluconate 30–50 mg/kg (up to 1000 mg), insulin 0.1 U/kg (up to 10 U), glucose (dextrose) 1–2 g/kg (up to 50 g), sodium bicarbonate 1 mEq/kg (up to 50 mEq), and inhaled beta agonists.

One of the side effects of large-volume transfusion is the accumulation of potassium. This can be worsened if the vigor of the transfusion results in hemolysis. Calcium helps stabilize the myocardium from the effects of hyperkalemia. Insulin, beta agonists, and possibly bicarbonate help push potassium back into the cells. Glucose (dextrose) should be given to prevent hypoglycemia from the insulin bolus. Diuresis with potassium-wasting diuretics like furosemide and hemodialysis once out of the OR can help clear the potassium out of the body.

- Hypocalcemia:

Treatment includes calcium chloride 10–20 mg/kg (up to 500 mg) or calcium gluconate 30–50 mg/kg (up to 1000 mg).

- Acute hemolytic reaction, transfusion-associated cardiovascular overload, or TRALI (see Chapter 19 on transfusion reactions for further details on treatment of these conditions)

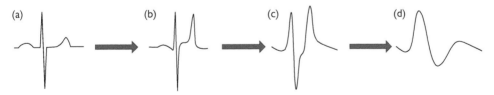

Figure 16.4 ECG signs of progressively worsening hyperkalemia. A: Normal ECG. B: Flattening P wave and peaked T wave. C: Widened QRS. D: Sine wave pattern.

9. Immediate postoperative management.

The surgeon might leave the abdomen temporarily closed if practicing "damage control surgery," requiring a return to the OR in the future for complete closure. Consider postoperative mechanical ventilation if the patient is hypothermic or has hemodynamic instability or a vasopressor requirement, or if concerns exist about increased work of breathing from large amounts of transfusions/intravenous fluids, extensive intra-abdominal/thoracic surgery, or other comorbidities. Transport the patient to ICU for postoperative care *or* to interventional radiology if the source of bleeding is still unclear and further evaluation is warranted.

>> **Tip on Technique:** Err on the side of continued postoperative ventilation if reestablishing the airway is higher risk.

Other Management Considerations

Patients with hemophilia A or B, von Willebrand disease, specific factor deficiencies, malignancy, and anticoagulant medications like warfarin or clopidogrel will bleed more easily. Traumas to the chest, abdomen, pelvis, long bones, or major vasculature are also more apt to hemorrhage.

Disorders like hemophilia A or B, von Willebrand disease, and specific factor deficiencies have treatments that replace the deficiency and can help improve coagulation. A history suggestive of cancer, particularly leukemia, may help point toward a thrombocytopenia. In addition, pharmacologic anticoagulation like that caused by warfarin or newer anticoagulants like dabigatran and apixaban also has specific reversal agents. Coagulation studies and discussion with a hematologist, if available, can help guide treatment in many of these cases.

Communication between the surgical and anesthesia teams about the status of the patient and hemorrhage control is vitally important. In addition, the team in the OR and the blood bank need to be in constant communication to ensure the appropriate availability of blood products, particularly while an MTP is in place.

Jehovah's Witness patients interpret certain Bible passages to mean that they should not receive blood products. Whole blood, cells, plasma, and platelets are generally considered to be unacceptable, and fractional components such as albumin, topical hemostatic agents, and clotting factors are matters of personal decision. It is common practice to review all the options for blood replacement and blood loss prevention prior to a procedure in these patients.

Trauma and pediatric patients pose two separate but related ethical issues in this population. A trauma victim who has become incapacitated cannot indicate refusal or acceptance of any treatment, including transfusion. In this case, it is reasonable to give the patient blood in the event that it would prevent loss of life or limb. Similarly, a pediatric patient does not have decision-making capacity, and therefore relies on the parent or guardian to consent. In the case of Jehovah's Witness patients, a parent cannot refuse transfusion for their minor child in the event that it would potentially save the child's life.[6]

References

1. Guerado, E., Medina, A., Mata, M.I., Galvan, J.M., and Bertrand, M.L. 2016. Protocols for massive blood transfusion: when and why, and potential complications. *European Journal of Trauma and Emergency Surgery*, 42(3), pp.283–295.
2. Olaussen, A., Blackburn, T., Mitra, B., and Fitzgerald, M. 2014. Shock index for prediction of critical bleeding post-trauma: a systematic review. *Emergency Medicine Australasia*, 26(3), pp.223–228.
3. Brenner, M., Teeter, W., and Hoehn, M. 2018. Use of resuscitative endovascular balloon occlusion of the aorta for proximal aortic control in patients with severe hemorrhage and arrest. *JAMA Surgery*, 153(2), pp.130–135.
4. Shakur, H., Roberts, I., Bautista, R., et al. 2010. Effects of tranexamic acid on death, vascular occlusive events, and blood transfusion in trauma patients with significant hemorrhage (CRASH-2): a randomized, placebo-controlled trial. *The Lancet*, 376(9734), pp.23–32.
5. Hauser, C.J., Boffard, K., Dutton, R., et al. 2010. Results of the CONTROL trial: efficacy and safety of recombinant activated Factor VII in the management of refractory traumatic hemorrhage. *Journal of Trauma*, 69, pp.489–500.
6. Waters, J., and Shander, A., eds. 2014. *Perioperative Blood Management,* 3rd Edition. Bethesda, MD: American Association of Blood Banks.

Chapter 17

Intraoperative Management of the Bleeding Patient

Renuka M. George and Loren R. Francis

Summary Page
Signs and Symptoms:

The following signs and symptoms can indicate blood loss.

- Signs
  - Tachycardia
  - Hypotension
  - Increased stroke volume variance
  - Decreased end-tidal carbon dioxide
  - Decreased mixed venous oxygen saturation
  - Underfilled ventricle on transthoracic echo or transesophageal echo
  - Decreased central venous pressure
- Symptoms
  - Pallor
  - Abnormal skin turgor
  - Thready pulse
  - Decreased urine output
  - Cold extremities
  - Dry mucous membranes

Differential Diagnosis:

- Neurologic
  - Intracranial herniation
  - Neurogenic shock
- Cardiac
  - Myocardial ischemia/infarction
  - Cardiac tamponade
- Pulmonary
  - Pulmonary embolism
  - Aspiration
  - Tension pneumothorax
- Systemic
  - Anaphylaxis
  - Distributive shock
  - Blood loss
  - Venous air embolism
- Anesthesia
  - Inappropriate anesthetic depth
  - Malignant hyperthermia

Introduction

A bleeding patient in the intraoperative setting can be complex to diagnose and manage. It is important for anesthesiologists to recognize signs and symptoms of bleeding, rule out differential diagnoses, and treat appropriately to optimize resuscitation. Ideal management starts in the preoperative setting with the goal of preparing the patient for surgery, followed by thorough evaluation and close monitoring on the day of surgery.

Utilization of both invasive and noninvasive monitors provides information about the patient's clinical picture in the intraoperative setting. In addition to traditional laboratory tests, newer point-of-care testing is available to efficiently diagnose complex coagulopathies. Perioperative management requires knowledge of commonly utilized blood products including packed red blood cells, fresh frozen plasma, platelets, and cryoprecipitate. The anesthesiologist must keep in mind the type of surgery, overall clinical picture, and laboratory results and understand that transfusion is not always the best answer.

Treatment

Blood management starts with communication between the surgeon, patient, and anesthesiologist to differentiate high-risk from low-risk surgical candidates. Use of preoperative erythropoietin, iron supplements, and intraoperative tranexamic acid can prevent need for transfusions.[1] Preoperative autologous blood donation can also help reduce transfusion requirements.[1]

Correct diagnosis of intraoperative bleeding requires recognition of a combination of symptoms, signs, laboratory values, and clinical picture. It is imperative to rule out life-threatening differential diagnoses prior to treating potential blood loss. Early diagnosis relies on communication with the surgeon and vigilance. Timely management ensures adequate organ perfusion and limits ischemia, which in turn avoids increased transfusion requirements later. Transfusing blood products is not always the best solution, and treatment should be individualized for the given patient, surgery, and situation.

Note: For acute hemorrhage, especially due to trauma, go to chapter 16 on acute hemorrhage.

WARNING!! If the patient is actively bleeding with hemodynamic instability, skip steps 1–5 and **PROCEED IMMEDIATELY** to step 6!

If the patient is stable but at risk for bleeding or is actively bleeding, follow the steps below in order.

Step by Step

1. **Assess the patient preoperatively for risk of bleeding.**

    Discuss the likelihood of bleeding with the surgeon preprocedure or during the "timeout."

    >> **Tip on Technique:** Early discussions with the surgeon can help predict blood management.

    Obtain baseline laboratory values and vital signs as well as relevant medical history that could affect oxygenation, perfusion, and coagulation. Discuss risks and benefits of transfusion and blood management with the patient should transfusion be warranted, and obtain consent for transfusion. Coordinate with the blood bank and utilize institutional electronic medical records to ensure blood is available to high-risk patients while decreasing unnecessary blood ordering and reducing cost to the institution.[2]

2. **Place appropriate monitors and lines.**

Place standard American Society for Anesthesiologists (ASA) monitors: pulse oximetry, electrocardiogram (ECG), noninvasive blood pressure (NIBP), end-tidal capnography, and temperature probe. Consider placement of additional invasive monitors in high-risk patients such as an arterial line, pulmonary artery catheter, or transesophageal echo probe.

The type of access placed should be based on the risk of bleeding. For high-risk patients, consider large-bore IV lines for resuscitation plus a central line if there may be a need for continuous vasopressor support. For low-risk patients, access should be placed based on estimated fluid requirements and needed infusions.

>> **Tip on Technique**: If the patient's arms are tucked and access to the patient is limited, consider placing increased or redundant vascular access.

3. **Optimize the patient.**

Optimize positioning to avoid unnecessary exposure that might increase heat loss, and check access to prevent impingement or kinking of IVs.

Avoid hypothermia less than 34 degrees with the use of forced air warmers, warmed IV fluids, and increased operating room temperature. Normothermia can prevent blood loss since body temperature less than 34°C significantly decreases fibrinogen synthesis and platelet function.[3]

Consider administering antifibrinolytic agents in high-risk patients: tranexamic acid (TXA) 1 gram IV over 10 minutes followed by 1 gram IV over 8 hours. TXA prevents clot breakdown and decreases intraoperative bleeding.

Calculate maximum allowable blood loss (Table 17.1).

Table 17.1 **Calculating Maximal Allowable Blood Loss**

ABL= [EBV x (Hi-Hf)]/Hi

Key:	EBV Values:
ABL: Allowable blood loss	Premature Neonates: 95 mL/kg
Hi: Initial Hematocrit	Full Term Neonates: 85 mL/kg
Hf: Final Hematocrit	Infants: 80 mL/kg
EBV: Estimated blood volume	Adult Men: 75 mL/kg
	Adult Women: 65 mL/kg

4. **Evaluate for blood loss.**

Communicate with the surgeon throughout the procedure to identify sources of bleeding.

Bleeding may be surgical versus nonsurgical (coagulopathy). Surgical bleeding can be managed by cauterization of the source, application of clamps to vessels, or packing of the site to tamponade the bleeding. If coagulopathy is the source of the bleeding, see steps 8 and 9 for evaluation and treatment of coagulopathies.

Quantify ongoing blood loss by looking at suction canisters, laparotomy pads, and gauze in the surgical field or after collection. One fully soaked gauze = 10 ml of blood loss, while one laparotomy pad (lap sponge) fully soaked = 100–150 ml of blood loss.

>> **Tip on Technique**: Talk to the surgeon or scrub technician about the amount of irrigation fluid used when looking at suction canisters to avoid overestimation of blood loss.

Check an arterial blood gas if an arterial line is in place to evaluate hemoglobin levels to help guide transfusion. An arterial blood gas can also identify any electrolyte imbalances that may exacerbate intraoperative bleeding. Treat imbalances to avoid acidosis of a pH <7.1 or hypocalcemia (an ionized calcium <0.7 mmol/L). Acidosis with a pH <7.1 decreases thrombin generation, platelet count, and fibrinogen levels. If the ionized calcium level is <0.7 mmol/L, there is an increased risk of coagulopathy due to calcium's involvement in fibrinogen protection, fibrin stabilization, platelet activity, and thrombin generation.[3]

>> **Tip on Technique:** Estimating blood loss can be difficult and takes experience. Clinical guides can help quantify the amount of blood loss when looking at surgical sponges.[4]

5. **Evaluate for hypovolemia.**
    Signs and symptoms of hypovolemia include:
   - Tachycardia and arrhythmias on ECG
   - Hypotension or decrease in mean arterial pressure
   - Stroke volume variance (SVV) >10–15% as measured via arterial line
   - Decrease in central venous pressure (CVP) from baseline or <2–6 mmHg
   - SVO_2 <70% and CO <4–8 L/min measured from pulmonary artery catheter
   - Decreased chamber size, hyperdynamic, or decreased inferior vena cava (IVC) diameter with increased collapsibility measured via transesophageal echo (TEE) or transthoracic echo (TTE)

>> **Tip on Technique:** Continuous NIBP monitoring (such as the Edwards Clearsight monitor) allows for earlier detection and management of hypotension.[5] Focused TTE is an increasingly important tool as well for hemodynamic assessment of patients intraoperatively.[6]

6. **Use temporizing measures.**
    Communicate blood loss concerns to the surgeon to coordinate management and discuss the need to alter surgical technique or use cell salvage (cell saver) to limit blood loss. While assessing blood loss, vasopressor support, minimizing oxygen requirements, and maximizing oxygen delivery serve as temporizing measures.

Use goal-directed fluid therapy to support organ perfusion while keeping in mind the possibility of developing hemodilution.

Administer vasopressor support as necessary to maintain perfusion and titrate to the desired blood pressure goal:

- Phenylephrine 80–160 mcg IV bolus or 10–200 mcg/min IV infusion
- Ephedrine 5–10 mg IV bolus
- Vasopressin 1–2 units IV bolus or 0.01–0.04 units/min IV infusion
- Norepinephrine 4–8 mcg IV bolus or 4–12 mcg/min IV infusion
- Epinephrine 4–8 mcg IV bolus or 0.05–0.2 mcg/kg/min IV infusion

Maximize oxygen delivery by adjusting ventilator settings as needed, including positive end-expiratory pressure (PEEP) and FiO_2 to target SPO_2 of 95–97% and PaO_2 of 70–100. An increase in PEEP increases alveoli recruitment but can also decrease cardiac output by decreasing preload due to increased thoracic pressure. Temporarily increasing FiO_2 to 1.0 will also help oxygenation, though continued hyperoxia can lead to free radical formation and cause organ damage.

Minimize oxygen demand by avoiding tachycardia, hypothermia, or hyperthermia if possible.

Caution! In extensive surgeries the combination of blood loss, factor consumption, dilution of factors, and fluid administration can cause a dilutional coagulopathy.[7]

---

7. **Transfuse blood as needed based on laboratory tests and hemodynamic status.**

Use monitors to ascertain hemodynamic instability and evaluate for fluid responsiveness using SVV, IVC size, and collapsibility on TTE/TEE if available. Evaluate continuing blood loss via discussion with the surgeon.

If the patient is hemodynamically unstable:

- Transfuse 1 unit of packed red blood cells (PRBCs).
- For severely unstable patients requiring massive transfusion, refer to Chapter 16 on massive transfusion.
- Continue with supportive and temporizing measures as previously listed.
- Reevaluate hemodynamics and lab values after transfusion of 1 unit PRBCs and at regular intervals throughout case.

If the patient is hemodynamically stable, use the following hemoglobin levels as transfusion triggers:

- Low risk of ischemia: 6–8 g/dl
- High risk of ischemia: <10 g/dl

Reassess hemodynamics and lab values regularly. Use blood tubing, filters, and warmers to prevent hypothermia and transfusion of any clots.

>> **Tip on Technique:** Hospitals often institute patient blood management protocols to optimize the efficacy of blood transfusion, maximize benefits, and minimize risk.[8–10] Overall, blood management should be individualized for each patient and situation.[10]

8. Evaluate for coagulopathy.

Check laboratory values to guide transfusion of blood products.
Normal values include:

- Platelet count: 140,000–450,000 cells per microliter
- Fibrinogen level: 175–433 mg/dl
- Prothrombin time (PT): 11.5–14.5 seconds
- Partial thromboplastin time (PTT): 24.5–35.2 seconds
- Use thromboelastography/rotational thromboelastometry (TEG/ROTEM) to assist in diagnosis (Figure 17.1 and Table 17.2)[11]

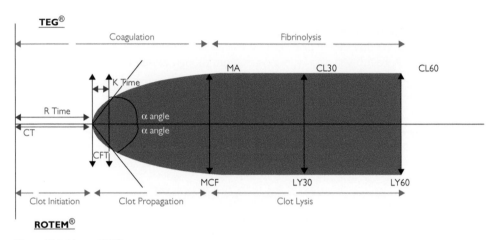

Figure 17.1 Normal TEG.

Table 17.2 **Comparing TEG and ROTEM**

TEG	ROTEM	Measurement
R Time	CT (clotting time)	Time from start to when waveform reaches 2 mm above baseline
K Time	CFT (clot formation time)	Time from 2 to 20 mm above baseline
α angle	α angle	Angle of tangent at 2 mm amplitude
MA (Max Amplitude)	MCF (Max Clot Formation)	Maximum strength

>> **Tip on Technique:** TEG has become practical as a fast point-of-care method of evaluating abnormal coagulation. Two TEG tests are available that give rapid information about the dynamics of clot development and stabilization: TEG and ROTEM tests (see Figure 17.1 and Table 17.2). TEG and ROTEM tests have identifiable shapes and patterns that correspond to deficiencies in fibrinogen, platelets, and coagulation factors. Narrow TEG/ROTEM profiles are present when fibrinogen and/or platelets

are deficient. If the patient is lacking coagulation factors, then the time until the beginning of the test profile will be prolonged. Refer to Figures 17.2–17.4 to help visualize these changes.

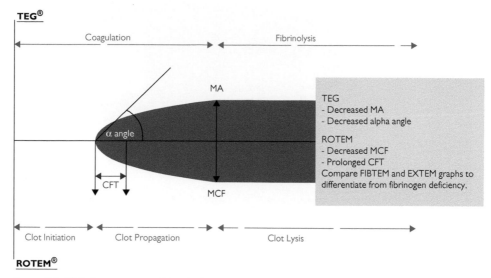

Figure 17.2 TEG showing impaired platelet function. Figure courtesy of author.

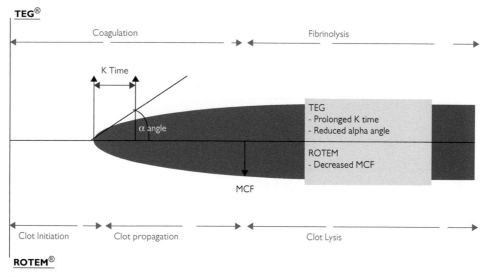

Figure 17.3 TEG showing hypofibrinogenemia. Figure courtesy of author.

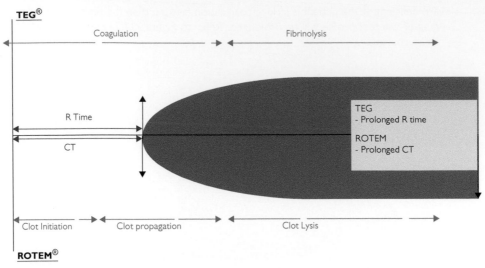

Figure 17.4 TEG showing deficit in coagulation factors. Figure courtesy of author.

9. **Transfuse additional blood products if needed.**

>>**Tip on Technique**: See Figures 17.2–17.4 for abnormalities seen on TEG/ROTEM to aid in the diagnosis and treatment of coagulopathies.

To treat thrombocytopenia (Figure 17.2):
- Transfuse 1 apheresis platelet.
- Consider transfusion if platelet count falls below 50,000/μl[7]
- Keep platelets at room temperature prior to transfusion and use platelet filter.

Transfuse 1 bag of cryoprecipitate for hypofibrinogenemia (Figure 17.3):
- Consider transfusion if fibrinogen level falls below 80–100 mg/dl.[12]
- Stored frozen and contains factor VIII, von Willebrand factor, and fibrinogen.
- Transfuse via blood tubing and warmer.

Transfuse 10–15 ml/kg fresh frozen plasma (FFP) for low coagulation factors (Figure 17.4):
- Consider transfusion if international normalized ratio is >2.0 or PRBC transfusion >70 ml/kg.
- Transfuse via blood tubing and warmer.

Other Management Considerations

Anesthesiologists have a wide arsenal of tools at their disposal and in high-risk patients can use more invasive measures including SVV monitoring via the arterial line, pulmonary artery pressures, and real-time TEE. Certain caveats apply; PEEP has a direct relationship with SVV that is enhanced in the setting of hypovolemia.[13] CVP as measured via a central line is more useful as a trend rather than a discrete number. Its variation has been shown to predict fluid responsiveness in patients after cardiac surgery.[14] Using thermodilution, a pulmonary artery catheter can measure mixed venous oxygenation. This dynamic measurement is typically superior to static measures such as CVP.[14]

Both crystalloids and colloids serve a purpose in goal-directed fluid therapy; avoid large boluses of crystalloid before reassessment of fluid status. Albumin is more beneficial in maintaining hemodynamics and avoiding hemodilution in trauma.[15]

Transfusion of any blood product should be approached systematically with an understanding of the effect of each type of product (Table 17.3). Cryoprecipitate is stored frozen and needs to be thawed prior to administration. It contains fibrinogen and coagulation factors. A reasonable goal is to maintain at least 30% of normal level of coagulation factors. Patients with immunological disease, sepsis, uremia, or liver impairment are at higher risk for baseline platelet dysfunction. Hypofibrinogenemia is often the first factor deficiency to occur during surgical bleeding.[12]

Table 17.3 Blood Product Dosages and Expected Impact

Blood Product	Strategy	Result (in Average-Sized Adult)
PRBC	1 unit	Each unit of PRBC increases hemoglobin approximately 1 g/dl
FFP	10–15 mL/kg	Each unit of FFP increases the level of each clotting factor by 2–3%
Platelet apheresis (pooled from 6 units)	1 apheresis	Increases platelet count by 30,000–60,000 cells per μl
Cryoprecipitate bag (pooled from 5 units)	1 bag	Increases fibrinogen by 50 mg/dl

References

1. Practice guidelines for perioperative blood management. *Anesthesiology*. 2015;122(2):241–275.
2. Frank SM, Oleyar MJ, Ness PM, Tobian AAR. Reducing unnecessary preoperative blood orders and costs by implementing an updated institution-specific maximum surgical blood order schedule and a remote electronic blood release system. *Anesthesiology*. 2014;121(3):501–509.
3. Lier H, Krep H, Schroeder S, Stuber F. Preconditions of hemostasis in trauma: A review. the influence of acidosis, hypocalcemia, anemia, and hypothermia on functional hemostasis in trauma. *J Trauma*. 2008;65(4):951–960.
4. Ali Algadiem E, Aleisa AA, Alsubaie HI, Buhlaiqah NR, Algadeeb JB, Alsneini HA. Blood loss estimation using gauze visual analogue. *Trauma Monthly*. 2016;21(2): e34131.
5. Maheshwari K, Khanna S, Bajracharya GR, et al. A randomized trial of continuous noninvasive blood pressure monitoring during noncardiac surgery. *Anesth Analg*. 2018;127(2):424–431.
6. Kratz T, Steinfeldt T, Exner M, et al. Impact of focused intraoperative transthoracic echocardiography by anesthesiologists on management in hemodynamically unstable high-risk noncardiac surgery patients. *J Cardiothorac Vasc Anesth*. 2017;31(2):602–609.
7. Innerhofer P, Kienast J. Principles of perioperative coagulopathy. *Best Pract Res Clin Anaesthesiol*. 2010;24(1):1–14
8. Wallace SK, Halverson JW, Jankowski CJ, et al. Optimizing blood transfusion practices through bundled intervention implementation in patients with gynecologic cancer undergoing laparotomy. *Obstet Gynecol*. 2018;131(5):891–898.
9. Rineau E, Chaudet A, Chassier C, Bizot P, Lasocki S. Implementing a blood management protocol during the entire perioperative period allows a reduction in transfusion rate in major orthopedic surgery: A before-after study. *Transfusion*. 2016;56(3):673–681.

10. Bou Monsef J, Figgie MP, Mayman D, Boettner F. Targeted pre-operative autologous blood donation: A prospective study of two thousand and three hundred and fifty total hip arthroplasties. *Int Orthop*. 2014;38(8):1591–1595.

11. Pape A, Weber CF, Stein P, Zacharowski K. ROTEM and multiplate—a suitable tool for POC? *ISBT Science Series*. 2010;5(1):161–168.

12. Franchini M, Lippi G. Fibrinogen replacement therapy: A critical review of the literature. *Blood Transfus*. 2012;10(1):23–27.

13. Kawazoe Y, Nakashima T, Iseri T, et al. The impact of inspiratory pressure on stroke volume variation and the evaluation of indexing stroke volume variation to inspiratory pressure under various preload conditions in experimental animals. *J Anesth*. 2015;29(4):515–521.

14. Cherpanath TG, Geerts BF, Maas JJ, de Wilde RB, Groeneveld AB, Jansen JR. Ventilator-induced central venous pressure variation can predict fluid responsiveness in post-operative cardiac surgery patients. *Acta Anaesthesiol Scand*. 2016;60(10):1395–1403.

15. Ansari BM, Zochios V, Falter F, Klein AA. Physiological controversies and methods used to determine fluid responsiveness: A qualitative systematic review. *Anaesthesia*. 2016;71(1):94–105.

Chapter 18

Post-Tonsillectomy Bleeding

Rhae Battles, Adrian Ching, Sandra Gonzalez, and Sonia Mehta

Summary Page

Symptoms:

- Bleeding, hemorrhage, clot formation in tonsillar fossa and/or oropharynx
- Airway obstruction/compromise
- Hypoxemia
- Hemoptysis
- Hematemesis
- Anemia
- Hypovolemia

Differential Diagnosis:

- Postoperative edema
- Gastrointestinal bleeding
- Bleeding/hemorrhage from nonoperative site

Introduction

Post-tonsillectomy hemorrhage is a potentially life-threatening complication after tonsillectomy and/or adenoidectomy that can be challenging to manage for even the most experienced anesthesia providers. The problem of post-tonsillectomy hemorrhage is multifaceted, and the anesthesiologist is often tasked with coordinating the management of the difficult airway, airway obstruction and respiratory compromise, potential aspiration, fluid resuscitation, hemodynamic instability, and maintaining effective lines of communication between the anesthesia team, surgeons, emergency department providers, nursing, and operating room staff.[1] While the problem of post-tonsillectomy hemorrhage primarily presents in the pediatric population, it can also occur in adult patients.

Post-tonsillectomy bleeding is a surgical emergency, with 75% of cases presenting within the first 6 hours postoperatively (primary bleeding). The incidence in pediatric patients is ~2%, while the incidence in adults is ~5%.[2]

Treatment (Figure 18.1)

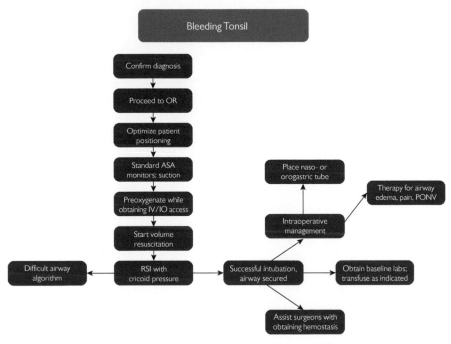

Figure 18.1 Algorithm for response to post-tonsillectomy hemorrhage. ASA = American Society of Anesthesiologists; PONV = postoperative nausea and vomiting.

Step by Step

1. Confirm the diagnosis of tonsillar hemorrhage.

Signs and symptoms of tonsillar hemorrhage include visible airway bleeding, hematemesis, hypotension, tachycardia, decreased capillary refill, agitation (seen mostly in children, less common in adults), and changes in mental status. Hypotension and tachycardia are often a late finding and reveal insufficient intravascular volume replacement, which is a priority.

Once the diagnosis is confirmed, arrange to bring the patient back to the operating room (OR) for surgical hemostasis.

2. **Send lab tests, if not already done.**

Lab tests should include a complete blood count (CBC) since the initial CBC before fluid resuscitation may underestimate the real hemoglobin/hematocrit [Hb/Hct], coagulation panel (Prothrombin/ Partial Thromboplastin Time [PT/PTT] or Thromboelastogram (TEG) if available), and type and cross-match to ensure blood availability.[3,4] The need for blood transfusion in adults with post-tonsillectomy bleeding is rare; therefore, cross-match is optional.

3. **Prepare the patient for induction of anesthesia and call for help.**

It is vital to have ear, nose, and throat (ENT) surgeons and extra anesthesia providers in the room for difficult airway assistance. DO NOT start induction of anesthesia before the surgeon is in the room! Patients with bleeding tonsils present with more airway edema and frank blood and may require difficult airway assistance.

Ensure all equipment and medications that are needed are available and ready to use.

Optimize patient positioning. For pediatric patients consider positioning upright or in lateral decubitus with Trendelenburg. For adult patients, position supine with Trendelenburg. Optimal positioning is important to optimize ventilation and reduce risk of pulmonary aspiration from swallowed blood.

Apply standard American Society for Anesthesiologists (ASA) monitors, including pulse oximetry, noninvasive blood pressure cuff, and electrocardiogram (ECG) leads. Ensure suction is available: both a hard (Yankauer) and soft suction device. Ideally two suction devices should be available.

>> **Tip on Technique:** For children, ensure that the correctly sized hard and soft suction tools are attached and readily available (Table 18.1). Suction size should be selected based on patient age.

4. **Ensure adequate intravenous or intraosseous (IO) access.**

DO NOT proceed with induction of anesthesia without IV/IO access. Adults will usually have an IV placed in the emergency department but children may not. If not placed yet, IV access must be obtained.

> **WARNING!!** If IV/IO access is difficult secondary to an uncooperative or hypovolemic patient, consider restraints or ketamine 4–5 mg/kg IM for sedation.

5. **Initiate volume resuscitation.**

This should ideally be performed PRIOR to induction.

For pediatric patients give 20 ml/kg of isotonic crystalloid solution (Plasma-Lyte A or normal saline). For adult patients, give a bolus of 20 ml/kg of crystalloid solution if there is no contraindication from a cardiac standpoint.

6. **Perform rapid sequence induction.**

Double check that suction devices are functional before starting.

Ensure that all needed airway equipment is available in the appropriate sizes, including face masks, oral airways, supraglottic airway devices, cuffed oral RAE (Ring,

Adair, and Elwyn) tubes, and laryngoscopy devices (see Table 18.1). Consider having a videolaryngoscope in the room, as well as supplemental difficult airway equipment.

Surgical airway instruments, flexible and/or rigid bronchoscopy, and direct and indirect laryngoscopy should be available for possible difficult airway. Refer to pediatric or adult difficult airway algorithms as appropriate.

Place the patient in supine sniffing position or lateral decubitus and preoxygenate with 100% FiO_2.

Table 18.1 Appropriate Sizing of Direct and Indirect Laryngoscopy Blades Based on Weight and Age

	Weight (kg)	Oral Airway (mm)	Suction Catheter (Fr)	ETT (Cuffed) (mm)	ETT @ Lips (cm)	Laryngo-scope Blade Size	Video-laryngo-scope	SGA
Neonate	<1	40	6	2.5	6	Miller 0	Mil 0	1
Neonate	1–2	40	6	2.5–3.0	7	Miller 0	Mil 0	1
Neonate	2–3	40	6	2.5–3.0	8	Mil 0/Mil 1	Mil 0/1	1
Neonate	>3	40	6	2.5–3.0	9-10	Mil 0/Mil 1	Mil 1	1
1–6 mo	4-6	40-50	8	2.5–3.0	11	Mil 1/Wis 1.5	Mil 1	1-1.5
6 mo–1 yr	6–10	50	8	3.0–3.5	11	Wis 1.5	Mil 1	1.5
1–2 yr	10–12	50	8	3.5–4.0	11–12	Wis 1.5	Mac 2	2
2–4 yr	12–16	60	8	4.5	13–14	Wis 1.5/Mac 2	Mac 2	2
4–6 yr	16–20	70	10	5.0	14–15	Wis 1.5/Mac 2	Mac 2	2
6–8 yr	20–30	80	10	5.5	15–16	Mil 2/Mac 2	Mac 2	2.5
9–12 yr	30–45	80	12	6.0–6.5	16–18	Mil/Mac 2-3	Mac 2/3	3
>12 yr	>50	80	12	6.5	20–22	Mil/Mac 2-3	Mac 3	4

>> **Tip on Technique**: Mask induction is NOT appropriate for a bleeding tonsil! Proceed only with IV induction. The surgeon MUST be present for induction, in case additional airway assistance or a surgical airway is needed!

Administer agents that preserve hemodynamics:
- Ketamine 1–2 mg/kg IO/IV *or* etomidate 0.2–0.3 mg/kg IO/IV
- Rocuronium 0.8–1 mg/kg IO/IV *or* succinylcholine 2 mg/kg IO/IV

Caution! Keep in mind that succinylcholine is a trigger agent for malignant hyperthermia. If used, simultaneously administer atropine 0.02 mg/kg IO/IV for succinylcholine-induced bradycardia. Ketamine is the preferred agent as etomidate can cause profound adrenal insufficiency after a single dose. Propofol 2–4 mg/kg IO/IV may be used, but it may exacerbate preexisting hypotension.

7. **Perform rapid sequence intubation.**

   Cricoid pressure should be applied in both adults and children. Intubate using conventional laryngoscopy or videolaryngoscopy, depending on available resources and the provider's experience. Have an appropriately sized cuffed endotracheal tube (ETT) (cuffed oral RAE tubes are preferable), plus additional sizes above and below the calculated ETT size (see Table 18.1 for recommended laryngoscope and tube sizes based on age). The airway must be managed by an experienced provider, and care must be taken to minimize trauma and to avoid dislodging a forming clot in the tonsillar bed. Once the airway is secured, confirm endotracheal intubation and ETT position with capnography and bilateral auscultation.[5]

WARNING!!   If intubation fails, proceed to initiate ventilation with bag-mask or supraglottic airway (SGA), although this may increase the risk of aspiration.

WARNING!!   If you are unable to ventilate or intubate, get the ENT surgeon to assist, and consider a surgical airway before the patient becomes profoundly hypoxemic. Be prepared for a difficult intubation!

!! **Potential Complication:** Cricoid pressure during intubation may make an already poor laryngoscopy view worse. If needed to obtain an adequate view, cricoid pressure may be released in order to secure the airway, although suction should be readily available.

   Place an orogastric or nasogastric tube after the airway is secured. Consider asking the surgeon to advance the orogastric tube, under direct vision, to evacuate any blood that may be present in the gastrointestinal tract.

Caution!   Blind insertion of an orogastric tube can cause further trauma and bleeding and is not recommended.

---

8. **Continue management of the patient's hemodynamics and ventilation.**

   If electrocautery is used, it is important to keep the FiO_2 <30% to reduce the risk of an airway fire.

   If bleeding is uncontrolled or the patient is anemic based on abnormal lab results, give:
   - 10–15 ml/kg IO/IV packed red blood cells (for Hgb <7, uncontrolled hemorrhage)
   - 10–15 ml/kg IO/IV fresh frozen plasma
   - 5–10 cml/kg platelets IO/IV, if platelets <50,000

   If bleeding is diffuse, consider coagulopathy and platelet function disorders as a possible differential diagnosis. Pediatric patients have a higher likelihood of need for transfusion of blood products compared to adults.[6]

9. **Emergence and postoperative care.**

   Administer agents to decrease airway swelling and prevent postoperative nausea and vomiting:
   - Dexamethasone 0.5 mg/kg IO/IV (no more than 12 mg)
   - Ondansetron 0.1–0.15 mg/kg IO/IV (no more than 4 mg)
   - Adult dosing: dexamethasone up to 10–12 mg IV and ondansetron 4 mg IV

> **Caution!** Do not use ondansetron in the presence of prolonged QT interval.

Give multimodal pain control, if tolerated hemodynamically. For pediatric patients, consider acetaminophen 10–15 mg/kg IO/IV (max 1 gram, assuming no liver issues or elevated liver enzymes) or fentanyl 2 mcg/kg IO/IV (titrate carefully). For adult patients, longer-acting narcotics can be used for postoperative analgesia. Titrate carefully. Avoid long-acting opioids as they may add to the risk of postoperative apneic events in these patients who are at increased risk of airway obstruction.

For emergence and extubation, verify that the surgeon has advanced the orogastric tube, that stomach contents have been suctioned, and that hemostasis has been satisfactory.

Discontinue volatile anesthetics, increase FiO_2 to 90–100%, and increase fresh gas flows.

Insert a soft bite block if one is not already in place. Assess routine extubation parameters such as adequate tidal volume and respiratory rate, and level of consciousness. Airway reflexes must be present, and patients should be alert and purposeful.

Make sure patients meet all extubation criteria. Consider keeping the patient intubated if there is any concern about airway patency, rebleeding (risk will depend on the primary reason for bleeding), or potential need for further resuscitation or intervention. Patients should be monitored for airway patency and hemodynamic status in an intensive care unit (ICU) setting postoperatively.

Position the patient in reverse Trendelenburg, or in lateral decubitus, for extubation to decrease risk of aspiration. If suctioning the oropharynx is necessary, carefully use a soft suction catheter, and insert it midline to avoid trauma to the tonsils. After extubating the trachea, verify airway patency and adequate respiratory pattern before transporting patient to the postanesthesia care unit.

Note: Emergence and extubation have been shown to be a critical time for hypoxia. Airway equipment must be readily available during extubation!! Airway procedures carry a higher risk of airway-related complications, and early detection and treatment of issues such as laryngospasm are critical for patient safety. Transfer to ICU level of care for close monitoring is recommended.

Other Management Considerations

While treatment in adults is similar to children (main focus is on initial resuscitation and control of bleeding source), there are some differences in regard to post-tonsillectomy bleeding in adults. In one study, incidence of post-tonsillectomy bleeding was higher for patients 16 years and older (4.9%) than in children 5–15 years old (3%) and children younger than 5 (1.9%). Over 50% of adults with post-tonsillectomy bleeding will require surgical hemostasis, but the need for blood transfusion is highly unlikely. In general, adults will routinely have IV access, are able to provide more information, and will be more cooperative than pediatric patients.

Pediatric patients may present with congenital (e.g., Goldenhar syndrome, Pierre-Robin sequence, trisomy 21) or acquired (e.g., postsurgical, radiation-induced changes, trauma) airway abnormalities, confounding an already potentially difficult airway in the presence of post-tonsillectomy hemorrhage. Obesity, obstructive sleep apnea, head and neck cancer, and previous trauma or surgery may further complicate airway management in both pediatric and adult patients. It is important to note that obstructive sleep apnea may persist after tonsillectomy, with risk factors including craniofacial/mandibular anomalies, obesity, neuromuscular disorders, preoperative severe obstructive sleep apnea, genetic disorders, and asthma. Difficult airway algorithms should be followed for an effective and organized approach. These patients should be treated concurrently with ENT surgeons, and proceeding to a surgical airway may be necessary in a cannot-ventilate/cannot-intubate scenario.

References

1. Fields RG, Gencorelli FJ, Litman RS. Anesthetic management of the pediatric bleeding tonsil. Paediatr Anaesth. 2010 Nov;20(11):982–986. doi: 10.1111/j.1460-9592.2010.03426.x. PubMed PMID: 20964765.
2. Lowe D, Van der Meulen J. Key messages from the national prospective tonsillectomy audit. Laryngoscope. 2007;117:717–724.
3. Wall JJ, Tay KY. Postoperative tonsillectomy hemorrhage. Emerg Med Clin North Am. 2018 May;36(2):415–426. doi: 10.1016/j.emc.2017.12.009. Epub 2018 Feb 10. Review. PubMed PMID: 29622331.
4. Myssiorek D, Alvi A. Post-tonsillectomy hemorrhage: an assessment of risk factors. Int J Pediatr Otorhinolaryngol. 1996 Sep;37(1):35–43. PubMed PMID: 8884405.
5. Barash PG (Ed.). *Clinical Anesthesia* (7th ed.). Philadelphia, PA: Wolters Kluwer Health/Lippincott Williams & Wilkins; 2013.
6. Miller, RD (Ed.). *Miller's Anesthesia* (7th ed.). Philadelphia, PA: Churchill Livingstone/Elsevier; 2010.

Chapter 19

Transfusion Reactions

Geoffrey D. Panjeton, Alex Coons, Jayme N. Looper, and Jeffrey D. F. White

Summary Page

Symptoms:

- Acute reactions (minutes to hours)
  - Symptoms evident under general anesthesia
    - Hypotension
    - Tachycardia
    - Rash
    - Fever
    - Flushed appearance
    - Wheezing (immunologic/allergic)
    - Hemoglobinuria and acute renal failure as evidenced by decreased urine output (hemolytic)
    - Diffuse bleeding (hemolytic)
  - Symptoms masked by general anesthesia
    - Dyspnea
    - Chills
    - Nausea/vomiting
    - Myalgia and headache (immuno-logic/allergic)
- Delayed reactions
  - Transfusion-related acute lung injury
  - Transfusion-associated cardiac overload

Differential Diagnosis:

- Anaphylaxis from other medications
- Rhabdomyolysis
- Flash pulmonary or cardiogenic edema
- Acute myocardial infarction
- Disseminated intravascular coagulation
- Septic versus hemorrhagic shock

Introduction

Blood product transfusions may be required during a variety of surgical procedures. Anesthesia providers must be vigilant and prepared to administer transfusion(s) of the correct blood components. Providers must be knowledgeable about the possible transfusion reactions that might subsequently occur, especially their various manifestations in the patient under general anesthesia. Providers must further be able to implement the necessary and appropriate treatment. The American Association of Blood Banks (AABB) reported that in 2013 the rate of adverse reactions following blood product transfusion was 0.25%, or 2.5 per 1000 units transfused. Therefore, the likelihood that an anesthesia provider will encounter a perioperative blood transfusion reaction during their career is very high.

Transfusion reactions can occur due to a variety of etiologies. Table 19.1 outlines the underlying pathophysiology of acute transfusion reactions, highlighting the reaction as well as the typical etiology.[1,2] The most devastating reactions within the setting of the operating room include hemolytic transfusion reactions due to ABO-incompatible blood administration. This would manifest under general anesthesia as acute-onset hypotension and progressive development of hemoglobinuria, and the process can progress to disseminated intravascular coagulation (DIC) and acute renal failure.

Table 19.1 Underlying Pathophysiology of Acute Transfusion Reactions, Including Reaction and Typical Etiology

Causes of Acute Transfusion Reactions		
Reaction		**Typical Etiology**
Caused by Antibodies in the Recipient • Mild allergic (1–3%) • Febrile nonhemolytic (0.1–1%) • Acute hemolytic (1:76,000) • Anaphylactic (1:20,000–1:50,000)	→	**Recipient Antibody Directed Toward Blood Donor . . .** • Plasma proteins • Leukocytes • ABO blood group (or certain other RBC antigens) • Immunoglobulin A
Caused by Antibodies from the Donor • Acute lung injury or TRALI (1:1200–1:190,000)	→	**Blood Donor Antibody Directed Toward Recipient . . .** • Leukocytes
Caused by Contamination of Blood Product • Bacterial contamination	→	**Bacteria from . . .** • Donor's blood or skin; product manipulation
Cause Not Intrinsic to the Unit of Blood • Volume overload (TACO) (<1%) • Hypothermia • Metabolic abnormalities	→	**Due to Transfusion to a Patient That Cannot . . .** • Tolerate extra fluid volume • Compensate for volume of cold blood • Metabolize blood product anticoagulants
Cause Intrinsic to the Unit of Blood • Bradykinin activation	→	**Due to Transfusion to a Patient That Cannot . . .** • Metabolize bradykinins normally (associated with ACE inhibitors)

Adapted and modified from Crookston KP, Koenig SC, Reyes MD. Transfusion reaction identification and management at the bedside. *J Infus Nurs* 2015;38(2):104–113; Fung MK, Grossman BJ, Hillyer CD, Westhoff CM. *Technical Manual.* 18th ed. Bethesda, Maryland: AABB; 2014.

Treatment

Blood transfusion reactions within the operating room can range in severity from minor to life-threatening, and presentation times can range from immediate (minutes to hours) to delayed (hours to days). The correct treatment plan can run the gamut from stopping the transfusion and observing the patient to instituting advanced cardiac life support (ACLS). Delayed transfusion reactions from transfusions given prior to surgery can present within the operating room as acute problems requiring acute diagnosis and treatment.

WARNING!! If at any point during the following steps cardiopulmonary arrest ensues, call a code and start ACLS protocols.

Step by Step

1. Identify signs of possible transfusion reaction (Figure 19.1).

General anesthesia can mask many of the signs of transfusion reaction. The anesthesiologist must be vigilant in identifying other possible signs of a transfusion reaction including hyperthermia, hemoglobinuria, microvascular bleeding, hypoxemia, increased peak airway pressures, urticaria, hypotension, and hypocalcemia.[3]

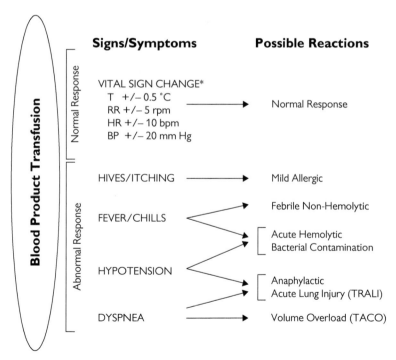

Figure 19.1 Highlights of normal and abnormal responses to blood product transfusion, with a correlation between presenting signs/symptoms and their possible diagnostic implication. T = temperature; RR = respiratory rate in respirations per minute (rpm); HR = heart rate in beats per minute (bpm); BP = either systolic or diastolic blood pressure in millimeters of mercury (mmHg). TACO = transfusion-associated circulatory overload. TRALI = transfusion-related lung injury. Reprinted with permission from Crookston KP, Koenig SC, Reyes MD. Transfusion reaction identification and management at the bedside. J Infus Nurs 2015;38(2):104–113.

WARNING!!	If the patient is in cardiovascular compromise, call a code and begin ACLS!
WARNING!!	IF THE PATIENT IS HEMODYNAMICALLY UNSTABLE, proceed directly to step 2.

For hemodynamically stable patients, proceed to step 8.

2. **Immediately stop the transfusion.**

    Maintain IV access and administer IV crystalloids to maintain hemodynamics. Keep all blood product bags and documentation, as they will be needed by the blood bank for further testing.

3. **Inform the team and call for additional help.**

    Alert the surgical (or intensive care unit team) and call for additional help to manage the patient. Inform the blood bank of a possible transfusion reaction and provide them the product bags for testing.

4. **Secure the airway if needed.**

    If the patient is already intubated, increase FiO_2 to 100%. If the patient is not already intubated, secure the airway if signs of airway compromise exist. Obtain difficult airway equipment/difficult airway cart in case of airway edema.

    >> **Tip on Technique:** Awake fiberoptic bronchoscopy should be attempted early as repeated attempts at laryngoscopy can cause further swelling and airway obstruction. Equipment for surgical airway including an emergency cricothyroidotomy kit should be readily available. Care should be taken as severe angioedema in this setting can make it difficult to identify superficial landmarks to guide the surgical airway. In these instances, ultrasound in the hands of a skilled operator may be a useful adjunct to help secure airway access.

Caution!	Anaphylactic reactions can cause edema of the tongue and pharyngeal tissues that can complicate laryngoscopy.

5. **Consider epinephrine to support hemodynamic status, especially if concerned for anaphylaxis.**

    Give epinephrine 10–50 mcg IV; repeat as necessary.

    >> **Tip on Technique:** Maintain a high suspicion for anaphylaxis, especially of concern in patients with IgA deficiency.

6. **Start volume resuscitation to support hemodynamics.**

    Give primarily isotonic crystalloid infusions (typically 1–2 L) to a goal mean arterial pressure >60 mmHg and central venous pressure (CVP) >8 mmHg (if central line in place to monitor CVP).

    >> **Tip on Technique:** Patient-specific characteristics such as depressed ejection fraction and decreased renal function may require less fluid administration. As such, fluid resuscitation should be guided using dynamic hemodynamic parameters such as pulse pressure variation responses to fluid challenges in mechanically ventilated patients. Patients with pulse

pressure variations >10% are typically considered fluid responsive. Echocardiography can also be useful to estimate left ventricle systolic function and volumes.

7. **If hypotension persists, administer vasopressors.**

Give vasopressin 0.5–2 units IV as a bolus or as an infusion at 0.01–0.04 units/min IV. Consider norepinephrine 0.01–3 mcg/kg/min IV if unresponsive to vasopressin. Decrease anesthetic doses as they can worsen hypotension.

>> **Tip on Technique**: Isolated hypotension after administration of blood products can also occur in patients on angiotensin-converting enzyme (ACE) inhibitor medications and is caused by bradykinin. In these patients, treat hypotension by discontinuing the transfusion and holding ACE inhibitors for 24 hours prior to transfusion.

8. **If clinical condition requires further transfusion, switch to units of O-negative packed red blood cells (PRBCs) or AB plasma.**

O-negative PRBCs are the universal donor for blood, and AB plasma is the universal donor if plasma is needed. If AB plasma is unavailable, the blood bank may have type A plasma with low titers of anti-B, and this is safe to be administered until the patient is stabilized.[4] However, this requires that a measurement of the anti-B titer be made prior to transfusion. In either case, the Rh type of plasma is not necessary.

9. **Assess and treat other symptoms.**

Closely monitor vitals for signs of hemodynamic instability including diminished urine output and bleeding. Patients are at high risk for development of shock, renal failure, and DIC. If wheezing is present, administer albuterol to decrease bronchospasm (1–2 puffs inhaled every 4–6 hours). If hives or urticaria is present, administer an H1 blocker (diphenhydramine 50 mg IV). Also consider administration of an H2 blocker (ranitidine 50 mg IV or famotidine 20 mg IV) and steroids (dexamethasone 8–20 mg IV or methylprednisolone 100 mg IV).

If hemoglobinuria is present, infuse 500 ml 0.9% NaCl per hour until hemoglobinuria decreases. Also consider low-dose dopamine infusion (2–3 mcg/kg/min IV), osmotic diuresis with mannitol 0.5–1.5 mg/kg IV, or alkalinizing the urine with sodium bicarbonate 50 mEq IV.

10. **Send blood and urine for laboratory analysis.**

Send complete blood count (CBC), basic metabolic panel (BMP), urinalysis, urine hemoglobin, prothrombin/partial thromboplastin time (PTT/PT), direct Coombs testing, haptoglobin, bilirubin, fibrin degradation products, and tryptase.

11. **Treat DIC if present.**

DIC presents clinically as diffuse oozing of blood, with the following corroborating laboratory findings: thrombocytopenia, low fibrinogen level, prolonged PT/PTT, and elevated D-dimer.

Treatment should include transfusing with fresh frozen plasma (FFP), pooled cryoprecipitate for fibrinogen, and/or platelet concentrates.

12. **If the patient exhibits oxygen desaturation, send brain natriuretic peptide (BNP) to rule out transfusion-associated cardiac overload (TACO) or transfusion-related acute lung injury (TRALI).** [5]

TRALI can manifest within 6 hours of blood transfusion and manifests as a noncardiogenic pulmonary edema with likely associated hypotension, fever, and leukopenia. TRALI will demonstrate a normal BNP.[5] Start mechanical ventilation with low tidal volumes and do NOT give diuretics. Consider fluid administration if the patient is hypotensive.

TACO is related to fluid overload, manifesting with cardiogenic pulmonary edema in the setting of increased pulmonary capillary wedge pressure, elevated BNP, and frequently hypertension. [5] Treat by removing fluid with either diuretics or phlebotomy.

>> **Tip on Technique**: TRALI is a diagnosis of exclusion. See Table 19.2 for how to differentiate between TACO and TRALI.[1]

Table 19.2 Key Factors Differentiating TACO and TRALI[5]

	TACO	TRALI
Pulmonary edema fluid	Transudative	Exudative
Blood pressure	Usually hypertensive	Usually hypotensive
Pulmonary capillary wedge pressure	High	Normal
Temperature	Normal	High
BNP	Elevated	Normal
Treatment	Diuresis	Supportive

13. Treat fever if present.

Treat fever with acetaminophen 15 mg/kg (IV or PO depending on available access) and change forced air and fluid warmers to cool, but do not give aspirin or steroids. Send blood cultures and start antibiotics with gram-negative (*Yersinia*) and gram-positive (*Staphylococcus*) coverage if there is likelihood of bacterial contamination (i.e., abnormal stat gram stain results). Monitor vitals for signs of impending sepsis and Modified Early Warning Score (MEWS) of 5 or higher. MEWS >5 is associated with increased risk of clinical deterioration and the need for transfer to a critical care unit.

>> **Tip on Technique**: Have a high suspicion for bacterial contamination, especially with platelet administration. Platelets are at highest risk of bacterial contamination (1:2000) because they are stored at room temperature, followed by red cell concentrates (1:500,000).[6]

!! **Potential Complications**: Aspirin inhibits platelet function, and steroids can mask the signs and symptoms of transfusion reactions and possibly delay recognition. Malaria and other bloodborne viruses may be spread via transfusion.[6]

14. Manage and treat delayed reactions.

If easy bruising and bleeding are present, check platelet count for thrombocytopenia. Maintain a high index of suspicion for posttransfusion purpura (alloimmunization against platelet antigens that results in thrombocytopenia) if the patient has received a platelet transfusion. If platelets are severely decreased, give immune globulin 0.5–1 g/kg IV as first-line treatment. Consider plasmapheresis or high-dose corticosteroids (2 mg/kg prednisolone IV or equivalent dose of alternative steroid) as second-line therapies.

If fever, malaise, or jaundice is present, have a high suspicion for delayed hemolytic reaction. These are typically caused by antibodies to minor antigens, such as Rh, Kidd, and others. Check hematocrit, direct Coombs test, urine hemoglobin, white blood cell count, bilirubin, haptoglobin, and lactose dehydrogenase (LDH). Treatment is supportive: IV hydration and monitoring of renal function and hemoglobin levels.

>> **Tip on Technique:** If the patient requires subsequent transfusion, ensure updated red blood cell matching to check for new antibodies and ensure that new blood products have been appropriately screened.

If fever, severe rash, and diarrhea are present, have a high suspicion for graft-versus-host disease, especially in immunocompromised patients. Check CBC and liver function tests. Transfusion-associated graft-versus-host disease (TA-GVHD) is a rare yet potentially fatal transfusion reaction that typically occurs within 2–30 days of transfusion.[7] It presents with an erythematous, maculopapular rash; fever; elevated liver enzymes; and gastrointestinal symptoms (nausea, vomiting, diarrhea).[7] TA-GVHD occurs due to viable T lymphocytes in the transfused product not being recognized as foreign by the transfusion recipient's immune system.[7] This permits the transfused T cells to survive and mount a vigorous immune response against recipient tissues, including bone marrow.[7] Treatment is supportive as there is no effective treatment for this condition.

>> **Tip on Technique:** To prevent this reaction in patients who are immunocompromised, administer irradiated and leukoreduced cellular components for transfusion.

Other Management Considerations

Massive transfusion of PRBCs can lead to citrate toxicity, the development of hypocalcemia, and severe hypotension. Calcium chloride or gluconate administration will reverse this, in distinction from acute (bradykinin-associated) hypotensive transfusion reactions where stopping of the transfusion resolves the hypotension rapidly. Additional transfusion reactions include immunologic nonhemolytic reactions, which may be masked under general anesthesia.

Delayed reactions can occur in patients undergoing chronic transfusions, such as trauma and other critical care patients who may have received prior transfusions during their hospital admission. In these circumstances, reviewing the medical record to identify previous blood transfusion, history of drug-induced coagulopathy, history of thrombotic events, and risk factors for organ ischemia along with a review of the patient's hematologic and coagulation profiles is an integral aspect of preoperative evaluation.[3]

Additional delayed transfusion reactions include transfusion-transmitted infection (TTI). TTI is becoming less common since the advent of screening for high-risk patient populations and viruses. New considerations for TTI include the transmission of endemic diseases based on possible exposure, such as West Nile virus, malaria, and Creutzfeldt-Jacob disease.[6]

Pediatric patients are at an increased risk of adverse outcome related to blood product transfusion.[8] Unfortunately, a majority of these adverse outcomes are related to human error, specifically overtransfusion.[3] Children require a weight-based dosing of blood, rather than whole units as administered for adults. There is a great deal of variability in the formula used or the ideal dosing for blood transfusion in children; however, a recent evidence-based recommendation is to administer 10 ml/kg.[9]

References

1. Crookston KP, Koenig SC, Reyes MD. Transfusion reaction identification and management at the bedside. *J Infus Nurs* 2015;38(2):104–113.
2. Fung MK, Grossman BJ, Hillyer CD, Westhoff CM. *Technical Manual.* 18th ed. Bethesda, Maryland: AABB; 2014.
3. American Society of Anesthesiologists Task Force on Perioperative Blood Management. Practice guidelines for perioperative blood management: an updated report by the American

Society of Anesthesiologists Task Force on Perioperative Blood Management. *Anesthesiology* 2015;122(2):241–275.

4. ACS TQIP Massive Transfusion in Trauma Guidelines. Available at: https://www.facs.org/-/media/files/quality-programs/trauma/tqip/transfusion_guildelines.ashx Accessed March 18, 2019.

5. Skeate RC, Eastlund T. Distinguishing between transfusion related acute lung injury and transfusion associated circulatory overload. *Curr Opin Hematol* 2007;14(6):682–687.

6. Clevenger B, Kelleher A. Hazards of blood transfusion in adults and children. *Cont Ed in Anaes Crit Care & Pain* 2014;14(3):112–118.

7. Fast LD. Developments in the prevention of transfusion-associated graft-versus-host disease. *Br J Haematol* 2012;158(5):563–568.

8. Lavoie J. Blood transfusion risks and alternative strategies in pediatric patients. *Paediatr Anaesth* 2011;21(1):14–24.

9. Davies P, Robertson S, Hegde S, Greenwood R, Massey E, Davis P. Calculating the required transfusion volume in children. *Transfusion* 2007;47(2):212–216.

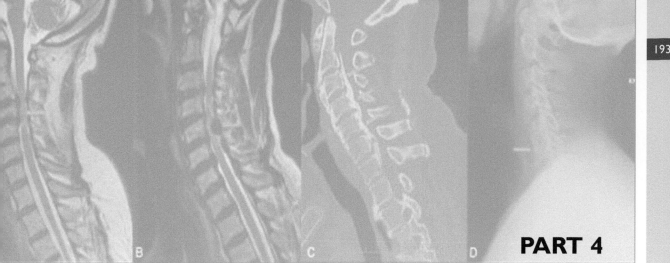

PART 4

NEUROLOGIC

Chapter 20

Management of the Unstable Cervical Spine

Peggy White and Christopher W. Maxwell Jr.

Summary Page

Symptoms:

- Neck pain
- Radiculopathy
- Altered mental status
- Coma
- Dysesthesias, paresthesias
- Dyspnea
- Shock
- Hypoxia

Differential Diagnosis:

- Intracerebral hemorrhage
- Ligamentous injury
- Atlantoaxial instability
- Atlantooccipital instability
- Odontoid fracture

Introduction

Spinal cord injury can occur due to trauma or secondarily by maneuvering the pathologic spine. Damage can be exacerbated when manipulating the airway with intubating devices, as well as with bag-mask ventilation. Remain cautious, even when a cervical collar is in place, as the spinal cord integrity is still at risk.

Despite decades of research on cervical column stability with the use of airway devices, there remains no clear evidence that supports the use of one device over the other. However, use of manual in-line stabilization has stood the test of time in rapidly providing safe intubating conditions. If time allows, a properly performed awake fiberoptic intubation is the preferred method if the patient is calm and cooperative.

Myriad other injuries can be associated with traumatic cervical spine injuries. One must have comprehensive knowledge of these to predict complications and treat accordingly. If the integrity of the spinal cord is disrupted, neurogenic and spinal shock can be an acute threat to life.

Treatment

Spinal cord injury may be caused by compression, contusion, laceration, or vascular damage. The force required to cause injury to the cervical spine can be significant and is often associated with other injuries. A Glasgow Coma Score (GCS) below 8 has been associated with cervical spinal cord injury.[1] Traumatic brain injury (TBI), facial fractures, and vertebral artery dissection can be associated with this type of injury. Other concerns based on mechanism of injury include large vessel rupture, pulmonary or cardiac contusion, long bone or pelvis fractures, and abdominal organ damage. The patient may present in shock and/or hypoxia. It is difficult to distinguish spinal cord contusion versus transection at initial presentation. Nonetheless, care of these patients should be focused on managing airway, breathing, and circulation while minimizing secondary injury.[2]

All trauma patients with a suspicious mechanism of injury should be placed in a cervical collar. Patients presenting as the result of a trauma often have altered mental status or distracting injuries or may be under the influence of drugs or alcohol. These circumstances may mask the evaluation of neck stability and should always be treated as an unstable cervical spine.

When there is cervical malalignment, patients may be placed in traction. It is important to ensure that in-line stabilization is maintained at all times. Supine or slight head elevation with manual in-line stabilization (MILS) are options for providing the most optimal intubating conditions. When performing an awake fiberoptic intubation, the best position is supine or sitting with the cervical collar in place.

Step by Step

1. **Evaluate the patient to ensure adequate oxygenation, ventilation, airway patency, and spontaneous ventilation.**

   Perform a baseline neurological assessment and assess for deficits. Place standard American Society for Anesthesiologists (ASA) monitors and assess for oxygenation and ventilation. Apply supplemental oxygen, preferably with positive pressure such as self-inflating bag with positive end-expiratory pressure (PEEP) valve, Mapleson, or, if available, high-flow nasal cannula. Noninvasive positive pressure ventilation can improve oxygen reserve.[3]

> **WARNING!!** If the patient is NOT adequately oxygenating or ventilating, PROCEED IMMEDIATELY TO INTUBATION (STEP 4)!

> **WARNING!!** A patient with an acute cervical fracture above C5 may present with respiratory failure due to injury to the phrenic nerve (originates from C3, C4, C5) and need emergent intubation. Patients with GCS <8 may also require immediate intubation for airway protection. If so, proceed immediately to step 4 with MILS and secure the airway efficiently with the least amount of cervical spine motion as possible.

2. Ensure adequate IV access.

Place at least one large-bore IV (16 gauge or larger) for rapid bolus of crystalloid or transfusion of blood products. Additional peripheral IVs are recommended for infusions of other medications (opioids, vasoactive agents).

Placement of an arterial line prior to intubation is recommended if time permits for closer monitoring of blood pressure (to maintain spinal cord perfusion) and blood gas sampling.

> **Caution!** Injuries to other vital organs (liver, spleen, heart, lungs) may require central venous access for rapid resuscitation and/or prolonged infusions of vasoactive agents. The preferred location for central venous access is the right internal jugular vein via ultrasound guidance. The presence of a cervical collar may necessitate subclavian central access. If there is concern for associated TBI and increased intracranial pressure, femoral vein access should be considered (to avoid the Trendelenburg position).

3. Manage hemodynamics; monitor for spinal or neurogenic shock.

It is important to distinguish between spinal or neurogenic shock and hemorrhagic shock, though each can be life threatening.[4,5] Management of hemorrhagic shock should be focused on restoration of blood volume, correction of coagulopathies, and control of bleeding.

Hemodynamic goals with spinal cord injury should be to maintain a mean arterial pressure goal of >85 mmHg for 7 days. To maintain hemodynamics, give vasopressors as needed.

Note: If repeated boluses are needed, consider starting an infusion:

- Phenylephrine 100–200 mcg IV and/or 0.1–1 mcg/kg/min IV infusion
- Vasopressin 1–2 units IV bolus and/or 0.02–0.04 units/hr IV infusion
- Norepinephrine 4 mcg IV and/or 0.01–0.20 mcg/kg/min infusion
- Ephedrine 5–10 mg IV
- Epinephrine 4 mcg IV and/or 0.01–0.20 mcg/kg/min infusion

Consider for bradycardia associated with spinal shock:
- Glycopyrrolate 0.2–0.4 mg IV
- Atropine 0.5–1 mg IV

>> **Tip on Technique**: Hemodynamics can be maintained by using phenylephrine, but patient factors such as heart rate and myocardial function may necessitate a different choice such as norepinephrine or epinephrine. Bradycardia can be managed with anticholinergics such as glycopyrrolate, but some cases may require pacing.[6,7]

> **WARNING!!** Neurogenic shock can occur with injury to the brain, brainstem, or upper cervical cord, affecting the cardioaccelerator fibers (C1–4), leading to hemodynamic instability.

4. Prepare airway equipment and select method of intubation.

Airway equipment should include a self-inflating bag, working suction, laryngoscopes and endotracheal tube loaded with stylet, alternate intubation devices such as videolaryngoscopes, flexible bronchoscopes, and airway adjuncts (gum elastic bougie, oral airway, tongue depressors). See Figure 20.1 for recommended airway equipment.

Airway device	Image	Pros	Cons
Video laryngoscope	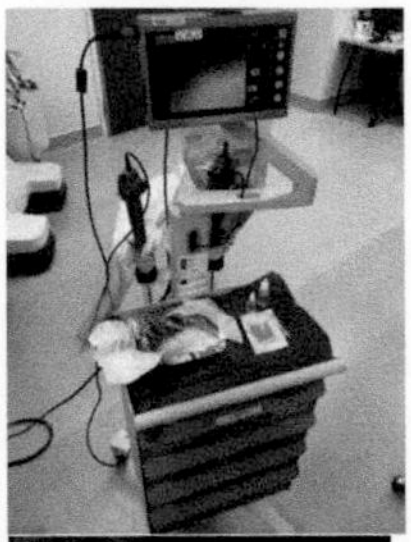 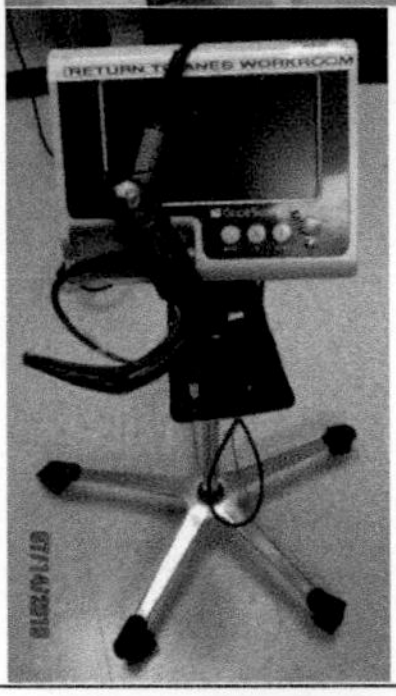	- Improved laryngoscopy view[9,10] - Less mouth opening required	- Similar amount of neck movement as DL - Increased neck movement than fiberoptic[11] - Not always available
Flexible bronchoscope	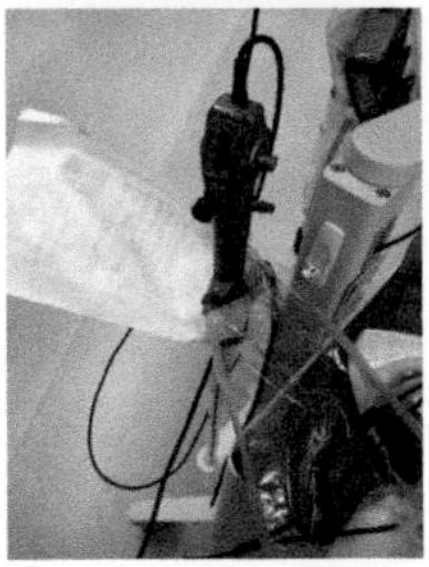	- Minimal/least neck movement[12,13] - Excellent for cooperative patients - Allows for documentation of neurologic exam before and after intubation[13] - Awake fiberoptic has not been shown to have superior neurologic outcomes compared to asleep[8]	- Relatively expensive - Longer time to perform - Requires experience and patient cooperation (awake technique) - Not always available

Figure 20.1 Common airway adjuncts.

Airtraq	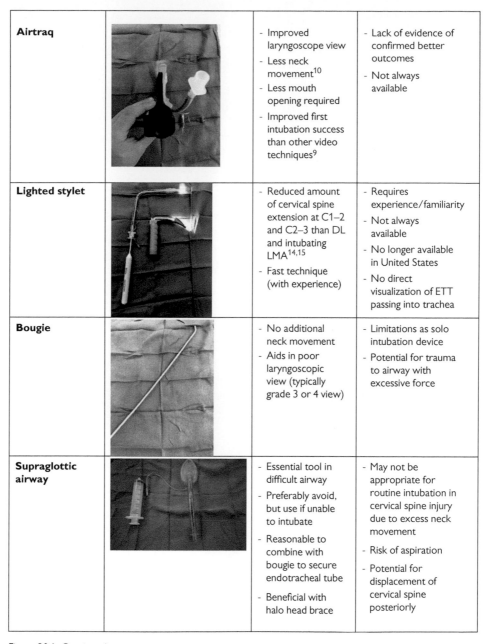	- Improved laryngoscope view - Less neck movement[10] - Less mouth opening required - Improved first intubation success than other video techniques[9]	- Lack of evidence of confirmed better outcomes - Not always available
Lighted stylet		- Reduced amount of cervical spine extension at C1–2 and C2–3 than DL and intubating LMA[14,15] - Fast technique (with experience)	- Requires experience/familiarity - Not always available - No longer available in United States - No direct visualization of ETT passing into trachea
Bougie		- No additional neck movement - Aids in poor laryngoscopic view (typically grade 3 or 4 view)	- Limitations as solo intubation device - Potential for trauma to airway with excessive force
Supraglottic airway		- Essential tool in difficult airway - Preferably avoid, but use if unable to intubate - Reasonable to combine with bougie to secure endotracheal tube - Beneficial with halo head brace	- May not be appropriate for routine intubation in cervical spine injury due to excess neck movement - Risk of aspiration - Potential for displacement of cervical spine posteriorly

Figure 20.1 Continued

>> **Tip on Technique:** There is no clear evidence in the literature to support one particular intubation technique. The goal is successful oral intubation with minimal to no neck movement.[1] Consider the need for postintubation neurological exam when selecting technique and medications. Assess the neurological exam as soon as possible after intubation. Options include a wake-up test and/or neuromonitoring (electrophysiological monitoring) if asleep intubation is selected.

Options include:

- Rapid sequence induction (RSI) with MILS if the patient is unstable, obtunded, or uncooperative (see steps 5–7)
- Awake flexible fiberoptic intubation if patient is cooperative and hemodynamically stable (see steps 8–11)

>> **Tip on Technique:** Glycopyrrolate 1–5 mcg/kg IV will limit oral secretions. Up to a maximum dose of 1 mg can be used if heart rate tolerates.[8] The usual onset of glycopyrrolate is approximately 5 minutes, so give early enough to take effect.

To perform RSI with MILS, follow steps 5–7.

5. **Remove ONLY the anterior portion of the cervical collar and apply MILS.**

   >> **Tip on Technique:** To perform MILS, remove the cervical collar and stabilize the neck as shown in Figure 20.2. Replace the cervical collar after intubation. Keeping the collar in place can limit mouth opening and make intubation more difficult.[16,17]

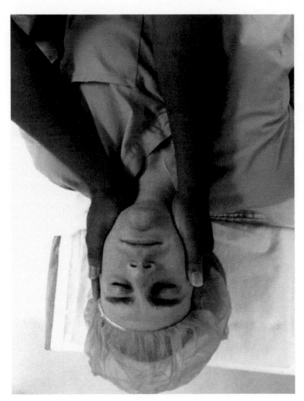

Figure 20.2 Manual in-line stabilization. Photo courtesy of author.

6. **Preoxygenate and give induction medications.**

   Continue with patient preoxygenation if spontaneously ventilating; otherwise, place an oral airway without manipulating the neck to gently mask ventilate.

> **Caution!** Be cautious with mask ventilation to reduce cervical spine movement. Oral airway placement is recommended to reduce the need for neck movement.

Recommended induction medications:

- Lidocaine 1 mg/kg IV
- Propofol 1–2 mg/kg IV
- Fentanyl 1–2 mcg/kg IV
- Succinylcholine 1.5 mg/kg IV

> **Caution!** Doses should be adjusted based on patient hemodynamics. Consider etomidate (0.3 mg/kg) and/or ketamine (2 mg/kg) if potential exists for hypovolemia/hemorrhage, spinal shock, or myocardial dysfunction related to other injuries. Be aware of the risk for adrenal suppression with etomidate use. Consider administering hydrocortisone 100 mg IV if using etomidate.
>
> **Caution!** Avoid succinylcholine if spinal cord injury is >24 hours old or if other risks exist for hyperkalemia. Proliferation of extrajunctional nicotinic acetylcholine receptors may lead to hyperkalemia with succinylcholine administration. Use rocuronium 1.2 mg/kg IV instead.

Closely monitor hemodynamics and supplement with vasoactive medications from step 3 as needed.

7. Perform direct or indirect laryngoscopy and intubation.

See Figure 20.1 for options. To minimize neck movement, consider the use of an adjunct such as a gum elastic bougie if visualization is difficult. Videolaryngoscopy or flexible fiberoptic bronchoscopy may be preferred to minimize neck movement and improve first-pass success.[9,10,12,13] Confirm placement of the endotracheal tube with end-tidal carbon dioxide on three consecutive breaths, as well as auscultation to confirm breath sounds bilaterally.

>> **Tip on Technique:** An RSI with direct or indirect laryngoscopy with MILS is preferred for emergent intubation.

To perform awake fiberoptic intubation, follow steps 8–11.

8. Preoxygenate patient and prepare equipment.

Continue with patient preoxygenation. Maintain cervical collar and elevate head of bed. Consider placing the patient in a sitting position.

Prepare the flexible bronchoscope with anti-fog solution and suction. Load the appropriately sized endotracheal tube over the flexible bronchoscope and secure with tape that is easy to remove.

9. Consider sedation.[8,12,14]

Options include:

- Dexmedetomidine infusion (0.5–1 mcg/kg IV over 10 minutes, followed by infusion at 0.2–0.7 mcg/kg/hr)
- Ketamine (0.1–0.2 mg/kg IV to a maximum of 1 mg/kg)

- Remifentanil (0.05–0.5 mcg/kg/min IV)
- Midazolam (0.05–0.1 mg/kg to a maximum of 5 mg IV)

Caution! Sedation can result in loss of airway reflexes and possibly airway obstruction, as well as disinhibition and loss of patient cooperation and ability to perform a neurological exam. Titrate carefully if using.

WARNING!! Excessive sedation can occur when combining opioids and benzodiazepines, particularly at moderate to high doses. Ketamine and dexmedetomidine are viable options to preserve spontaneous ventilation. Additionally, sedation with awake intubation may prevent the ability to obtain a neurological exam and should be used only as necessary.

10. Topicalize the airway.

This is important to allow the patient to tolerate the intubation with minimal neck movement. Start with lidocaine nebulization. Have the patient gargle and swallow viscous lidocaine solution or spray lidocaine past the tongue.

Consider performing nerve blocks for oral awake flexible bronchoscopic intubation.[8,12,14] All three of the blocks listed below should be performed to ensure adequate topicalization for intubation.

1. Glossopharyngeal nerve block: Inject 2–5 ml 2% lidocaine to the base of the posterior tonsillar pillars bilaterally, *or* place pledgets soaked with viscous 2% lidocaine at the base of posterior tonsillar pillars bilaterally (Figure 20.3).

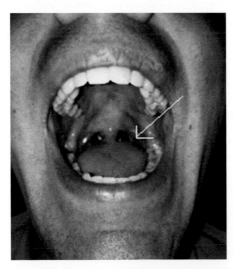

Figure 20.3 Target for glossopharyngeal nerve block at the base of the posterior tonsillar pillars. Left tonsillar pillar is marked by the white arrow. This is the target for the glossopharyngeal nerve block. Photo courtesy of author.

2. Superior laryngeal nerve block: Inject 3–5 ml of 2% lidocaine at the lateral aspect of the greater cornu of the hyoid bone bilaterally, *or* spray 15 ml of viscous 2% lidocaine to the base of the tongue or have patient swallow it, *or* deliver nebulized 4% preservative-free lidocaine.

3. Recurrent laryngeal nerve block: Inject 3–5 ml of 2% lidocaine transtracheally by advancing a small-gauge needle or angiocatheter on a syringe through the cricothyroid membrane until air is aspirated. Caution: The patient will cough.

Topicalization alternatives to performing airway blocks:
- Place an epidural catheter through the side port of the flexible bronchoscope and spray the vocal cords with 3–5 ml 2% lidocaine.
- Deliver nebulized 4% preservative-free lidocaine via facemask.
- For nasal intubation, apply vasoconstrictors and local anesthesia to the nasal passages and dilate the nasal passages with nasal airways.

>> **Tip on Technique:** For the nasal approach, consider 4% cocaine via nasal spray topically to provide local anesthesia and vasoconstriction. Total dose should not exceed 200 mg in adults. Avoid in patients with ischemic heart disease, uncontrolled hypertension, preeclampsia, or pseudocholinesterase deficiency, and in those taking monoamine oxidase inhibitors.[8]

Caution! The maximum dose of lidocaine without epinephrine is 4.5 mg/kg.[9] Calculate the patient's maximum dose in advance.

---

11. Perform awake intubation.

Oral flexible bronchoscopic intubation is often the preferred approach, although the nasal route may have the least amount of neck movement.[18] Consider placing an oral airway to guide the flexible bronchoscope. Ensure the endotracheal tube fits through the oral airway.

Pass the flexible bronchoscope orally past the tongue or nasally to the base of the oropharynx and visualize the cords. Consider passing an epidural catheter through the sampling line of the scope to further topicalize the cords with lidocaine.

Pass the flexible bronchoscope through the vocal cords into the trachea until the carina is visualized, and then advance the endotracheal tube over the scope, visualizing the endotracheal tube in the trachea. Confirm placement of the endotracheal tube with end-tidal carbon dioxide on three consecutive breaths and listening to breath sounds bilaterally.

Caution! Pay attention to hemodynamics during intubation, as coughing or bucking can greatly increase intracranial pressure. Treat hemodynamics with beta blockers (esmolol or labetalol) if needed.

---

12. Transfer of care and decision to extubate.

The decision to extubate postoperatively in patients with cervical spine injury should be made carefully.

Extubation criteria for the intensive care unit include:

- Rapid shallow breathing index (RSBI) <100 (RSBI = respiratory rate/tidal volume (RR/TV) in liters)
- Vital capacity ≥15 ml/kg
- Negative inspiratory force more negative than −20 cm H_2O
- Presence of endotracheal tube cuff leak
- Ability to follow commands
- Ability to manage secretions/protect airway
- Adequate oxygenation (PaO_2:FiO_2 ratio >300)

> **Caution!** Spinal cord edema peaks at 3 to 6 days after injury. Consider postponing extubation until edema is resolved. The need for reintubation after cervical fixation may pose a significant challenge for the intensivist or anesthesiologist.[6,8]

Other Management Considerations

Mask ventilation caused the most displacement of the cervical spine (2.93 mm) in a study by Hauswald et al., followed by oral intubation (1.51 mm), with nasal intubation causing the least displacement (1.20 mm).[19] Therefore, be cautious with mask ventilation while preoxygenating. Narrowing of the space available for the spinal cord can occur with jaw thrust, chin lift, and cricoid pressure, even with the cervical collar in place.[1]

MILS provides better cervical stability but impairs the Cormack-Lehane view. Nevertheless, when MILS is utilized, the incidence of neurologic impairment due to endotracheal intubation is extremely rare.[8] Laryngoscope insertion has been shown to cause minimal movement, but blade elevation results in significant extension of all cervical segments, especially the atlanto-occipital and atlanto-axial joints.[20] The gum elastic bougie can be used with good success.[16,20]

The use of direct laryngoscopy for intubation with cervical spine injury is recommended with MILS, even though there is a decreased Cormack-Lehane view.[8] Videolaryngoscopy has been shown to improve the grade view.[9,10] The technique with the least amount of neck movement is nasal flexible bronchoscopic intubation;[14] however, oral intubation is optimal for prolonged intubation.

References

1. Crosby ET. Airway management in adults after cervical spine trauma. *Anesthesiology*. 2006;104(6):1293–1318.
2. Kwon BK, Tetzalff W, Grauer JN, et al. Pathophysiology and pharmacologic treatment of acute spinal cord injury. *Spine*. 2004;4(4):451–464.
3. Monro-Somerville T, Sim M, Ruddy J, et al. The effect of high-flow nasal cannula oxygen therapy on mortality and intubation rate in acute respiratory failure: a systematic review and meta-analysis. *Crit Care Med*. 2017;45(4):e449–e456.
4. Mataliotakis G, Tsirikos AI. Spinal cord trauma: pathophysiology, classification of spinal cord injury syndromes, treatment principles and controversies. *J Orthop Trauma*. 2016;30(5):440–449.
5. Lee J, Thumbikat P. Pathophysiology, presentation and management of spinal cord injury. *Surgery (Oxford); Orthopaedics II: Spine and Pelvis*. 2015;33(6):238–247.

6. Hadley MN, Walters BC, Grabb PA, et al. Blood pressure management after acute spinal cord injury. *Neurosurgery*. 2002;50(3 Suppl):S58–S62.

7. Bilello JF, Davis JW, Cunningham MA, et al. Cervical spinal cord injury and the need for cardiovascular intervention. *Arch Surg*. 2003;138(10):1127–1129.

8. Barash PG, Cullen BF, Stoelting RK, Cahalan MK, Stock MC, Ortega R. *Clinical Anesthesia*. 7th edition. Philadelphia, PA: Wolters Kluwer Health/Lippincott Williams & Wilkins, 2013; Chapter 27: Airway Management, 789–790; Chapter 36: Anesthesia for Neurosurgery, 1020–1024.

9. Murray M, Harrison B, Mueller J, Rose S, Wass C, Wedel D. *Faust's Anesthesiology Review*. 4th edition. Philadelphia, PA: Elsevier Saunders, 2015; Chapter 117: Toxicity of Local Anesthetic Agents, 272.

10. Hirabayashi Y, Fujita A, Seo N, et al. A comparison of cervical spine movement during laryngoscopy using the Airtraq or Macintosh laryngoscopes. *Anaesthesia*. 2008;63(6):635–640.

11. Nolan JP, Wilson ME. Orotracheal intubation in patients with potential cervical spine injuries. An indication for the gum elastic bougie. *Anaesthesia*. 1993;48(7):630–633.

12. Johnston KD, Rai MR. Conscious sedation for awake fibreoptic intubation: a review of the literature. *Can J Anesth*. 2013;60(6): 584–599.

13. Aziz M. Airway management in neuroanesthesiology. *Anesthesiol Clin*. 2012;30(2): 229–240.

14. Mingo O, Ashpole K, Irving C, Rucklidge M. Remifentanil sedation for awake fiberoptic intubation with limited application of local anesthetic in patient for elective head and neck surgery. *Anaesthesia*. 2008 Oct;63(10):1065–1069.

15. Wendling AL, Tighe PJ, Conrad BP, et al. A comparison of 4 airway devices on cervical spine alignment in cadaver models of global ligamentous instability at c1-2. *Anesth Analg*. 2013;117(1):126–132.

16. Goutcher CM, Lochhead V. Reduction in mouth opening with semi-rigid cervical collars. *Br J Anaesth*. 2005;95(3):344–348.

17. Prasarn ML, Conrad B, Del Rossi G, et al. Motion generated in the unstable cervical spine during the application and removal of cervical immobilization collars. *J Trauma Acute Care Surg*. 2012;72(6):1609–1613.

18. Swain A, Sahu S, Swain BP. Cervical spine movement during intubation. *J Neuroanaesthesiol Crit Care*. 2017;4(Suppl S1):76–80.

19. Hauswald M, Sklar DP, Tandberg D, et al. Cervical spine movement during airway management: cinefluoroscopic appraisal in human cadavers. *Am J Emerg Med*. 1991;9(6):535–538.

20. Austin N, Krishnamoorthy V, Dagal A. Airway management in cervical spine injury. *Int J Crit Illn Inj Sci*. 2014;4(1):50–56.

Chapter 21

Emergent Craniotomy

Nelson N. Algarra and Taylor Johnson

Summary Page

Symptoms:

- Altered mental status
- Posturing
- Elevated intracranial pressure
- Bradycardia
- Hypertension
- Loss of consciousness with or without a period of lucidity
- Hemiparesis
- Pupillary changes

Differential Diagnosis:

- Traumatic brain injury
- Subarachnoid hemorrhage
- Cerebral vascular accident
- Concussion
- Meningitis/encephalitis
- Nonconvulsive status epilepticus/ postictal state
- Wernicke's encephalopathy
- Reaction syndromes (psychiatric)
- Delirium
- Alcohol intoxication
- Sedatives/hypnotics
- Hepatic encephalopathy
- Hypoglycemia

Introduction

Patients present for emergency craniotomy for a variety of reasons: evacuation of blood from a bleeding aneurysm, arteriovenous malformation, stroke or traumatic brain injury (TBI), or treatment of malignant edema due to tumor or sequelae of TBI. Patients pose a special challenge as they often have comorbid conditions that require special attention. You can expect them to have a full stomach, possible cervical spine injury, increased intracranial pressure (ICP), multiorgan trauma, or shock. Patients usually have exhausted the compliance in the cranial vault and the increased pressure compromises vital central nervous system (CNS) functions. Physiologic adaptations to intracranial hypertension help to maintain supplies of oxygen, substrate, and blood flow to vital areas of the CNS. The preparation and conduction of proper anesthetic aim to maintain appropriate cerebral perfusion pressure (CPP), maximize exposure for the surgeon, and provide for a neurological examination promptly after surgery.

The most common causes for emergent craniotomy include TBI with severe edema, intracranial bleed with blood accumulation, skull fractures, or malignant increases in ICP refractory to treatment (Figure 21.1). The primary mode of diagnosis includes neurological examination and emergent noncontrast computed tomography.

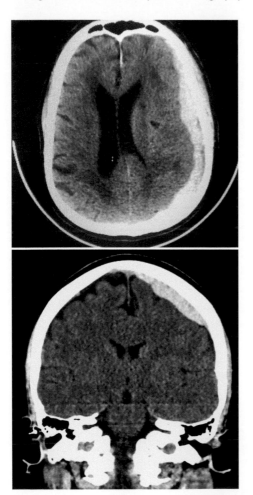

Figure 21.1 Noncontrast computed tomography images of the head showing an acute subdural hematoma along the left frontal and parietal regions. Courtesy of the author.

Management

Many large facilities have subspecialty trained neuroanesthesiologists who manage neurosurgical cases. Emergent craniotomies are managed by on-call staff familiar with the management of emergency craniotomies in most places.

Step by Step

1. Prepare the room prior to patient arrival.

Prepare standard American Society for Anesthesiologists (ASA) monitors. Prepare for arterial line placement and indwelling urinary catheter, and set up IV lines for volume and infusion of vasopressors.

Review the most recent lab results including arterial blood gas (ABG), sodium, basic metabolic panel, complete blood count, and osmolarity.

Note: Indications for arterial line placement include repeated ABG measurements, partial pressure of carbon dioxide ($PaCO_2$) management, glucose management, and osmolarity calculation. Indications for an indwelling urinary catheter include monitoring urinary output, especially with administration of dehydration agents such as mannitol, and monitoring body temperature.

2. Perform a neurologic assessment.

Evaluate the patient and assess for current or prior motor, sensory, or speech deficits. If unable to evaluate the patient in person, ask for a report from the receiving unit, paramedics, emergency department staff, or surgeon. It is important that you know the baseline neurological status.

Assess for signs and symptoms of increased ICP such as headache, nausea, vomiting, papilledema, focal neurological deficits, altered consciousness, or vital signs that indicate increased ICP such as bradycardia and hypertension.

>>Tip on Technique: Inspect all lines for patency and ease of access as the arms may be tucked and away from you during the procedure. Assess for presence of an external ventricular drain (EVD) and whether it is open or closed. Always monitor ICP when possible.

3. Discuss the plan for management with the surgical team.

Note: This is a critical step in patient management that should always be performed.

Discuss medication management and hemodynamic targets.
Discussion should include, but not be limited to, the following:
- Antiepileptic medications to be given
- Potential interventions to control ICP
- If steroids should be given
- Dosing and timing of antibiotics
- CPP and mean arterial pressure (MAP) goals
- $PaCO_2$ target

Note: Establishing a $PaCO_2$ target with the surgical team is a crucial step. $EtCO_2$ is not an adequate target as ventilation will affect the individual patient gradient and $EtCO_2$ may not be equivalent to $PaCO_2$.

Note: See steps 6 and 7 for medication dosing and specific hemodynamic targets.

4. **Induce anesthesia and secure the airway.**

Preoxygenate the patient to avoid hypoxemia.

> **Caution!** Hypoxemia is associated with increased mortality and poor neurologic outcome in patients with TBI.

Induce anesthesia and perform intubation. Place a bite block since the head will not be accessible during the procedure.

The following medications can be used for induction:

- Fentanyl 1–5 mcg/kg IV
- Propofol 1–2.5 mg/kg IV
- Etomidate 0.2–0.6 mg/kg IV
- Succinylcholine 1–2 mg/kg IV
- Rocuronium 0.6–1.2 mg/kg IV
- Esmolol 0.5–2 mg/kg IV

> **WARNING!!** Direct laryngoscopy and intubation are very stimulating. Be sure to ensure an adequate depth of anesthesia prior to intubation.

> **Caution!** Rapid induction and intubation are paramount. While the actual induction technique can vary, the goal should be to avoid increasing ICP or compromising cerebral blood flow from inadequate anesthetic depth. Both hypertension and hypotension are deleterious. Securing the airway is paramount, and the transient increase in ICP from succinylcholine, if used, can be compensated by rapid hyperventilation following a gentle laryngoscopy.

> **WARNING!!** A patient with a TBI will usually have a cervical collar because concomitant cervical injuries are likely. In this case, remove the front of the collar to allow mouth opening and chin displacement. An assistant should maintain manual in-line stabilization during laryngoscopy and intubation. Be prepared to have rescue airway equipment ready for use. (See Chapter 20 on management of the unstable cervical spine for more details.)

Maintain PaO_2 >100 mmHg and avoid desaturation.

5. **Position the patient for surgery and place additional lines.**

The patient's head will be placed in the Mayfield head holder and turned to one side.

Turn the patient's body as a unit, aligning the shoulders and maintaining the head in neutral position with the body. Ensure sufficient shoulder, hip, and knee support. Refer to Figure 21.2 for positioning options.

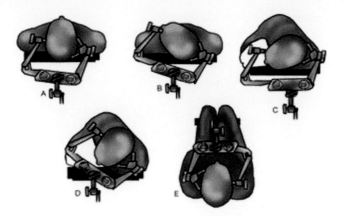

Figure 21.2 Five images of the head pinned in a Mayfield clamp in comparison to the body. A: Supine with head in neutral position, pinned for a unilateral or bilateral frontal craniotomy. B: Supine with head in turned position, pinned for a frontotemporal craniotomy. C: Lateral position, pinned for a suboccipital craniotomy. D: Lateral position, pinned for a more midline suboccipital craniotomy. E: Semi-sitting position, pinned for midline suboccipital craniotomy. With permission from Sekhar, L. *Atlas of Neurosurgical Techniques: Brain*, 1st ed., Chapter 1. Thieme, 2006.

Caution! Positioning is critical to assist in proper jugular venous drainage and reduction of ICP. Lateral or prone position may be required for some procedures.

>> **Tip on Technique:** Anticipate hemodynamic changes, such as an increased heart rate and blood pressure, with Mayfield pin placement. Consider managing hemodynamic response by deepening inhalational agent, giving an IV bolus of propofol, administering IV narcotics (fentanyl, hydromorphone, or remifentanil), and/or giving esmolol 0.5 mg/kg IV.

Ensure that an arm can be accessed even after surgical draping to place invasive monitors and obtain additional intravenous access. Obtain at least two large-bore peripheral intravenous lines.

Caution! Do not delay surgery to place an arterial line. Place the transducer at the level of the external auditory meatus to best estimate CPP.

Caution! While a central line is a valuable monitor and provides access to the central circulation, placement is not without risk and technically can be difficult and time consuming in a trauma patient. If placed, a femoral line is preferred as the patient cannot be placed in the Trendelenburg position, and the head cannot be turned for placement.

If the patient has an EVD, level it at the external auditory meatus. Confirm with the neurosurgical team the settings for draining cerebrospinal fluid and make sure you are familiar with the EVD system.

6. Administer critical medications.

Give antibiotics, anticonvulsants, and dehydrating agents, if indicated. Anticonvulsants include:[1]

- Midazolam 2–4 mg IV bolus, may repeat in 5 minutes
- Diazepam 10–20 mg IV, no faster than 5 mg/min
- Lorazepam 4 mg IV bolus, may repeat in 5 minutes
- Pentobarbital 20 mg/kg IV
- Valproate 20–30 mg/kg IV, infusion rate 6 mg/kg/min
- Phenytoin 15–20 mg/kg IV, rate no faster than 50 mg/min
- Levetiracetam 20–30 mg/kg IV bolus, max dose 2 g

Dehydrating agents to reduce ICP include:[2]

- Mannitol 20% or 25% 0.5–1.5g/kg initial IV bolus
- 3% hypertonic saline (HTS) 150–250 mL IV bolus
- 7.5% HTS 4 ml/kg IV (max 250 ml)
- 23.4% HTS 30 ml IV bolus

> **WARNING!!** Rapid infusion of phenytoin increases the risk of cardiovascular complications. It is best to infuse <50 mg/min. Phenytoin blocks voltage-gated sodium channels, which shortens cardiac action potentials and increases the refractory period in between. This can lead to dysrhythmias, sinoatrial/atrioventricular nodal blockade, hypotension, and even cardiac arrest if administered too quickly.

7. Maintain hemodynamic targets.

Obtain a baseline ABG measurement. Ensure that there is adequate cerebral perfusion by monitoring and maintaining mean arterial blood pressure and ICP.

Guidelines for blood pressure and ICP management as recommended by the 2018 Brain Trauma Foundation for patient with a TBI include:[3]

- Maintain systolic blood pressure (SBP) >100 mmHg for patients 50–69 years of age
- Maintain SBP >110 mmHg for patients 15–49 and above 70 years of age
- Follow ICP and actively treat values higher than 22 mmHg

>> **Tip on Technique:** Obtain a baseline ABG in every patient and correlate the $PaCO_2$ to the $EtCO_2$. In stable patients, obtain ABG measurements at least every 2 hours. In bleeding patients, a full coagulation profile and complete blood count should be sent at the beginning of the surgery and then hourly. If there is massive bleeding, inform the blood bank and begin massive transfusion protocols (see Chapter 16 for more details on massive transfusion).

Note: Cerebral Perfusion Pressure (CPP) = Mean Arterial Pressure (MAP) – Intracranial Pressure (ICP). If the brain is not being perfused, then cerebral ischemia can occur. This may result from the MAP being too low or the ICP being too high.

> **Caution!** Allowing $PaCO_2$ in a hyperventilated patient to abruptly return to normal may cause a rebound increase in CBF and ICP.

8. **Decrease ICP to maintain CPP.**

   >> **Tip on Technique:** To decrease ICP, set the EVD to drain at the level of the external auditory meatus. Administer dehydration agents that remove water from the brain such as mannitol or hypertonic saline (see step 6). Promote venous return by positioning the head in a neutral position with the head of the bed at a 30-degree angle. To temporarily reduce ICP, hyperventilate the patient. Adjust ventilator settings based on $PaCO_2$ between 30 and 35 mmHg.

9. **Protect the brain by decreasing the cerebral metabolic rate of oxygen ($CMRO_2$)**
   All of the following medications can reduce $CMRO_2$:[4]
   - Propofol 1 mg/kg IV bolus followed by infusion 10–50 mg/kg/min IV
   - Dexmedetomidine[5] 1 mcg/kg over 10 minutes then 0.4 mcg/kg/hr IV
   - Etomidate[6] 0.2–0.6 mg/kg IV
   - Pentobarbital 20 mg/kg IV may be used for refractory increases in ICP to decrease $CMRO_2$ by burst suppression of electroencephalogram
   - Fentanyl 1–5 mcg/kg IV
   - Sufentanil 1–5 mcg/kg IV followed by infusion 0.1–0.5 mcg/kg/hr IV
   - Remifentanil 0.5–1 mcg/kg IV followed by infusion 0.05–0.5 mcg/kg/min IV
   - Sevoflurane 2–3% inhaled
   - Isoflurane 0.75–1.2% inhaled
   - Vecuronium 0.1 mg/kg or rocuronium 0.1 mg/kg IV bolus stops muscle activity

10. **Anticipate critical parts of surgery.**
    There can be significant stimulation and blood loss with skin incision and periosteal elevation. At this time, mannitol and adjustment for mild hyperventilation may be required.
    At the removal of the bone flap there is an increased risk of a venous air embolism as the operative site is above the level of the heart.

    >> **Tip on Technique:** Prior to opening the dura, discuss the need for brain relaxation with the neurosurgical team to improve surgical exposure in the setting of swelling.

    Consider administration of the following to improve brain relaxation:
    - Dehydrating agents (see Step 6)
    - Furosemide 10–20 mg IV
    - Dexamethasone 10 mg IV
    - Hyperventilation to $PaCO_2$ 30–35 mmHg
    - Elevating the head of the bed to promote venous drainage

11. **Prepare the patient for extubation.**
    The goal is emergence from anesthesia smoothly with minimal coughing.
    The risk of postoperative seizures should be discussed with the surgical team.

WARNING!!   Coughing may worsen intracranial hemorrhage or cerebral edema.

>> **Tip on Technique:** Remifentanil infusion (0.05–0.5 mcg/kg/min IV) is an ideal maintenance/emergence medication as it does not increase ICP, provides hemodynamic protection, and allows for a predictable wake-up and neurologic examination.

> **Caution!** Do not attempt to wake up the patient while the patient's head is positioned in the Mayfield head holder. If the patient moves while in pins, this could lead to neck or cranial injuries as well as lacerations to the scalp. Delay emergence and extubation until the Mayfield pins are removed.

Extubation should be based on standard extubation criteria and the patient should be hemodynamically stable:

- Adequate oxygenation: SpO_2 >92%
- Adequate ventilation: Vt >5 mL/kg, respiratory rate 8–24 breaths per minute, $EtCO_2$ <50 mmHg, $PaCO_2$ <60 mmHg
- Full reversal of muscle relaxation and demonstrating full strength: sustained tetany, sustained 5-second head lift or hand grasp
- Neurologically intact: follows verbal commands, intact cough/gag reflex
- Normothermia
- Consider airway edema, aspiration risk, acid-base status

‼ Potential Complication: Patients with delayed awakening and/or unable to elicit a postoperative neurological exam may need to go directly to computed tomography to rule out bleeding, stroke, or hydrocephalus. Consider also reversal of narcotic agents to rule out narcotic overdosing as a cause of delayed emergence.

Other Management Considerations

There is an absolute contraindication for intranasal probes or nasotracheal tubes in head trauma patients with a suspected or known basilar skull fracture.

Check the fingerstick blood glucose on all patients even if they are not known diabetics; the sympathetic response will increase glucose levels and the steroids will further exacerbate hyperglycemia. Maintain a serum glucose <180 gm/dl.

Many TBI patients will develop a Takotsubo cardiomyopathy–like state (signs of heart failure, ventricular arrhythmias, severe mitral regurgitation, left ventricular outflow obstruction). If required, use norepinephrine as a first-line vasopressor.

Most patients will present with hypertension and tachycardia mediated by an intense sympathetic response. Upon induction of anesthesia or when the dura is open, expect blood pressure and heart rate to decrease. The brain is very susceptible to secondary insults from cerebral or systemic hypotension and decreased oxygen availability in at-risk areas in the brain.

Maintain normothermia, normal osmolality, and normal acid-base balance.

Hypothermia can decrease $CMRO_2$ and have a protective effect on the brain. However, the risk of pulmonary sequela and coagulopathy may outweigh any benefits. The Brain Trauma Foundation and the American Foundation of Neurological Surgeons issued only a level III recommendation for the use of hypothermia in adults with TBI.[3,7]

Further Reading

Ayrian, E., Kaye, A. D., Varner, C. L., Guerra, C., Vadivelu, N., Urman, R. D., et al. (2015). Effects of anesthetic management on early postoperative recovery, hemodynamics and pain after supratentorial craniotomy. *Journal of Clinical Medicine Research*, 7(10), 731.

Honeybul, S., & Ho, K. M. (2011). Long-term complications of decompressive craniectomy for head injury. *Journal of Neurotrauma*, 28(6), 929–935.

Aarabi, B., Hesdorffer, D. C., Ahn, E. S., Aresco, C., Scalea, T. M., & Eisenberg, H. M. (2006). Outcome following decompressive craniectomy for malignant swelling due to severe head injury. *Journal of Neurosurgery*, *104*(4), 469–479.

References

1. Yasiry, Z., & Shorvon, S. D. (2014). The relative effectiveness of five antiepileptic drugs in treatment of benzodiazepine-resistant convulsive status epilepticus: a meta-analysis of published studies. *Seizure*, *23*(3), 167–174.
2. Strandvik, G. F. (2009). Hypertonic saline in critical care: a review of the literature and guidelines for use in hypotensive states and raised intracranial pressure. *Anaesthesia*, *64*, 990–1003.
3. Brain Trauma Foundation Guidelines: https://braintrauma.org/guidelines/guidelines-for-the-management-of-severe-tbi-4th-ed#//:guidelines
4. Kaisti, K. K., Långsjö, J. W., Aalto, S., Oikonen, V., Sipilä, H., Teräs, M., et al. (2003). Effects of sevoflurane, propofol, and adjunct nitrous oxide on regional cerebral blood flow, oxygen consumption, and blood volume in humans. *Anesthesiology: The Journal of the American Society of Anesthesiologists*, *99*(3), 603–613.
5. Drummond, J. C., Dao, A. V., Roth, D. M., Cheng, C. R., Atwater, B. I., Minokadeh, A., et al. (2008). Effect of dexmedetomidine on cerebral blood flow velocity, cerebral metabolic rate, and carbon dioxide response in normal humans. *Anesthesiology: The Journal of the American Society of Anesthesiologists*, *108*(2), 225–232.
6. Renou, A. M., Vernhiet, J., Macrez, P., Constant, P., Billeerey, J., Khadaroo, M. Y., & Caille, J. M. (1978). Cerebral blood flow and metabolism during etomidate anaesthesia in man. *BJA: British Journal of Anaesthesia*, *50*(10), 1047–1051.
7. Peterson, K., Carson, S., & Carney, N. (2008). Hypothermia treatment for traumatic brain injury: a systematic review and meta-analysis. *Journal of Neurotrauma*, *25*(1), 62–71.

Chapter 22

Perioperative Complications of Neuraxial Anesthesia

Richa Wardhan and Adejuyigbe Olusegun Adaralegbe

Summary Page

Signs/Symptoms:

High/Total Spinal:

- Nausea
- Hypotension
- Bradycardia
- Cardiac arrest
- Respiratory insufficiency
- Anxiety
- Weakness
- Loss of consciousness

Spinal/Epidural Hematoma:

- Neck or back pain
- Radicular paresthesia
- Sudden or gradual paralysis

Differential Diagnosis:

High/Total Spinal:

- Systemic toxicity
- Concurrent administration of sedatives
- Seizure disorder
- Cerebrovascular accident
- Cardiac arrest from other causes
- Hypoglycemia
- Embolism

Spinal/Epidural Hematoma:

- Cerebral infarction
- Acute coronary syndrome
- Brown Sequard syndrome
- Subdural placement of local anesthetic in case of thoracic epidural

Introduction

Spinal and epidural anesthesia is commonly referred to as neuraxial anesthesia. Neuraxial anesthesia is a routinely performed anesthetic procedure for a variety of surgical procedures. There are numerous advantages of neuraxial anesthesia including decreased bleeding, lower risk of deep vein thrombosis, decreased risk of nausea and vomiting, and minimal risk of postoperative cognitive dysfunction. However, neuraxial anesthesia can be associated with some major and minor complications. The major complications are high/total spinal, systemic toxicity, and epidural hematoma. High/total spinal can lead to cardiac arrest and death, while epidural hematoma can result in debilitating paraplegia.

It is important to note that high or total spinal can develop regardless of the technique, method of administration, or type of local anesthetic.[1,2]

Common risk factors for this complication include:

- High dose of local anesthetic administered via unrecognized intrathecal administration in a planned epidural or redosing of a subclinical epidural block.
- Spinal block placed at unintended higher lumbar levels (L1–2 or higher).
- Faster rate of administration of medication in the neuroaxis without careful aspiration while injecting. Faster injection utilizes higher injection pressure, which leads to erratic spread of the medication.
- Patient position during and after injection of local anesthetic.[3,4] A steep Trendelenburg position will increase the incidence of high/total spinal especially in a patient receiving spinal anesthetic due to the medication traveling rapidly in the cerebrospinal fluid.
- Pregnancy modifies the spread of local anesthetics injected in the neuroaxis. In pregnant patients, the volume of local anesthetic administered must be reduced by at least 30%.

The diagnosis and management of a high/total spinal, systemic toxicity, and epidural hematoma will be discussed separately. Systemic toxicity is also covered in more detail in Chapter 25.

High Spinal/Total Spinal Anesthesia

Treatment

A high spinal is defined as the spread of local anesthetic above the T4 level and is considered a total spinal when loss of consciousness with apnea and/or aphonia occurs. When a high or total spinal occurs, apnea can also occur without loss of consciousness. Expect respiratory insufficiency to follow once the patient starts developing symptoms of cervical blockade including upper extremity weakness and paresthesia.

Step by Step

1. Evaluate the patient and assess for total spinal anesthesia.

> **WARNING!!** If the patient is hemodynamically unstable, call a code and start advanced cardiac life support (ACLS) (step 3).

Assess vital signs and airway patency and check level of spinal blockade. Shoulder weakness could signal impending weakness of the diaphragm, resulting in difficulty breathing and hypoxemia.[3] Signs and symptoms of a high spinal include nausea and vomiting, hypotension, bradycardia, mydriasis, and dysarthria if cranial nerves are involved.

>> **Tip on Technique:** Recognize early signs and symptoms (nausea, dyspnea, hypoventilation, inability to raise voice, anxiety, etc.) and check vitals before assessing for level of spinal blockade.

Cranial nerve involvement in a total spinal may resemble but should not be confused with a stroke. Cranial nerve involvement may be evidenced by symptoms like mydriasis and dysarthria.[4,5] These are expected to resolve as the spinal anesthetic wears off.

> **WARNING!!** During procedures under sedation or general anesthesia, early signs may be more difficult to assess. Apnea or cardiac arrest may be the first presenting signs. Tinnitus, lingual anesthesia, and perioral paresthesia are common early signs of systemic toxicity.

> **Caution!** Loss of consciousness can be the first sign of total spinal.[5]

2. **Manage ventilation and hemodynamics.**

Increase inhaled O_2 to 100%. Call for help and pause the procedure. Call a code if appropriate.

If the patient is bradycardic, give atropine to a maximum total dose of 3 mg but restrict the total dose to 0.03–0.04 mg/kg in patients with ischemic heart disease. If the patient is hypotensive, give ephedrine 5–10 mg IV or phenylephrine 100 mcg IV and titrate to effect. Discontinue anesthetic agents, if appropriate.

> **WARNING!!** If the patient is hemodynamically unstable, call a code and start ACLS (step 3).

3. **Initiate ACLS if the patient is in cardiac arrest.**

Initiate cardiopulmonary resuscitation immediately if the patient is in cardiac arrest regardless of cause.

4. **Manage the airway if needed.**

> **Caution!** Cardiac arrest warrants immediate intubation.

>> **Tip on Technique:** A high/total spinal may present with apnea without cardiac collapse or loss of consciousness. If a high spinal or total spinal is present with acute respiratory insufficiency, intubate immediately as a high spinal can progress to a total spinal with loss of consciousness and apnea very quickly.

> **Caution!** If the patient is unconscious and severely hypotensive (total spinal), then emergent intubation is necessary without medications. Loss of consciousness from a total spinal is usually accompanied by obtundation of most reflexes including gag reflexes.

If the patient is awake but with respiratory insufficiency, medications will be required to facilitate placement of an endotracheal tube. Induce anesthesia with propofol 2 mg/kg IV bolus and succinylcholine 1 mg/kg IV.

If a high spinal is present without acute respiratory insufficiency, provide supplemental oxygen via nasal cannula or facemask and consider cautious sedation with midazolam 0.1–0.2 mg/kg IV.

5. Manage seizures, if present.

If seizures are present with airway compromise, give a loading dose of midazolam 0.2 mg/kg IV and then induce anesthesia with propofol 2 mg/kg IV bolus and succinylcholine 1 mg/kg IV and intubate the patient.

If seizures are present without airway compromise, give a loading dose of midazolam 0.2 mg/kg IV. A propofol 0.25–0.5 mg/kg IV bolus can be used if midazolam is not immediately available.

6. If a high spinal is present but the patient is hemodynamically stable, provide supportive care.

Support hemodynamics if needed and provide supportive care. For bradycardia, give atropine up to a maximum total dose of 3 mg IV but restrict total dose to 0.03–0.04 mg/kg in patients with ischemic heart disease. For hypotension give ephedrine 5–10 mg IV or phenylephrine 100 mcg IV. For nausea and vomiting give ondansetron 4–8 mg IV.

Patients may have difficulty coughing or taking deep breaths due to the high spinal level of the block. Reassure the patient that their condition is temporary and symptoms will lessen when the neuraxial block starts to recede. Provide supplemental oxygen via nasal cannula or facemask as needed. Consider careful administration of midazolam 0.2 mg/kg IV to allay anxiety.

Caution! Many of the symptoms seen with high spinal can also be seen with an evolving cerebrovascular event. If a stroke is suspected, send the patient emergently for a computed tomography (CT) scan and stroke workup.

Other Management Considerations

How to prevent high spinal/total spinal during placement of spinal anesthesia:

- Choose the appropriate local anesthetic dose per patient's height and weight.
- Choose the appropriate spinal level for placement of the neuraxial block.
- Ensure that the operating room table is in neutral position prior to positioning the patient.
- Avoid fast injection through the syringe.

>> **Tip on Technique:** The spinal cord ends at L1–2. It is safe to place a spinal anesthetic past that level. An epidural can be placed anywhere along the lumbar and thoracic spine; however, local anesthetic dose should be modified accordingly. In the lumbar spinal location, the epidural can be dosed in aliquots of 5 ml at a time to a maximum of 15–20 ml of local anesthetic depending on the type, concentration, and dose of the local anesthetic. The lower thoracic epidural level (T8–12) can be similarly loaded with 10–15 ml of local anesthetic. At high thoracic levels (T7 and higher), dosing should be made even more carefully since the block of the cardioaccelerator fibers arising from T1–4 control heart rate and contractility, and their absence can lead to excessive vagal reflexes, which can produce sinus arrest.

Management of Local Anesthetic Toxicity (Also See Chapter 25 on Local Anesthetic Systemic Toxicity)

Treatment

Systemic toxicity occurs with intravascular administration of local anesthetics. Symptoms can resemble those of a high/total spinal with cardiovascular collapse, loss of consciousness, and seizure. It is more likely with epidural or caudal blockade than with spinal blockade, due to the larger doses of local anesthetics used in those blocks.

Consider intralipid emulsion even at the slightest suspicion for local anesthetic toxicity (see Chapter 25 for more details of the steps listed below on how to manage local anesthetic systemic toxicity (LAST)).

>> **Tip on Technique**: LAST is more common with epidural blocks. LAST is less common with spinal blocks since the amount of local anesthetic placed in the intrathecal space is very small.

Note: Local anesthetic toxicity usually unfolds in two stages: an excitatory initial phase with symptoms of numbness of the face or tongue, metallic taste, and tinnitus, followed by confusion or agitation and generalized seizures. These symptoms may then lead to depression with coma and respiratory depression.

Caution! Patients with metabolic acidosis are at higher risk for neurological complications of local anesthetic toxicity even if the dose is adequate.

Step by Step

1. **Call for help and stop administration of the local anesthetic.**

2. **If the patient is in cardiovascular collapse, call a code and begin ACLS.**

3. **Confirm adequate ventilation and oxygenation.**

   Increase inhaled O_2 to 100%. Call for help and pause the procedure. Call a code if appropriate.

4. **Treat seizures, if present.**

   If seizures are present with airway compromise, give a loading dose of midazolam 0.2 mg/kg IV and then induce anesthesia with propofol 2 mg/kg IV bolus and succinylcholine 1 mg/kg IV and intubate the patient.

   If seizures are present without airway compromise, give a loading dose of midazolam 0.2 mg/kg IV. A propofol 0.25–0.5 mg/kg IV bolus can be used if midazolam is not immediately available.

5. **Start lipid emulsion therapy as soon as possible.**

   Give lipid emulsion (Intralipid) 20% 1.5 ml/kg as an IV bolus followed by 25 ml/kg/min until cardiac arrhythmias abate. Repeat bolus dosing for persistent cardiac collapse.

Diagnosis and Management of Spinal/Epidural Hematoma

Epidural hematoma (Figure 22.1) is a rare but potentially devastating complication of neuraxial anesthesia with an incidence, according to a recent 10-year closed claims analysis, of 1:775,000.[6,7]

Risk factors include female gender, advanced age, traumatic and multiple attempts, vascular malformations, anticoagulation therapy, and hypertension.[8]

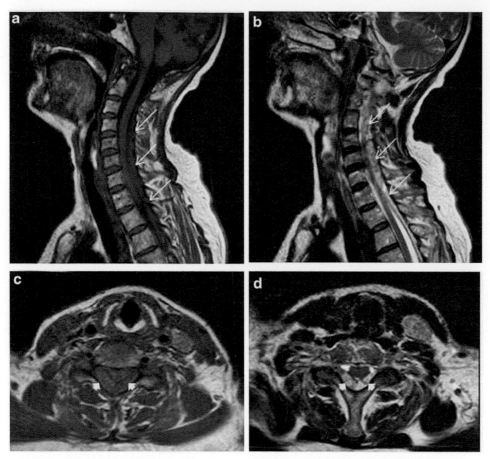

Figure 22.1 MRI findings of epidural hematoma in the setting of a previously unknown vascular malformation. A: T1-weighted sagittal image showing an intermediate signaling mass, corresponding to an epidural hematoma (arrows). B: T2-weighted image showing a hyperintensive signaling mass depicting an abnormal clustering of vessels corresponding to a vascular malformation (arrows) and the hematoma. C and D: T1- and T2-weighted axial images of the upper cervical spine showing the epidural hematoma (arrows) compressing posteriorly the spinal cord toward the vertebral bodies. Reprinted by permission from Springer Nature: *Spinal Cord*, Delayed spinal epidural hematoma following spinal anesthesia, far from needle puncture site, Makris A, Gkliatis E, Diakomi M, Karmaniolou I, Mela A, 52 Suppl 1:S14–16, Copyright 2014.

Treatment

Step by Step

1. Diagnose the presence of a spinal/epidural hematoma.

Spinal/epidural hematoma can present as percussion tenderness in the back, radicular pain, lower motor paresis/loss of motor function in the extremities, or cauda equina syndrome. Compression of the L5–S1 nerve root bundle by an epidural hematoma can lead to loss of bowel and bladder control, numbness around the anus, and low back pain.

2. Discontinue the neuraxial infusion.

> **WARNING!!** DO NOT remove the neuraxial catheter.

3. Evaluate the patient's neurological status.

Perform a complete neurologic exam and assess Glasgow Coma Score.

4. Call for a neurosurgery consult emergently and send for a CT scan of the thoracic and lumbar spine.

If the CT scan shows an epidural hematoma, the patient may need surgical decompression versus conservative therapy with steroids. Surgical treatment involves taking the patient to the operating room for immediate decompression.

> **Caution!** Time is of the essence, since within 12 hours after first symptoms, 88% of cases have good or very good results from surgical decompression. After 24 hours, only 40% have complete recovery, although in all cases surgery must be attempted, since complete recovery is also possible after 48 hours.

>> **Tip on Technique:** Magnetic resonance imaging (MRI) is more specific than CT for epidural hematoma, but an epidural catheter may not be MRI safe.

Other Management Considerations

Certain patients are at higher risk of developing epidural hematoma, such as those with HELLP syndrome (hemolysis, elevated liver enzymes, and low platelets, seen in pregnancy), obvious spinal deformity, or paresthesias on administration of local anesthetic in the epidural or spinal space.[6]

How to avoid a spinal or epidural hematoma from neuraxial anesthesia:

- Avoid placement in patients on anticoagulants or a disease process that may affect coagulation.
- Avoid multiple attempts during placement.

>> **Tip on Technique:** Optimize the position (sitting or lateral) well before starting the procedure. This will increase the rate of successful placement while avoiding multiple needle passes. A neuraxial block can be placed in sitting or lateral decubitus position depending on the patient's comfort level and safety. If the patient is pregnant, the left decubitus position can help improve preload.

>> **Tip on Technique:** After placing a neuraxial block, placing the patient in reverse Trendelenburg may help slow ascension of the spinal block. On the other hand, Trendelenburg position may cause the spinal block to spread higher, leading to more hypotension.

References

1. Foster LA, Deutz CK, Hutchins JL, Allen JA. Total spinal and brainstem anesthesia as complication of paravertebral ropivacaine administration. *Neurol Clin Pract*. 2017;7(5):430–432.

2. Beyaz SG, Özocak H, Ergönenç T, Erdem AF, Palabıyık O. Total spinal block after thoracic paravertebral block. *Turk J Anaesthesiol Reanim*. 2014;42(1):43–45.

3. Poole M. Management of high regional block in obstetrics. *Update in Anaesthesia*. 2009;25(2): 55–59. https://www.e-safe-anaesthesia.org/e_library/13/High_regional_block_in_obstetrics_Update_2009.pdf

4. Newman B. Complete spinal block following spinal anaesthesia. Anaesthesia Tutorial of the Week 180 24th May 2010. *World Federation of Societies of Anaesthesiologist*. https://resources.wfsahq.org/atotw/complete-spinal-block-following-spinal-anaesthesia/

5. Chan YK, Gopinathan R, Rajendram R. Loss of consciousness following spinal anaesthesia for Caesarean section. *BJA*. 2000;85(3):474–476.

6. Maddali P, Walker B, Fisahn C, et al. Subdural thoracolumbar spine hematoma after spinal anesthesia: a rare occurrence and literature review of spinal hematomas after spinal anesthesia. *Cureus*. 2017;9(2):e1032.

7. Makris A, Gkliatis E, Diakomi M, Karmaniolou I, Mela A. Delayed spinal epidural hematoma following spinal anesthesia, far from needle puncture site. *Spinal Cord*. 2014;52(Suppl 1):S14–S16.

8. Kreppel D, Antoniadis G, Seeling W. Spinal hematoma: a literature survey with meta-analysis of 613 patients. *Neurosurg Rev*. 2003;26(1):1–49.

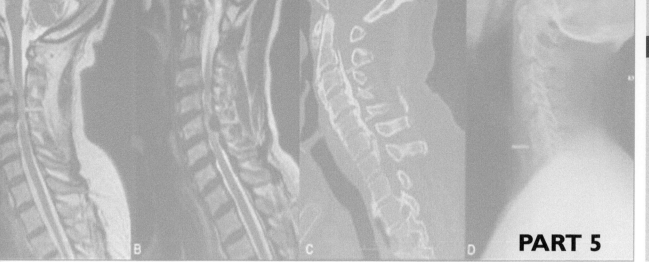

PART 5

ALLERGIC REACTION, TOXICITY

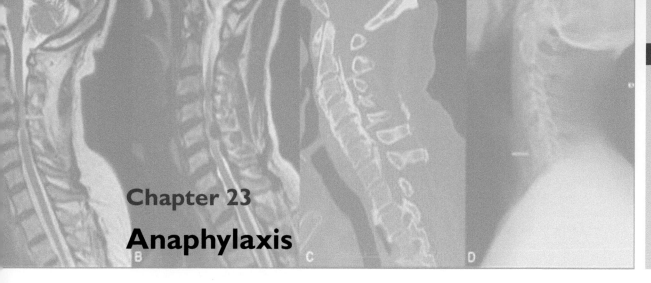

Chapter 23

Anaphylaxis

Richa Sutaria and Cosmin Guta

Summary Page

Symptoms:
- Rash (hives/urticaria)
- Hypotension
- Tachycardia
- Bronchospasm/wheezing
- Hypoxia/tachypnea
- Mucosal membrane swelling
- Cardiac arrest

Differential Diagnosis:
- Septic shock
- Myocardial ischemia
- Bronchospasm
- Transfusion reaction
- Tension pneumothorax
- Pulmonary embolism
- Venous air embolism/fat embolism/amniotic fluid embolism

Introduction

Anaphylaxis is a life-threatening, type 1 hypersensitivity reaction that occurs with reexposure to an antigen, eliciting an IgE-mediated response, which triggers a widespread mediator release of mast cells and basophils (Figure 23.1). The top causative agents of anaphylaxis during the perioperative period are neuromuscular blockers, antibiotics, and latex.[1,2] However, with the increased use of sugammadex, the overall incidence of anaphylaxis in patients under general anesthesia has been reported to be increased by one-third.[3–5] Symptoms can progress rapidly and involve multiple organ systems. During the perioperative period, anaphylaxis can be more severe with higher mortality rates as patients are unable to report their symptoms. For many cases, the initial detection of anaphylaxis occurs with severe airway obstruction and/or cardio-vascular collapse. The symptoms of anaphylaxis can be more difficult to recognize in sedated or anesthetized patients, requiring vigilant oversight by the anesthetic provider. Prompt recognition of these symptoms and initiating treatment of anaphylaxis are key as clinical deterioration can occur rapidly. It is of utmost importance to initiate early cardiopulmonary resuscitation with epinephrine administration and fluid resuscitation. Obtaining serum tryptase levels in a timely fashion can confirm the diagnosis.

Certain patient populations are at increased risk of anaphylaxis: patients with a history of drug or food allergies; multiple past surgeries/procedures; other allergic conditions like asthma, eczema, or hay fever; hereditary angioedema; or mast cell disorders.

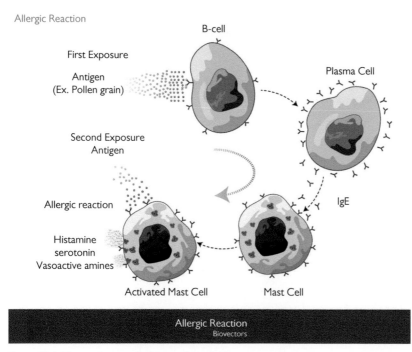

Allergic Reaction

B-cell

First Exposure

Antigen
(Ex. Pollen grain)

Plasma Cell

Second Exposure
Antigen

Allergic reaction

IgE

Histamine
serotonin
Vasoactive amines

Activated Mast Cell

Mast Cell

Allergic Reaction
Biovectors

Figure 23.1 The mechanism of allergy and anaphylaxis.

Treatment

For proper anaphylactic management, it is key to recognize the symptoms early. Some symptoms may be more difficult to detect in patients undergoing general anesthesia. In patients under general anesthesia, symptoms such as bronchospasm and hemodynamic instability may present as the first signs and can have a variety of causes in addition to anaphylaxis, although many of the treatments will be the same.

For severe anaphylaxis, follow the steps in order below. For patients with minor symptoms, it may be appropriate to skip to step 6 or 7.

Step by Step

1. Identify anaphylaxis.

If anaphylaxis is identified, immediately alert the team.

The initial presenting symptoms may differ depending on the level of anesthesia the patient is receiving.

Patients who are conscious or under moderate sedation may experience symptoms of anxiety ("feeling of doom") as well as cutaneous symptoms (hives, itching, urticaria, erythema), angioedema, shortness of breath, wheezing, nausea or vomiting, headaches, or confusion.

In patients under general anesthesia, anaphylaxis is more likely to present as hypotension, bronchospasm, decrease or loss of end-tidal CO_2, angioedema, or cardiovascular collapse.

> **Caution!** Cutaneous symptoms may be missed in patients undergoing general anesthesia due to draping, suboptimal lighting (dim lights for laparoscopic cases), and lack of patient report.

See Table 23.1 for the signs and symptoms of anaphylaxis.

Table 23.1 Signs and Symptoms of Anaphylaxis

Organ System	Signs and Symptoms	Presentation Under General Anesthesia
Cutaneous	Flushing, pruritis, urticaria, hives, erythema, angioedema	Angioedema, hives
Gastrointestinal	Nausea/vomiting, diarrhea	Possibly vomiting if unsecured airway
Respiratory	Laryngeal edema, wheezing, shortness of breath, stridor, bronchospasm, decreased SpO_2	Increased peak inspiratory pressures, increased $EtCO_2$, bronchospasm, wheezing, decreased SpO_2
Cardiovascular	Hypotension, palpitations, chest pain	Hypotension, decreased cardiac output, tachycardia, arrhythmias, cardiac arrest
Renal	Decreased urine output	Decreased urine output, acute tubular necrosis
Hematologic	DIC	DIC

DIC, disseminated intravascular coagulation.

Note: If symptoms are severe and the patient is hemodynamically unstable, steps 2–6 should be performed simultaneously if possible.

WARNING!!   If the patient is pulseless (in cardiac arrest), follow the advanced cardiac life support (ACLS) algorithm.

---

2. Call for help and consider aborting the procedure.

Call for help and obtain additional personnel and equipment, such as a code cart and difficult airway cart if needed, to allow for steps 2–6 to be performed simultaneously.

Whether or not to abort the surgical procedure will depend on the severity of the allergic reaction and the stability of the patient. Anaphylaxis has several different grades of severity (Table 23.2).[6] The procedure can most likely be continued for grade 1 and grade 2 anaphylaxis but should be cancelled for grade 4. Decisions regarding grade 3 anaphylaxis will depend on the type of procedure and the patient condition.

Table 23.2 Grades of Anaphylaxis, Adapted from Ring and Messmer Grading Scale

Grade	Summary	Signs and Symptoms	Proceed with Surgery?
1	Mucocutaneous signs	Erythema Urticaria Angioedema	Yes
2	Mild multiorgan signs	Mucocutaneous signs Bronchospasm Hypotension	Yes
3	Severe multiorgan signs	Pulselessness Desaturation Arrhythmia Bronchospasm Cardiovascular collapse	Depends on type of procedure and patient condition
4	Cardiopulmonary arrest	Cardiac arrest	No

Adapted from Ring J. Messmer K. Incidence and severity of anaphylactoid reactions to colloid volume substitutes. Lancet. 1977;1:466–469.

3. Stop the administration of any new medications.

Immediately stop any medications if they are potentially the source of the anaphylaxis, if they are still infusing. Often this is not possible as the reaction may occur several minutes after administration.

The most common agents that cause anaphylaxis in the operating room (OR) are muscle relaxants, antibiotics, and latex. There has been less anaphylaxis with latex as the routine use of latex is declining in modern operating rooms. [1,2] Other agents that may trigger anaphylaxis include blood products (see Chapter 19 on transfusion reactions), IV contrast, and IV dyes.

>> **Tip on Technique**: During anesthesia, 70% of the anaphylactic reactions were due to neuromuscular-blocking agents and 20% were caused by latex products.[1,2]

With the increased use of sugammadex (anaphylaxis risk of 1:4000) in ORs, the overall incidence of intraoperative anaphylactic events in patients undergoing general anesthesia has been reported to have increased by one-third.[3–5]

4. **Manage the airway and ensure adequate oxygenation and ventilation.**

    Administer 100% O_2. If the patient is not already intubated, assess the airway and use clinical judgment based on the patient's symptoms. Call for a difficult airway cart if this has not been done already.

    -   If the patient has mild to no respiratory symptoms, start with close observation.
    -   If the patient starts to have wheezing, stridor, or respiratory distress, start racemic epinephrine (0.5 ml of 2.25% epinephrine diluted in 3 ml of normal saline delivered via nebulizer) and consider early intubation.

    >> **Tip on Technique:** Perform intubation early if there are signs of marked stridor or angioedema. If there is increased mucosal membrane swelling, use videolaryngoscopy if possible, and have a low threshold for performing a surgical airway. In an emergent situation, consider using a supraglottic airway (SGA) for ventilation while trying to establish a secured airway.

> **WARNING!!** In the presence of increased supraglottic or glottic swelling, an SGA may not be adequate for ventilation or for long-term airway management. In that situation, consider endotracheal intubation.

If the patient is already intubated, ensure adequate oxygenation and ventilation and treat bronchospasm if present (see steps 5 and 7).

5. **Give epinephrine if the patient is hemodynamically unstable or severe bronchospasm is present.**

    Give epinephrine 10–100 mcg IV as needed for hypotension or severe bronchospasm unresponsive to bronchodilators. Infusions of epinephrine may be needed (0.02–0.2mcg/kg/min IV). This is one of the most important treatments for anaphylaxis and should be given right away as soon as anaphylaxis is suspected if symptoms are severe.

    If the patient is still hypotensive despite epinephrine, consider adding vasopressin 1–2 units IV, repeating as needed for hemodynamic stability.

    If hypotension does not respond to epinephrine or vasopressin, consider methylene blue 1.5 mg/kg IV.[7,8] Methylene blue has been used successfully in the treatment of anaphylaxis resulting from protamine infusion.[7,8]

    >> **Tip on Technique:** Invasive monitors can help guide treatment. Consider insertion of an arterial line or central venous access if not already in place, as well as transesophageal echocardiogram/transthoracic echocardiogram (TEE/TTE) to assess heart function and fluid status. Turn down/off inhalational anesthetics as they can worsen hypotension. Use other amnestic agents as needed. Place the patient in Trendelenburg position if hypotensive. Increasing preload to the heart will help hemodynamic status.

> **WARNING!!** If the patient is pulseless (in cardiac arrest), follow the ACLS algorithm.

Note: Racemic epinephrine can also be given to treat stridor or respiratory distress. The dosage is 0.5 ml of 2.25% epinephrine diluted in 3 ml of normal saline delivered via nebulizer over 15 minutes for adults and children 4 years and older.

See Table 23.3 for the mechanisms of action of epinephrine.

Table 23.3 Mechanisms of Action of Epinephrine with Anaphylaxis

Agonist Effects of Epinephrine with Anaphylaxis	
Alpha 1-adrenergic	Increased peripheral vascular resistance and decreased mucosal edema (i.e., in upper airway)
Beta 1-adrenergic	Increased inotropy and chronotropy
Beta 2-adrenergic	Decreased release of mediators of inflammation from mast cells and basophils and increased bronchodilation

6. **Give fluids for resuscitation.**

For adequate resuscitation 1–10 L of crystalloids may be needed. Consider Plasma-Lyte or lactated Ringer (LR) if giving high amounts of fluids.

!! **Potential Complication**s: Lactated Ringer solutions can potentially contribute to metabolic alkalosis, although large volumes of normal saline can cause hyperchloremic metabolic acidosis.

> **Caution!** Children should receive normal saline in boluses of 20 ml/kg, each over 5–10 minutes, repeated as needed.

7. **Administer bronchodilators for bronchospasm.**

Give albuterol 5–10 puffs as needed orally via inhaler or via the endotracheal tube, may repeat as necessary.

!! **Potential Complications:** Side effects of albuterol can include hypokalemia, tachycardia, and palpitations.

Terbutaline 0.25 mg can be injected subcutaneously into the lateral deltoid area. If there is no clinical improvement within 15–30 minutes, you may administer an additional 0.25 mg subcutaneous dose.

> **Caution!** The total dose of terbutaline within 4 hours should not exceed 0.5 mg. Side effects of terbutaline include tocolysis in pregnant women, palpitations, tremors, and tachycardia.

8. **Administer histamine antagonists.**

Give diphenhydramine 50 mg IV (H1 receptor antagonist) and ranitidine 50 mg IV (H2 receptor antagonist). Histamine stimulates vasodilation and increases vascular permeability, heart rate, and secretions. Histamine antagonists can counteract this response.

9. **Administer corticosteroids.**

Give hydrocortisone 0.25–1 g IV or methylprednisolone 30–35 mg/kg IV.

Corticosteroids are useful in attenuating late-phase reactions that can occur 12–24 hours after anaphylaxis.

Methylprednisolone may be useful in catastrophic pulmonary vasoconstriction after protamine reaction.

10. **Obtain blood samples to send for testing.**

Send basic metabolic panel (BMP), complete blood count (CBC), arterial blood gas (ABG), histamine levels, and mast cell tryptase to confirm the diagnosis.

>> **Tip on Technique:** Serum tryptase has a half-life of approximately 2 hours. The optimal time to collect tryptase levels is within 15 minutes up to 2 hours after onset of symptoms. This is the most widely used marker to identify anaphylaxis.[9]

>> **Tip on Technique:** Histamine levels only remain elevated for 30–60 minutes. The optimal time to collect histamine levels is within 5–10 minutes of symptoms.[9]

Caution! Elevated serum tryptase is considered to be highly suggestive of anaphylaxis, although normal levels do not exclude the diagnosis.

---

11. **Stabilize the patient and transport to the intensive care unit (ICU) for further care.**

Once the patient is stabilized, transport to the ICU for further management and observation, as anaphylaxis can be biphasic.[10,11]

Interventions that can be performed when the patient is stable:

- Verify serum tryptase and histamine levels (peak <60 minutes after event).
- Consider keeping the patient intubated if the reaction was severe.
- Monitor the patient for 24 hours after recovery.
- Refer the patient for postoperative allergy testing.

Note: The reaction can be prolonged for up to 32 hours and biphasic reactions occur in 20% of the cases.[9]

Note: Patients who experience true anaphylaxis should be referred to an allergy specialist to undergo skin testing. This way the cause of anaphylaxis can be identified and recommendations can be made for alternative agents that can be used for the future.[9]

Other Management Considerations

Anaphylaxis can also occur in different areas of the hospital where help and resources are not immediately available; for example, allergies to IV contrast can occur in radiology suites and the anesthesiologist may be called to assist.

Anaphylaxis vs anaphylactoid reactions:[12]

- Anaphylaxis is a type 1 hypersensitivity reaction that occurs when there is reexposure to an antigen that elicits an IgE-mediated response, which triggers mast cell mediator release.
- Anaphylactoid reactions are non-IgE-mediated reactions in which the mast cell membrane is triggered by complement activation. Although the mechanisms of action differ with anaphylaxis and anaphylactoid reactions, they cannot be distinguished clinically.

References

1. Levy JH, Ledford DK. Perioperative Anaphylaxis: Clinical Manifestations, Etiology, and Management. UpToDate. 2019. https://www.uptodate.com/contents/perioperative-anaphylaxis-clinical-manifestations-etiology-and-management

2. Meng J, Rotiroti G, Burdett E, Lukawska JJ. Anaphylaxis During General Anaesthesia: Experience from a Drug Allergy Centre in the UK. ACTA Anaesthesiologica Scandinavica. 2017;61(3):281. doi: 10.1111/aas.12858

3. Corda D, Gravenstein N. Sugammadex: The Anaphylactic Risk. Anesthesia Patient Safety Foundation Newsletter. Circulation. 2018;33:1.

4. Takazawa T, Katsuyuki M, Sawa T, et al. Current Status of Sugammadex Usage and the Occurrence of Sugammadex-Induced Anaphylaxis in Japan. Anesthesia Patient Safety Foundation Newsletter. Circulation. 2018;33:1.

5. Miyazaki Y, et al. Incidence of Anaphylaxis Associated with Sugammadex. Anesthesia and Analgesia. 2018;126(5):1505–1508. doi: 10.1213/ANE.0000000000002562

6. Ring J, Messmer K. Incidence and Severity of Anaphylactoid Reactions to Colloid Volume Substitutes. The Lancet. 1977;309(8009):466–469. doi:10.1016/S0140-6736(77)91953-5.

7. Bauer CS, Vadas P, Kelly KJ. Methylene Blue for the Treatment of Refractory Anaphylaxis Without Hypotension. American Journal of Emergency Medicine. 2013;31(1):264. doi: 10.1016/j.ajem.2012.03.036

8. Sheth SS, Del Duca D, Ergina P, Clarke AE. Methylene Blue as a Treatment for Refractory Anaphylaxis. Journal of Allergy and Clinical Immunology. 2007;119(1):S33. doi: 10.1016/j.jaci.2006.11.149

9. Campbell R, Kelso J. Anaphylaxis: Acute Diagnosis. UpToDate. 2019. https://www.uptodate.com/contents/anaphylaxis-acute-diagnosis

10. Tole JW, Lieberman P. Biphasic Anaphylaxis: Review of Incidence, Clinical Predictors, and Observation Recommendations. Immunology and Allergy Clinics of North America. 2007;27(2):309–326.

11. Sadlier PHM, Clarke RC, Bozic B, Platt PR. Consequences of Proceeding with Surgery After Resuscitation from Intra-operative Anaphylaxis. Anaesthesia. 2018;73(1):32–39. doi: 10.111/anae.14106.

12. Pattanaik D, Yataco J, Lieberman P. Anaphylactic and Anaphylactoid Reactions. In: Hall JB, Schmidt GA, Kress JP. Principles of Critical Care, 4e. New York, NY: McGraw-Hill; 2014. Chapter 128: 1269–1279.

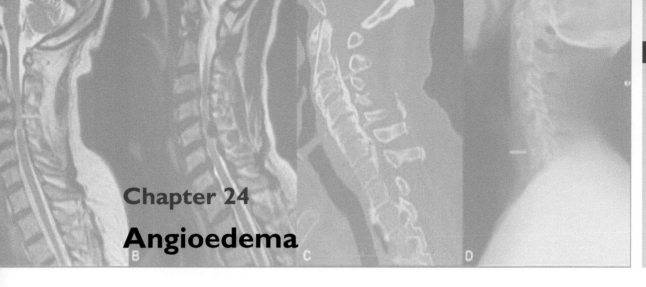

Chapter 24

Angioedema

Alberto Bursian and Yury Zasimovich

Summary Page

Symptoms:

- Nonpitting edema of the face, larynx, tongue, extremities, bowel, trunk, airway, and genitalia
- Hemodynamic instability (tachycardia, hypotension)
- Airway obstruction
- Urticaria
- Erythema

Differential Diagnosis:

- Anaphylaxis
- Contact dermatitis
- Superior vena cava syndrome
- Autoimmune disease

Introduction

Angioedema is a rare but potentially life-threatening event that can occur in the perioperative setting. Angioedema causes tissue swelling and edema usually within the skin but that can also affect mucosal surfaces, bowel, and the larynx. Signs and symptoms of angioedema are rapid nonpitting edema of tissue, hemodynamic instability, urticaria, erythema, and pruritis. Early recognition and appropriate treatment can be lifesaving.[1,2]

There are two main types of angioedema: histamine mediated (allergic, idiopathic) and bradykinin mediated (hereditary angioedema and drug-induced angioedema). Idiopathic angioedema is recurrent without any explanation. Hereditary angioedema (HAE) is due to C1 inhibitor deficiency. Drug-induced angioedema is often secondary to angiotensin-converting enzyme (ACE) inhibitors and resolves when the ACE inhibitor is discontinued. It is important to distinguish between these two types since progression of the symptoms as well as response to therapy will differ.

Histamine-mediated angioedema is mediated by immunoglobulin IgE antibodies, and symptoms appear quickly (within an hour) after exposure to an offending agent and resolve faster (after several hours), and are often associated with urticaria. Causes include drugs, foods, latex, and insect bites.

Hereditary and ACE inhibitor–induced angioedema is usually bradykinin mediated and is not associated with urticaria. Swelling attacks in bradykinin-mediated angioedema progress much slower (over a few hours) but last longer (typically 2–5 days without treatment) and are characteristically unresponsive to epinephrine, corticosteroids, and antihistamines.

Treatment

Appropriate treatment includes removal of the offending agent, supportive care, airway management, epinephrine, antihistamines, steroids, and administration of bronchodilators.

Have a high suspicion if the patient history is suggestive of allergic response: allergies to foods, latex, drugs, insects, etc.; familial history of hereditary angioedema; or use of ACE inhibitors.

Management of perioperative angioedema is similar to management of angioedema outside of the operating room with the following considerations: presentation and progression of signs and symptoms as well as physical exam findings may be more difficult to recognize intraoperatively.

Step by Step

> **WARNING!!:** If signs of acute airway obstruction/respiratory compromise are present, **proceed directly** to step 3 and secure the airway!

1. **Verify the diagnosis.**

    Signs and symptoms include nonpitting edema of any structures, tachycardia, hypotension, bronchospasm, rash, airway swelling/angioedema, and difficulty breathing (Figures 24.1 and 24.2).

    Halt the administration of any agents (IV or inhalational) that may potentially be triggering the reaction. Common offending agents include ACE inhibitors, antibiotics, nonsteroidal anti-inflammatory drugs (NSAIDs), latex, certain foods, and insects.

    Obtain labs: C4 and tryptase.

Angioedema:

non-pitting edema of the face, tongue, airway, bowel, extremities, trunk, and genitalia, frequently with urticaria, erythema, and pruritis

Frequently Affected Areas:

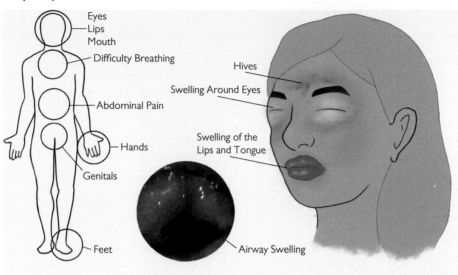

Figure 24.1 Angioedema and rash locations.

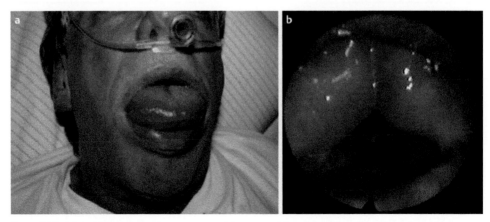

Figure 24.2 ACE inhibitor–induced angioedema of the tongue (A) and the larynx (B). Source: Bas, Murat. (2016). Evidence and evidence gaps of medical treatment of non-tumorous diseases of the head and neck. GMS Current Topics in Otorhinolaryngology, Head and Neck Surgery. 15. 10.3205/cto000129. available via license: CC BY 4.0

> **Caution!** These labs should be considered to assist in the diagnosis of hereditary angioedema and angioedema associated with anaphylaxis, respectively. However, the results will not be available for 24 hours. Although this information is important for future follow-up and management, it is not helpful in the acute phase.[3]

2. **Call for help and notify surgeon.**

   Call for crash cart and difficult airway cart with flexible bronchoscope. Ask the surgeon to halt the procedure. Symptoms may progress rapidly, leading to severe airway compromise (step 3).

   Ask the team to be prepared to perform a surgical airway: identify and mark the cricothyroid membrane and prepare surgical instruments.

3. **Manage the airway.**

   Increase FiO_2 to 100%. Confirm that the airway is patent and the patient is breathing. If the airway is NOT PATENT, intubate the trachea immediately!

> **WARNING!!** Oxygen saturation and capnography may remain close to normal until edema is advanced and intubation becomes difficult. Flexible bronchoscopic evaluation to assess for laryngeal and base of the tongue edema needs to be performed early in patients with head and neck angioedema or any signs of respiratory compromise. Consider the use of nasal trumpets, noninvasive continuous positive airway pressure (CPAP), and bag-mask ventilation as temporizing measures until the airway can be secured with an endotracheal tube.

Pearl: Inspiratory stridor and inability to swallow saliva suggest severe angioedema and impending respiratory failure.

> **WARNING!!** Blood and secretions can make intubation more challenging. Make every attempt to minimize airway trauma during airway instrumentation.

>> **Tip on Technique:** Consider a smaller endotracheal tube if laryngeal edema is suspected/present. Nasal flexible bronchoscopic intubation may be the only option if the tongue is significantly swollen. Maintaining spontaneous ventilation and performing an awake intubation are recommended if the patient is stable and maintaining oxygenation. Do not hesitate to perform a surgical airway (tracheostomy versus cricothyroidotomy) if unable to intubate.

!! **Potential Complication:** Rapid progression of airway edema in response to airway manipulation can lead to respiratory compromise and make following intubation attempts more difficult.

> **Caution!** Blind nasotracheal intubation is contraindicated in the patient with angioedema because airway distortion makes passage of the endotracheal tube extremely unlikely and localized trauma may induce further swelling. Severe edema may not allow passage of an endotracheal tube through the glottic opening, even with advanced flexible bronchoscopic or video techniques. Cricothyrotomy will be required if this is the case. If this is anticipated, the location of the cricothyroid membrane should be marked prior to any airway instrumentation being attempted. Having a surgeon experienced with surgical airway placement on standby is always warranted.

If the patient has a stable airway with adequate oxygenation and ventilation, perform a flexible bronchoscopic evaluation of the airway to assess for edema.

Note: The decision to intubate should be based on clinical signs and symptoms, other comorbidities, airway anatomy, and the results of flexible bronchoscopic evaluation.

> **Caution!** Airway edema may rapidly progress to complete airway obstruction. If the patient is stable, close monitoring is essential!

4. **Manage hemodynamics.**

Treat hypotension with normal saline fluid boluses 10–30 ml/kg IV. Discontinue any anesthetic agents. Give epinephrine 10–100 mcg IV or 0.2–0.5 mg SQ if hypotension is nonresponsive to fluid bolus. If an infusion is required, start at 0.02–0.2 mcg/kg/min and titrate to effect.

Give steroids: methylprednisolone 60–120 mg IV. If the patient has an allergy to other corticosteroids, dexamethasone 12 mg IV is the preferred agent. Give antihistamines to reduce swelling: diphenhydramine 50 mg IM/IV.

For bronchospasm, give bronchodilators:
- Salbutamol 2.5–5 mg via nebulizer
- Aminophylline 0.5 mg/kg/hr IV (in elderly give 0.3 mg/kg/hr)
- Magnesium sulfate 1–2 g IV over 20 minutes

If the patient is refractory to the above treatments, consider giving 2 units of fresh frozen plasma (FFP).[4]

Pearl: Patients with bradykinin-mediated angioedema will not respond to antihistamines, corticosteroids, or epinephrine, and while this therapy is not contraindicated, targeted therapy for HAE (or FFP) must be implemented to alleviate the symptoms.

For known acute attacks of HAE, use specific targeted therapy:
- Berinert (plasma-derived C1-INH) 20 units/kg IV
- Ecallantide (plasma-kallikrein inhibitor) 30 mg SQ
- Icatibant (Bradykinin 2-receptor antagonist) 30 mg SQ
- Ruconest (recombinant C1-INH) 50 units/kg IV

Analgesics and antiemetics should be prescribed as needed to alleviate the pain and nausea frequently manifested by HAE patients presenting with an acute abdominal attack. In mild HAE attacks, analgesics and antiemetics may be all that is needed; however, use of targeted therapies may mitigate the need for narcotics and result in more rapid resolution of the pain.

5. **Admit patient to the intensive care unit (ICU) for observation and further workup.**

The patient should be admitted to the ICU until symptoms resolve.

If intubation was required, the decision to extubate should be made with caution. Airway edema should be resolved prior to extubation. Repeat flexible bronchoscopic examination may be useful to assess for resolution of edema.

After stabilization, patients should be discharged with an epinephrine autoinjector kit until seen by an angioedema specialist who can confirm their diagnosis and the need for specific therapy.

Patients with ACE inhibitor–induced angioedema should discontinue their ACE inhibitor. An alternative antihypertensive agent should be started.

Other Management Considerations

Airway edema can develop perioperatively despite a normal airway examination at the time of intubation. If lip or tongue swelling is present at the conclusion of the procedure and angioedema is suspected, extubation should be delayed until swelling resolves.

If the patient presents with angioedema in the preoperative phase, surgery should be reconsidered based on patient disposition and urgency of surgery.

Certain patient comorbidities increase the likelihood of this type of event occurring:[5–7]

- Allergies to foods, latex, drugs, insects, etc. (this history may be present in allergic, histamine-mediated angioedema).
- ACE inhibitor use: African Americans and patients on immunosuppressors are at higher risk, especially if ACE inhibitor therapy was initiated within the last 30 days. This reaction commonly manifests as edema of the lips and tongue.
- NSAID use: Angioedema is associated with inhibition of cyclooxygenase, leading to an accumulation of leukotriene mediators as seen with reactions to NSAIDs. Patients with this condition usually manifest with urticaria and facial swelling upon exposure to the drug, but can present with swelling only.
- Familial history of HAE: HAE is due to a mutation of the gene encoding the C1 inhibitor, which is inherited in an autosomal dominant pattern, and that leads to overproduction of bradykinin.
- Lymphoreticular disorders, autoimmune disease, and other malignancies that lead to an acquired C1 esterase deficiency due to excessive C1 inhibitor catabolism.

References

1. Hoyer, Catharina, Matt R. Hill, and Edward R. Kaminski. "Angio-oedema: an overview of differential diagnosis and clinical management." *Continuing Education in Anaesthesia, Critical Care & Pain* 12.6 (2012): 307–311.
2. Misra, Lopa, Narjeet Khurmi, and Terrence L. Trentman. "Angioedema: classification, management and emerging therapies for the perioperative physician." *Indian Journal of Anaesthesia* 60.8 (2016): 534.
3. Moellman, Joseph J., et al. "A consensus parameter for the evaluation and management of angioedema in the emergency department." *Academic Emergency Medicine* 21.4 (2014): 469–484.

4. Jacob, Cherian, and Todd Sheppard. "Fresh frozen plasma (FFP) in angiotensin converting enzyme (ACE) inhibitor induced angioedema." *B56. Critical Care Case Reports: ICU Toxicology.* American Thoracic Society, 2017. A3813–A3813.

5. Williams, Anesu H., and Timothy J. Craig. "Perioperative management for patients with hereditary angioedema." *Allergy & Rhinology* 6.1 (2015): ar-2015.

6. Bas, Murat, Thomas K. Hoffmann, and Georg Kojda. "Evaluation and management of angioedema of the head and neck." *Current Opinion in Otolaryngology & Head and Neck Surgery* 14.3 (2006): 170–175.

7. Stojiljkovic, Ljuba. "Renin-angiotensin system inhibitors and angioedema: anesthetic implications." *Current Opinion in Anesthesiology* 25.3 (2012):356–362.

Chapter 25

Local Anesthetic Systemic Toxicity (LAST)

Timothy V. Feldheim and Rene Przkora

Summary Page

Signs/Symptoms:

- Sedation
- Confusion
- Dizziness
- Perioral numbness
- Tinnitus
- Visual disturbances
- Movement disorder
- Agitation/restlessness
- Seizure
- Coma
- Respiratory depression
- Bradycardia
- Tachycardia
- Hypertension (initially)
- Hypotension
- Atrioventricular conduction blockade
- Ventricular arrhythmia (ventricular tachycardia, ventricular fibrillation, torsades de pointes)
- Asystole
- Cardiac arrest

Differential Diagnosis:

- Anaphylaxis
- Anxiety
- Other sodium channel blocker toxicities (cyclobenzaprine, flecainide, procainamide)
- Cocaine toxicity
- Alcohol withdrawal
- Other cause of seizure (epileptic, neurogenic)
- Myocardial infarction

Introduction

Local anesthetic systemic toxicity (LAST) is a rare but serious complication that can occur in the setting of patients receiving or having recently received local anesthetics (LAs) for myriad reasons, but most often for nerve blockade. The symptoms of LAST can range from mild, such as drowsiness, perioral numbness, or tinnitus, to severe, involving the central nervous system (CNS) (such as seizure) and cardiovascular system (such as arrhythmia or cardiac arrest), and can even result in patient fatality. Several risk factors place a subset of patients at higher risk of developing LAST, such as small size, acidosis, and baseline cardiac conduction abnormalities. Careful and vigilant administration can help avoid the complication altogether, such as the use of ultrasound and aspiration prior to injection of LAs. Patients should always be observed with proper monitoring equipment while receiving and after injection of LAs. The treatment for LAST includes prompt recognition of symptoms, securement of the airway, administration of intravenous 20% lipid emulsion, treatment of other symptoms such as pharmacological ablation of seizures if present, advanced cardiac life support (ACLS) if needed, and supportive care as clinically warranted.

Certain patients are at increased risk of LAST. Since LAST is based on toxic doses of anesthetic, smaller patients, both infants or pediatric patients and smaller adults, are at an increased risk of developing the condition.[1] Other patient populations at increased risk are those with advanced age, heart failure, ischemic heart disease, arrhythmias and conduction abnormalities, liver disease, and metabolic diseases. [2] Patients with acidosis, who have low plasma protein concentrations, or who are already on medications that inhibit sodium channels (such as flecainide) are also at increased risk.[1,2] Pregnant patients have also been shown to have a lower threshold for the cardiotoxic effects of bupivacaine as well.[3,4]

Treatment

The first management step should always be removal of the offending agent. Signs and symptoms of LAST may occur while the LA is still being injected but can also be delayed. It is important to realize that LAST may present 30 minutes to hours after patients have been exposed to LAs, especially in patients who have received tumescent anesthetic.[1,5] It is also important to note that the less severe symptoms (drowsiness, agitation, confusion, perioral numbness, tinnitus, etc.) may not be able to be appreciated because patients may already be sedated or under general anesthesia. Because of this, the first signs of LAST may be the more serious symptoms (arrhythmia, seizure, hemodynamic instability).

Early administration of lipid emulsion therapy is a key aspect to treatment, while managing cardiovascular symptoms and seizures, if present. The American Society of Regional Anesthesia (ASRA) has published a LAST Checklist (Figure 25.1) that can be accessed via their website.[6]

>> **Tip on Technique**: Whenever possible, lipid emulsion therapy (step 6) should be started concurrently with all of the other steps listed below as early as possible to halt the reaction. Lipid emulsion therapy can also be started prior to signs of severe LAST if clinically warranted (i.e., worsening symptoms).

Step by Step

1. **Recognize signs/symptoms of LAST and stop injection of LA if still being injected.**[1,5]

WARNING!!	If the patient presents with cardiovascular collapse, call a code and initiate ACLS!

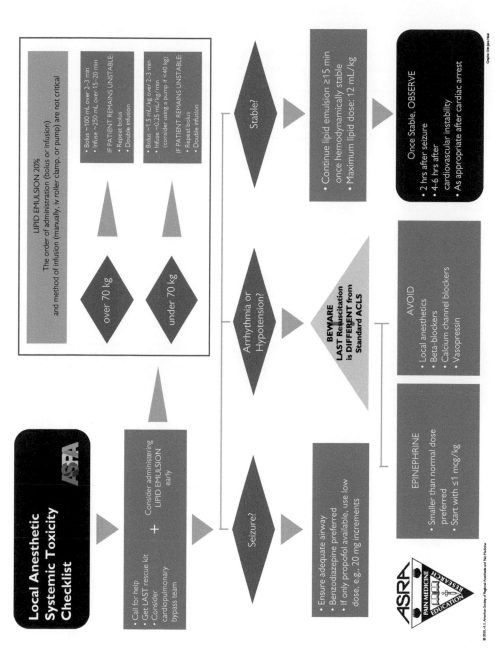

Figure 25.1 The ASRA Local Anesthetic Toxicity Checklist. Courtesy of ASRA. Copyright 2020 American Society of Regional Anesthesia and Pain Medicine. Used with permission. All rights reserved.

CNS symptoms are usually experienced first: perioral numbness, metallic taste, dizziness, sedation, confusion, and agitation, which can then progress to obtundation, apnea, coma, and seizures.

Cardiovascular symptoms then follow: rhythm abnormalities on electrocardiogram, hemodynamic instability, and cardiovascular collapse.

>> **Tip on Technique:** Patients do not always have a set progression of symptoms and may have initial presentation of seizure or even cardiovascular collapse.[1]

Caution! If the patient displays severe symptoms, start lipid emulsion therapy as quickly as possible (step 6) in concurrency with steps 2–5.

---

2. Call for help.

WARNING!! If the patient presents with cardiovascular collapse, call a code and initiate ACLS (step 5)!

If available, call for a LAST rescue kit (Figure 25.2). It is recommended that anywhere where LA is used, a LAST kit containing 20% lipid emulsion should be available.[1,5]

Alert the nearest emergency response and/or cardiopulmonary bypass team as resuscitation efforts have the potential to be extended.[6]

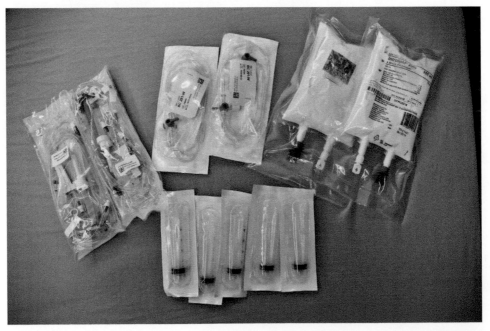

Figure 25.2 The components of an ASRA recommended LAST Rescue Kit, which includes 1 liter of 20% lipid emulsion, IV tubing, and syringes. Although not included in this photo, the ASRA LAST checklist (Figure 25.1) is recommended to be included with the kit.[6] Photo courtesy of Carolyn Witman, MD.

> **Caution!** If the patient displays severe symptoms, start lipid emulsion therapy as quickly as possible (step 6).

If the patient is hemodynamically stable and protecting their airway, consider skipping steps 3–5 and continue to step 6 if clinically warranted.

3. Establish adequate ventilation/oxygenation.

Patients should be ventilated with 100% oxygen.[1,5] Reducing hypoxemia and acidosis may relegate progression of neurological and cardiovascular symptoms, as well as help accelerate resuscitation.[8] Hyperventilation should be avoided as respiratory alkalosis may worsen effects of LA toxicity.[1,2,9] Airway adjuncts, advanced airways (supraglottic airways or endotracheal tubes), or surgical airways should be considered in patients unable to be ventilated via mask.

4. Ablate seizures pharmacologically if present.

Give lorazepam 0.1 mg/kg IV bolus at a maximum rate of 2 mg/min, to a maximum dose of 4 mg IV.[10] The dose may be repeated once in 5–10 minutes if the seizure has not subsided after the first dose. Lorazepam is the first-line drug, but if unavailable, diazepam 0.15 mg/kg IV can be given at a maximum rate of 5 mg/min, up to 10 mg per dose. [10]

If no IV access is present, IM midazolam can be administered (10 mg for adult >40 kg).[10]

>> **Tip on Technique:** Benzodiazepines are the preferred medication as they are less likely to cause further hemodynamic instability.[9]

> **Caution!** Propofol is not suggested for seizure management. The lipid portion of propofol is <20% (usually around 10%), so it is NOT recommended as a replacement for the use of 20% lipid emulsion.[1,7] Propofol's cardiac depressant effects can often worsen the hemodynamic instability that may develop as a result of LAST, so it should be used cautiously for seizure ablation.[1,9] If propofol is the only medication available to ablate a seizure, use a low dose (20-mg increments).[6]

>> **Tip on Technique:** If seizures do not resolve with benzodiazepines, small doses of succinylcholine or another short-acting neuromuscular blocker can be considered to reduce hypoxemia and acidosis.[1]

5. Treat cardiovascular symptoms.

> **WARNING!!** If the patient is pulseless, initiate cardiopulmonary resuscitation.[1,5]

Initiate ACLS protocols for appropriate ventricular arrhythmias. Treat hypotension with fluids and vasopressors as needed. Amiodarone is the medication of choice for ventricular arrhythmias.[1]

> **Caution!** Reduce epinephrine doses to ≤1 mcg/kg boluses as standard doses can often lead to ineffectual lipid emulsion therapy.[1] Avoid vasopressin for hypotension as the increase in afterload may put more strain on cardiac function.[7]
>
> **Caution!** Avoid beta blockers or calcium channel blockers for hypertension or arrhythmias as they may worsen the cardiac effects of LA.[3]

> **WARNING!!** If there is no response to lipid emulsion therapy and vasopressor therapy, cardiopulmonary bypass may be required. Alert the cardiopulmonary bypass team early in case they are needed.

6. Start lipid emulsion therapy.

>> **Tip on Technique**: Whenever possible, lipid emulsion therapy should be started concurrently with all of the previous steps as early as possible to halt the reaction. Lipid emulsion therapy can also be started prior to signs of severe LAST if clinically warranted (i.e., worsening symptoms).

If not started at the first sign of a serious LAST event, 20% lipid emulsion should at least be considered:[1,5,6]

- For patients >70 kg (lean body weight)
- 100 ml IV bolus over 2–3 minutes
- 200–250 mL IV infusion over 15–20 minutes
- For patients <70 kg (lean body weight)
- 1.5 ml/kg rapid IV bolus over 2–3 minutes
- 0.25 mL/kg IV infusion over 15–20 minutes

If the patient remains unstable after the initial dose:
- May repeat bolus once or twice[1]
- May double infusion rates[1]

>> **Tip on Technique:** Continue lipid emulsion therapy for at least 15 minutes after the patient becomes hemodynamically stable.

> **Caution!** Do not exceed a maximum dose of 12 ml/kg of lipid emulsion.[1,5,6] Well-known effects of lipid emulsion therapy are electrolyte imbalances, hypertriglyceridemia, allergy, fat embolism, infection, thrombophlebitis, and acute pancreatitis. Patients should not receive more than the recommended dosing (<12.5 mL/kg ideal body weight in 24 hours) to avoid adverse effects.[11]

A LAST Rescue Kit (see Figure 25.2) should be available for anywhere LA is routinely used. According to ASRA, components of a rescue kit should include:[1,5,6]

- Lipid emulsion 20% (1 L)
- Several large syringes and needles
- Standard IV tubing

7. Provide follow-up care once the patient is stabilized.

Patients should be monitored for at least 2–12 hours, depending on the severity of the event.

Patients who have had neurological symptoms should be observed for at least 2 hours.[1]

Patients who have had cardiovascular symptoms should be observed for at least 6 hours.[1]

Monitoring should take place in an area where American Society for Anesthesiologists (ASA) monitors are available, just as they would be monitored for any block procedure.[1]

Patients may also need higher levels of care, such as intensive care unit supportive care, especially for those requiring intubation and assisted ventilation; therefore, transfer to different units or admission to the hospital may be warranted. Patients may also require admission to the hospital from either the perioperative area or outpatient surgical centers, depending on the clinical scenario, for further observation or support.

If the patient was having the block performed for a surgical intervention, a discussion with the surgical team should take place as to whether it is safe to proceed with surgery that day or if it should be postponed.[9]

Other Management Considerations

LAST can develop anywhere where LA is being utilized, and up to several hours after administration. This includes in the operating room in patients under general anesthesia (GA). Because the patient is under GA, seizure or cardiac arrhythmias may be the only signs that may be present. Lipid emulsion should still be promptly administered, and seizure ablation/ACLS should be administered as warranted.[1]

Attentive and careful administration of LA is key to prevention. Using ultrasound during and aspirating the syringe prior to injection of LA help to prevent intravascular administration.[1] A test dose with a pharmacologic indicator, such as a small amount of LA with diluted epinephrine, may help identify intravascular injection as well.[8] The smallest dose of LA needed to obtain a block that is both sufficient in extent and length should be administered to reduce the risk of toxicity.[1]

Certain areas of the body absorb LA at different rates, leading to higher serum concentrations. The rate of absorption is proportional to the vascular supply of the area. Intrapleural injections have the highest rate of absorption, followed by intercostal blocks, caudal blocks, paracervical blocks, epidural blocks, brachial plexus/femoral nerve blocks, peripheral nerve blocks, and finally subcutaneous injection.[9,12] However, it is also important to realize that the amount of LA used in each block usually varies, and the same amount of LA given for a one block (e.g., intercostal) is often not used for other blocks (femoral nerve block).

References

1. Neal JM, Barrington MJ, Fettiplace MR, Gitman M, Memtsoudis SG, Mörwald EE, et al. The Third American Society of Regional Anesthesia and Pain Medicine Practice Advisory on Local Anesthetic Systemic Toxicity. *Regional Anesthesia and Pain Medicine*. 2018;43(2):113–123.
2. El-Boghdadly K, Pawa A, Chin KJ. Local anesthetic systemic toxicity: current perspectives. *Local and Regional Anesthesia*. 2018;11:35–44. Published 2018 Aug 8.

3. Dillane D, Finucane BT. Local anesthetic systemic toxicity. *Canadian Journal of Anesthesia/Journal Canadien Danesthésie*. 2010;57:368.

4. Bern S, Weinberg G. Local anesthetic toxicity and lipid resuscitation in pregnancy. *Current Opinion in Anaesthesiology*. Jun 2011;24(3):262–267.

5. Neal JM, Woodward CM, Harrison TK. The American Society of Regional Anesthesia and Pain Medicine checklist for managing local anesthetic systemic toxicity: 2017 Version. *Regional Anesthesia and Pain Medicine*. 2018;43:150–153.

6. https://www.asra.com/guidelines-articles/guidelines/guideline-item/guidelines/2020/11/01/checklist-for-treatment-of-local-anesthetic-systemic-toxicity

7. Weinberg GL. Treatment of local anesthetic systemic toxicity (LAST). *Regional Anesthesia and Pain Medicine*. 2010;35(2):188–193. 10.1097/AAP.0b013e3181d246c3.

8. Mahajan A, Derian A. Local anesthetic toxicity. In: *StatPearls* [Internet]. Treasure Island, FL: StatPearls Publishing; 2018 Jan [Updated 2018 Apr 29].

9. El-Boghdadly K. Local anesthetic systemic toxicity: continuing professional development. *Canadian Journal of Anesthesia/Journal Canadien Danesthésie*. 2016;63(3):330–349.

10. Brophy GM. Guidelines for the evaluation and management of status epilepticus. *Neurocritical Care*. 2012;17:3.

11. Bryan D. Systematic review of clinical adverse events reported after acute intravenous lipid emulsion administration. *Clin Toxicol*. 2016;54(5):365–404.

12. Tucker GT, Moore DC, Bridenbaugh PO, Bridenbaugh LD, Thompson GE. Systemic Absorption of Mepivacaine in Commonly Used Regional Block Procedures. *Anesthesiology*. 1972;37(3):277–287.

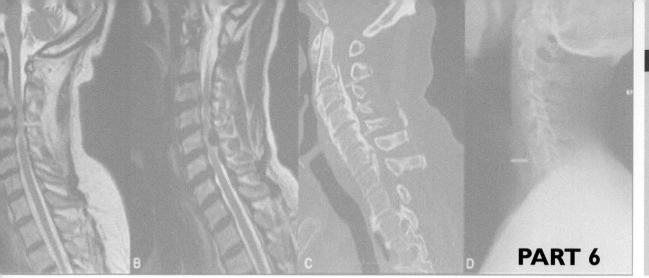

PART 6

METABOLIC

Chapter 26

Malignant Hyperthermia

Cameron R. Smith

Summary Page

Symptoms:

- Unexplained tachycardia
- Hypercapnia that DOESN'T resolve with increased ventilation
- Increasing oxygen consumption
- Masseter or other muscle spasm or rigidity, especially in the face of adequate neuromuscular blockade
- Tea- or cola-colored urine
- Increase in body temperature

Differential Diagnosis:

- Serotonin syndrome
- Neuroleptic malignant syndrome
- Acute stimulant intoxication (such as cocaine)

Introduction

Malignant hyperthermia (MH) is a rare but life-threatening condition that manifests almost exclusively as a result of exposure to volatile anesthetics such as sevoflurane or isoflurane, or succinylcholine.[1] MH results when a genetically susceptible individual is exposed to select drugs—in this case volatile anesthetics and/or succinylcholine. It is, at its core, a situation of hypermetabolism intrinsic to the muscle, resulting in signs and symptoms such as tachycardia, hypercapnia, increasing oxygen consumption, muscle rigidity, dark-colored urine, and rising core temperature.[2,3] Successful treatment requires prompt action.[4]

The clinical syndrome of MH results from malfunction of the ryanodine receptor and uncontrolled release of calcium from intracellular stores in the sarcoplasmic reticulum within muscle cells.[1,3] This results in direct activation of the contractile elements, causing uncoordinated muscle contraction independent of signaling from the nervous system.[1–3] This uncoordinated muscle activity causes greatly increased oxygen requirements and CO_2 production and results in a wide variety of signs such as tachycardia, hypercapnia, increased oxygen consumption (which may be so high as to cause a decrease in SpO_2), and increasing core body temperature.[5]

Successful treatment requires prompt action. A large number of people will be required, so call for help early. Early focus should be directed at preparation and administration of dantrolene, the only treatment available for MH, as each 30-minute delay in administration nearly doubles the rate of complications including death. Once this has been completed, care shifts to more supportive measures, such as correcting lab abnormalities and cooling. Additional support with diagnosis and treatment can and should be sought from the MH Hotline, which is staffed by MH experts at all times.

Management

Have a high index of suspicion. If the diagnosis and/or treatment of MH is significantly delayed, the prolonged hypoxic and hypermetabolic state could lead to hemodynamic disturbances such as arrhythmias and even cardiac arrest.[6]

MH can be subtle in its early presentation. Have a high index of suspicion if any of the following signs are present after exposure to inhalational anesthetics: unexplained tachycardia, unexplained or difficult-to-control hypercapnia, increasing difference between inspired and expired oxygen, presence of muscle rigidity, or increasing requests for neuromuscular blockade.[4,5]

Formal diagnosis of MH requires testing performed on a live muscle biopsy, but MH should be clinically suspected when a patient displays some or all of the following:

- Unexplained tachycardia
- Hypercapnia that DOESN'T resolve with increased ventilation—if minute ventilation has more than doubled from baseline, even in laparoscopic cases, either CO_2 is being insufflated somewhere it doesn't belong or CO_2 production has increased
- Increasing oxygen consumption—most easily detected as an increasing difference between inspired and expired oxygen
- Masseter or other muscle spasm or rigidity, especially in the face of adequate neuromuscular blockade
- Tea- or cola-colored urine—indicating likely rhabdomyolysis
- Increasing body temperature

> **Caution!** Muscle rigidity despite effective doses of neuromuscular blockers should not be taken lightly and should add MH to your differential diagnosis.[7–9]

Early MH signs and symptoms can be subtle and may mimic many other conditions. Nonetheless, early recognition and initiation of treatment are directly related to favorable outcomes.

Step by Step

1. Call for help.

Gather help and assign specific roles. Call for the MH cart immediately! Management of an acute MH event will require many people: anesthesiologists to manage the patient AND the MH event plus ADDITIONAL team members to draw up and administer dantrolene, actively cool the patient, and obtain additional supplies and medications as needed.[10–12]

> **WARNING!!** MH events are likely to require 10 or more people who will be actively involved, including a MINIMUM of 3 people to prepare and administer dantrolene, plus additional personnel to obtain supplies, cool the patient, and communicate with the team.

>> **Tip on Technique:** Two anesthesia teams are beneficial—one to manage the PATIENT and one to manage the MH EVENT. Have someone get the MH cart, and designate people to prepare and administer dantrolene. Be specific in designating roles and use closed-loop communication. For example, do NOT request "someone" to get the MH cart; clearly direct a specific individual to a task, ideally by name. You should expect them to communicate back to you that they have understood and are going to perform the assigned task.

2. Discontinue triggering agents.

Stop any triggering agents (volatile anesthetic agents, succinylcholine) and switch to total intravenous anesthesia (TIVA): propofol 200–300 mcg/kg/min IV, titrated to individual patient needs. Discontinuing volatile anesthetics without initiating TIVA will result in patient emergence from anesthesia and increase the risk of recall.

Discontinue the surgical procedure as quickly as possible and alert the surgeons of the diagnosis.[11,12]

3. Provide high-flow oxygen and increase ventilation.

Very high oxygen flow rates (approximately three times minute volume or greater) may be necessary to supply enough oxygen to all the active muscle elements. Very high minute ventilation may be needed to try to control hypercapnia and consequent acid-base disturbances.[4,11]

>> **Tip on Technique**: If adequate minute ventilation is difficult to achieve with mechanical ventilation, consider manual ventilation. This will require assigning an additional person to this task alone and increases the risk of pulmonary barotrauma.

!! **Potential Complication**: In some circumstances it is possible that the minute volume required to control hypercapnia may exceed the delivery capacity of the available ventilation equipment. This may result in overly large tidal volumes, pressures, or breath-stacking, which can put the patient at risk for pulmonary injury.

> **WARNING!!** If the gas flow needed to support the required minute volume exceeds the oxygen delivery capacity of your anesthesia machine, carefully consider adding air to the mixture. While this will increase the total fresh gas flow, it will also decrease the fraction of inspired oxygen.

4. Administer dantrolene 2.5 mg/kg IV.

Once an MH event is suspected, it is important to prepare and administer the initial dantrolene dose as quickly as possible. The incidence of complications increases 1.7-fold for every 30-minute delay in dantrolene administration after initial symptom presentation.[2,4]

Two commercially available preparations exist for dantrolene. One version, Revonto or Dantrium, is available in 20-mg vials that MUST be reconstituted in 60 ml of STERILE WATER and must be agitated for 4–7 minutes to properly dissolve the contents. For an average-sized adult patient at least 5 vials will be required for a single dose. Several providers will be required to prepare an entire dose in a timely fashion.

> **Caution!** Dantrolene CANNOT be administered until the solution is a uniform, translucent yellow with no remaining particulate matter (Figure 26.1).

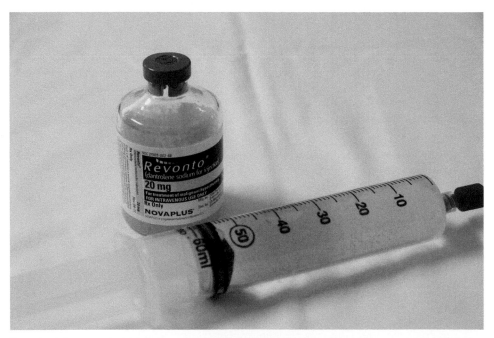

Figure 26.1 Revonto which has been completely dissolved. The contents of the syringe are a transparent yellow with no remaining particulate matter, which is easily distinguished from the hazy contents of the bottle, which is not yet properly dissolved. Each properly prepared 60 ml contains 20 mg of dantrolene.

!! Potential Complication: Failure to properly dissolve dantrolene will result in thrombophlebitis and will likely require larger doses, since the full dose of medication will not be delivered.

A newer preparation, Ryanodex, is available in 250-mg vials that are reconstituted in 5 ml of STERILE WATER and only requires 1–2 minutes of agitation for complete dissolution. This allows an entire dose to be administered with a single vial.

>>Tip on Technique: When properly prepared, the suspension will be opaque and bright orange in color (Figure 26.2).

If symptoms reemerge, redose dantrolene as needed to control symptoms. This may require cumulative doses as high as 10 mg/kg or more. Patients may require total doses exceeding 10 mg/kg.

>> Tip on Technique: Patients with fulminant MH events can quickly consume very large amounts of dantrolene. Consider seeking out additional supplies of dantrolene early.

WARNING!!   Both preparations of dantrolene MUST be prepared in STERILE WATER for injection. Substituting a balanced salt solution such as normal saline will result in approximately 40% of the dantrolene failing to dissolve.

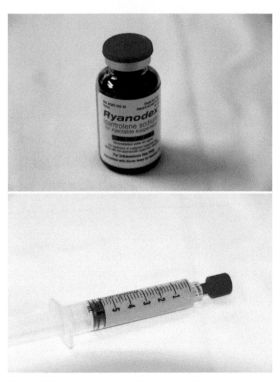

Figure 26.2 A. Ryanodex vial. B: A syringe filled with properly prepared Ryanodex. Please note the much smaller volume (5 ml versus 60 ml) of the contents of a single vial and that when properly prepared in sterile water, Ryanodex is an opaque, bright orange suspension. Each properly prepared 5 ml contains 250 mg of dantrolene.

5. **Add activated charcoal filters to the circuit or change the anesthesia machine.**

   Add activated charcoal filters to the anesthesia machine circuit on both the inspiratory and expiratory limbs (Figure 26.3). If activated charcoal filters are not available, consider replacing the entire anesthetic gas machine rather than just the circuit tubing and CO_2 absorbent cannister.[6,11,12]

   >> **Tip on Technique**: Addition of activated charcoal filters will make changing the circuit and CO_2 absorbent unnecessary. If filters are not available, the CO_2 absorbent canisters and circuit tubing should be changed when possible, but this will be time-consuming and should not be done at the expense of providing adequate oxygenation and ventilation.

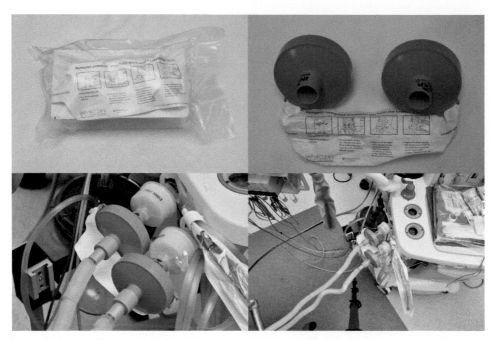

Figure 26.3 Vapor-Clean activated charcoal filters are an easy, inexpensive solution that remove anesthetic gases from the circuit within approximately 90 seconds of their application when used as directed.

6. **Consider ACTIVE COOLING.**

   This can be achieved using any combination of cold IV fluids; ice packed around the head, axillae, and/or groin; external surface cooling; and gastric, peritoneal, bladder, and/or rectal irrigation with cold fluids. Invasive methods such as peritoneal irrigation are not recommended except in circumstances where they are immediately available without any additional steps such as open abdominal surgeries.[11,12]

| **WARNING!!** | STOP cooling efforts when body temperature drops below 38°C to decrease risk of hypothermia. |

7. Monitor and correct lab disturbances. Treat hemodynamics if necessary.

Send labs: arterial blood gas (ABG), electrolytes, serum creatine kinase (CK), urine myoglobin. Monitor the patient for hyperkalemia and treat as needed. Given the mass of muscle relative to other tissues, potassium levels will require frequent monitoring. Consider placing an arterial line to monitor hemodynamics and for frequent lab draws.

If clinical signs of hyperkalemia (peaked T waves, arrhythmias) are present, administer as needed:

- Calcium 500–1000 mg IV
- Insulin 1–5 units IV
- Dextrose 24–50 grams IV

Administer bicarbonate as needed to control pH. A typical dose is 1–2 mEq/kg up to 50 mEq per dose.

Place a Foley catheter, if not already in place, to allow observation of urine volume and color, collection of urine lab tests, and bladder irrigation with cold fluids for active cooling. If urine is dark, tea, or cola colored, or if urine tests positive for myoglobin, consider administration of a diuretic and aggressive hydration for renal protection.[13]

WARNING!! If the diagnosis and/or treatment of MH is significantly delayed, the prolonged hypoxic and hypermetabolic state can lead to hemodynamic disturbances such as arrhythmias and even cardiac arrest.

‼ **Potential Complication**: Myoglobin released from injured myocytes can deposit in renal tubules, resulting in renal failure.

8. Arrange for an intensive care unit bed as soon as possible.

Dantrolene is a calcium channel blocker and may cause weakness sufficient to delay extubation. Even if this is not the case, patients who experience suspected MH events should be closely monitored for up to 72 hours for reemergence of symptoms.

Other Management Considerations

Additional support with diagnosis and treatment can and should be sought from the MH Hotline, which is staffed by MH experts at all times. The MH Hotline is staffed 24 hours per day, 7 days per week by physicians experienced in the management of MH. This service is free of charge.

MALIGNANT HYPERTHERMIA HOTLINE: 1-800-644-9737

Or 001-209-417-3722 outside US/Canada

Once the acute event is complete, please report the event to the North American Malignant Hyperthermia Registry by phone at 888-274-7899 or on the web at https://anest.ufl.edu/namhr/ so that your event can be added to the data repository, helping further MH research and understanding.

Reports to the registry can be made online or by telephone. The report can be made either by the patients themselves or by their treating physician. Ideally both are involved, providing the most complete data possible. Even incomplete data is highly valuable to the study of MH.

References

1. Hopkins PM. Malignant hyperthermia: pharmacology of triggering. *British Journal of Anaesthesia* 107: 48–56, 2011.

2. Larach MG, Gronert GA, Allen GC, Brandom BW, Lehman EB. Clinical presentation, treatment, and complications of malignant hyperthermia in North America from 1987 to 2006. *Anesthesia and Analgesia* 110: 498–507, 2010.

3. Wappler F. Malignant hyperthermia. *European Journal of Anaesthesiology* 18: 632–652, 2001.

4. Glahn KP, Ellis FR, Halsall PJ, Muller CR, Snoeck MM, Urwyler A, Wappler F, European Malignant Hyperthermia G. Recognizing and managing a malignant hyperthermia crisis: guidelines from the European Malignant Hyperthermia Group. *British Journal of anAesthesia* 105: 417–420, 2010.

5. Rosenberg H, Davis M, James D, Pollock N, Stowell K. Malignant hyperthermia. *Orphanet Journal of Rare Diseases* 2: 21, 2007.

6. Wappler F. Anesthesia for patients with a history of malignant hyperthermia. *Current Opinion in Anaesthesiology* 23: 417–422, 2010.

7. Littleford JA, Patel LR, Bose D, Cameron CB, McKillop C. Masseter muscle spasm in children: implications of continuing the triggering anesthetic. *Anesthesia and Analgesia* 72: 151–160, 1991.

8. Parness J, Bandschapp O, Girard T. The myotonias and susceptibility to malignant hyperthermia. *Anesthesia and Analgesia* 109: 1054–1064, 2009.

9. Rosenberg H. Trismus is not trivial. *Anesthesiology* 67: 453–455, 1987.

10. Pinyavat T, Wong C, Rosenberg H. Development and evolution of the MHAUS cognitive aid for malignant hyperthermia. *BMC Anesthesiology* 14: A25, 2014.

11. Goldhaber-Fiebert SN, Austin N, Sultan E, Burian BK, Burden A, Howard SK, Gaba DM, Harrison TK. Stanford Anesthesia Cognitive Aid Program. Emergency Manual: Cognitive aids for perioperative crises, Version 4, 2021. http://emergencymanual.stanford.edu

12. Schneiderbanger D, Johannsen S, Roewer N, Schuster F. Management of malignant hyperthermia: diagnosis and treatment. *Therapeutics and Clinical Risk Management* 10: 355–362, 2014.

13. Petejova N, Martinek A. Acute kidney injury due to rhabdomyolysis and renal replacement therapy: a critical review. *Critical Care* 18: 224, 2014.

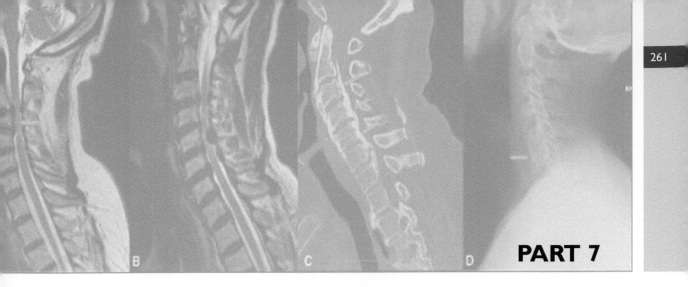

PART 7

OB, NEONATAL

Chapter 27

Amniotic Fluid Embolism

Adam Wendling and Brandon Lopez

Summary Page

Symptoms:

- Acute hypoxia and hypotension
- Cardiac arrest
- Coagulopathy
- Fetal distress
- Rarely, prodromal anxiety or "sense of doom"
- Rarely, altered mental status or seizures may be the presenting symptom

Differential Diagnosis

- Pulmonary embolism
- Placental abruption
- Septic shock
- Cardiomyopathy of pregnancy
- Anaphylactic shock
- Local anesthetic toxicity
- High neuraxial block

Introduction

Childbirth is expected to be a normal, joyful transition in life among a mostly young and healthy population, making the rare instance of severe maternal morbidity and even mortality all the more devastating. Yet, by all measures, maternal mortality and severe morbidity in the United States is increasing. While fortunately rare, amniotic fluid embolism (AFE) causes 5.5% of maternal mortalities in the United States (for context, anesthetic-related maternal mortality represents 0.4%).[1] Incidence varies by inclusion criteria from as low as <2 out of 100,000 pregnancies to as high as 1 out of 8000 with a mortality rate from 10% to 60% depending on inclusion criteria and initial presentation.[2–15] Of those that survive, as many as 85% suffer severe disability.[14,15]

Pathophysiology of the condition remains largely unknown. AFE was first described in the 1940s where autopsy findings after maternal cardiovascular collapse found squamous cells of presumed fetal origin in the maternal pulmonary circulation.[2,16,17] Since that time, the predominant theory used to explain sudden hypoxia, maternal cardiovascular collapse, and coagulopathy close to the time of delivery was amniotic fluid and other fetal debris entering maternal circulation and causing an embolic phenomenon in the maternal pulmonary circulation as well as activation of the coagulation cascade leading to cardiopulmonary collapse and consumptive coagulopathy. Although more recent evidence does not support this theory, the term "amniotic fluid embolism" persists for this syndrome.[2,16,17]

Risk factors include cesarean section, assisted second stage of labor, induction of labor, preeclampsia, multiple gestation, advanced age, and placenta previa.[7–9] These historical factors are so common they are unhelpful. The etiology of AFE remains unknown, but the leading theory is a fetal trigger in vulnerable women that leads to unregulated inflammation, shock, and coagulopathy similar to systemic inflammatory response and anaphylaxis[10] (Figure 27.1).

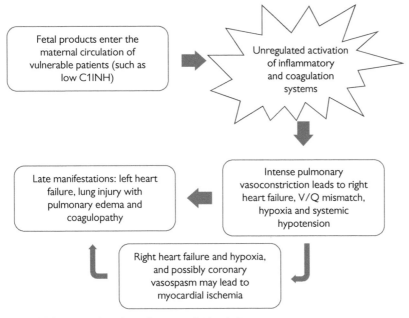

Figure 27.1 Proposed etiology of amniotic fluid embolism.

Treatment

Approximately 70% of AFEs occur during labor and 30% occur soon after delivery.

Therefore, many of these events will be first recognized in a labor room.

If cardiac arrest is the presenting symptom, it is generally recommended that the initial resuscitation occurs in the labor room, at least through perimortem cesarean delivery (see step 3 below).

If hemorrhage and disseminated intravascular coagulation (DIC) or significant hypotension and respiratory compromise are the presenting symptoms, strongly consider moving the patient to the operating room (OR). If available, consider the use of a trauma OR or hybrid OR where interventional radiology procedures such as embolization or REBOA placement could be pursued during the course of resuscitation.

>> **Tip on Technique:** All other elective activities on the labor and delivery floor should be held whenever possible. Labor inductions or augmentation should be temporarily withheld until the crisis is over.

Step by Step

1. **Recognize the event.**[18]

   The classic presentation is acute cardiopulmonary collapse, cardiac arrest, or severe hypoxia and hypotension, occasionally preceded by anxiety or a "sense of doom," followed later by coagulopathy, heart failure, and lung injury. Less commonly, coagulopathy may be the predominant symptom. Rarely, neurologic manifestations like seizures can precede the cardiopulmonary collapse.

   Signs and symptoms include:

   - Sudden severe hypoxia and hypotension (the most common initial presentation)
   - Cardiopulmonary arrest or significant hypotension (systolic blood pressure <90)
   - Respiratory compromise despite intensive medical therapy
   - Unexplained hemorrhage or DIC
   - Occasionally, DIC may be the predominant symptom with less prominent pulmonary and cardiovascular compromise
   - Uncommonly, nonspecific symptoms of anxiety, agitation, or a "sensation of doom" may precede significant hemodynamic collapse
   - Rarely, altered mental status and seizures could be the presenting symptom

   If **cardiac arrest** is the presenting symptom, do not move the patient! Resuscitate them where they are (step 3)! If the patient is stable enough to be moved, consider further management in the OR.

   Expect the patient to decompensate. Activate team members: anesthesiology, respiratory therapy, maternal-fetal medicine, critical care medicine, and neonatal resuscitation team (if AFE occurs prior to delivery). Activate massive transfusion protocol or obtain necessary blood products if needed.

   IF THE PATIENT PRESENTS WITH CARDIOPULMONARY COMPROMISE: GO TO STEP 3.

   IF THE PATIENT PRESENTS PREDOMINANTLY WITH DIC BUT IS STABLE: GO TO STEP 4. IF THEY HAVE DIC BUT ARE UNSTABLE: GO TO STEP 3.

3. **Perform high-quality cardiopulmonary resuscitation (CPR)/advanced cardiac life support (ACLS) if the patient is in cardiopulmonary compromise or arrest.**[18–21]

   CPR is the cornerstone for cardiac arrest due to AFE.

   Key areas of focus include:

   - Rapid chest compressions and complete recoil between compressions (100–120/min)
   - Chest compression depth 2–2.4 inches (5–6 cm)
   - Minimize interruptions in chest compressions
   - Early defibrillation for ventricular fibrillation (VF)/ventricular tachycardia (VT)
   - Resume chest compressions immediately after defibrillation
   - Switch the person doing chest compressions every 2 minutes
   - Consider not pausing chest compressions for intubation
   - Avoid prolonged pulse checks (<10 seconds)

   If AFE occurs prior to delivery, there are a few considerations for CPR in the pregnant patient:

   - Relief of caval compression by the gravid uterus. The patient should remain supine while a provider applies manual left uterine displacement.
   - Consider early endotracheal intubation. The physiologic changes associated with pregnancy lead to increased oxygen consumption, decreased oxygen reserves, and increased risk of aspiration.
   - Perimortem cesarean delivery should be pursued as soon as possible in settings of cardiac arrest with a potentially viable fetus (≥23 weeks' estimated gestational age).
   - Do not move the patient to an OR for perimortem cesarean delivery—bring the team and equipment to the patient.

WARNING!! The outcome for mother and baby are serious, with most registries reporting maternal mortality rates with AFE exceeding 20%.

---

4. **Secure the airway if necessary.**

   Intubation may be necessary even without cardiac arrest due to progression toward DIC, hemorrhage, and heart failure.

   Anticipate difficult intubation and consider the use of videolaryngoscopy:

   - Increased incidence of difficult intubation in pregnancy
   - Reduced pulmonary reserve and increased oxygen consumption
   - Increased risk of bleeding due to coagulopathy (nasal intubation has higher risk)

   >> **Tip on Technique:** Videolaryngoscopy may be the best option in a likely difficult situation. Second-generation supraglottic airways may be a temporizing effort but are unlikely to be sufficient for long in the evolving critically ill patient.

5. **Place additional IVs and invasive monitors.**

   Place large-bore IV access and an arterial line.

   >> **Tip on Technique:** Ultrasound guidance may minimize trauma associated with multiple attempts at IV and arterial line placement in a hemodynamically unstable patient who either has or will likely develop DIC. Consider central venous access if peripheral IV access is inadequate or if vasopressors are needed.

6. **Perform point-of-care ultrasound (POCUS) or transesophageal echocardiography (TEE).**[22]

POCUS or TEE can rule out other causes of instability and guide resuscitation, assist with line placement, and guide volume replacement. TEE can identify right ventricle (RV) strain or bulging of the intraventricular septum into the left ventricle (LV), or an underfilled LV.

7. **Provide right ventricular support if needed with medications.**[18]
   - Norepinephrine infusion (0.05 mcg/kg/min IV) is the preferred vasopressor for inotropic support
   - Consider dobutamine (0.5–20 mcg/kg/min IV) or milrinone (0.375–0.75 mcg/kg/min IV with or without loading dose of 50 mcg/kg) infusion as secondary agents
   Pulmonary vasodilators may also offer benefit:
   - Inhaled nitric oxide at 5–20 parts per million
   - Inhaled or possibly IV prostacyclin (epoprostenol) at 10–50 ng/kg/min inhaled or 1–2 ng/kg/min IV

   >> **Tip on Technique:** Many patients who die from AFE do so in the early phase when pulmonary hypertension with resultant right heart failure, hypoxia, and systemic hypotension is predominant.

   > **WARNING!!** Positive pressure ventilation may worsen venous return and increase pulmonary vascular resistance.

8. **Prepare and administer blood products as needed.**[23–25]

   Administer blood products until bleeding is controlled and lab values (fibrinogen, thromboelastogram (TEG)) are normalized. Give cryoprecipitate or fibrinogen concentrates early as fibrinogen <200 mg/dL is associated with worse outcomes.

   >> **Tip on Technique:** Use a higher fresh frozen plasma (FFP)–to–red blood cell (RBC) ratio transfusion (closer to 1 unit of FFP to 1 unit of RBC) because FFP contains C1 esterase inhibitor, an enzyme found to correlate to the incidence and severity of AFE.

   >> **Tip on Technique:** Treatment of uterine atony and bleeding includes careful examination for cervical or vaginal lacerations, surgical correction of bleeding with uterine tamponade, B-lynch sutures, hysterectomy, or pelvic packing.

   !! **Potential Complication:** Fluid overload and worsened heart function may occur in the setting of heart failure. Limit other volume replacement.

   Thromboelastography can monitor coagulopathy and response to transfusion (Figure 27.2).

   If hyperfibrinolysis is suspected, consider tranexamic acid 1 gram IV or epsilon aminocaproic acid 100 mg/kg IV.

   > **Caution!** Recombinant factor VIIa (NovoSeven) should be used only as a last resort.

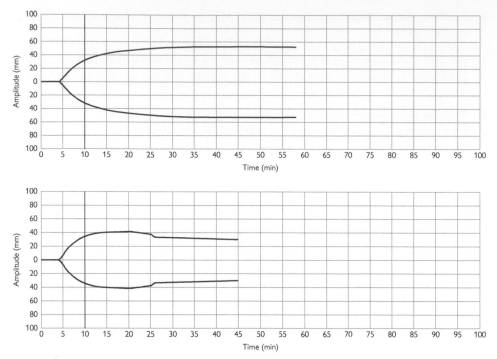

Figure 27.2 Thromboelastograph of normal coagulation (top) and fibrinolysis (bottom).

9. Consider other medications and possible treatments.

- Extracorporeal CPR (ECPR), more commonly known as extracorporeal membrane oxygenation (ECMO), as a bridge to recovery in refractory cardiac arrest has been used successfully in AFE patients.[22,26-29] Access to ECMO equipment may be limited to high-acuity, subspecialty hospitals.

- Hemofiltration: Continuous arteriovenous hemofiltration may remove inciting agents that led to the collapse. There is a limited body of evidence supporting this technique along with other hemodynamic support modalities.[30,31]

- C1 esterase inhibitor concentrates (C1INH) 500–1500 units IV. C1INH activity level has been found to correlate with incidence and severity of AFE, with lower C1INH activity associated with fatal AFE.[32,33] It may be hard to acquire.

- High-dose corticosteroids: hydrocortisone 500–1500 mg IV.

- A-OK: Atropine 0.2 mg IV, ondansetron 8 mg IV, and ketorolac 15 mg IV. These medications may block some of the downstream proinflammatory, vasodilatory reactions.[34,35] Caution: While evidence of efficacy of these agents is extremely limited, the ease of use and lack of serious side effects may make these agents worthwhile.

- Intralipid IV lipid emulsion therapy: 1.5 mL/kg bolus, then 0.25 mL/kg/min infusion.[36]

>> **Tip on Technique:** If ECPR is considered, the team necessary to accomplish this complex task needs to be mobilized early.

‼ **Potential Complication:** ECMO typically requires some degree of anticoagulation, which is complicated in these patients who frequently develop DIC.

> **Caution!** Hydrocortisone can suppress the inflammatory response, and its use is controversial with no obvious improvement in outcome.

Other Management Considerations

Perimortem cesarean delivery should be pursued as soon as possible in settings of cardiac arrest with a potentially viable fetus (≥23 weeks' estimated gestational age).[20] It can save the neonate and improve the mother's condition through the relief of caval compression, increase in preload, and increase in systemic vascular resistance associated with delivery. Despite the risk of surgery in the setting of coagulopathy, in a parturient in cardiac arrest, it is unlikely to worsen her condition.

Do not move the patient to an OR for perimortem cesarean delivery; bring the surgical team and equipment to the location of the arrest, whether that be a labor suite, a triage room, or an antepartum room. In most facilities, moving a parturient even under perfect conditions takes minutes, thereby reducing the likelihood of neonatal rescue. However, as uterine atony and DIC with resultant massive hemorrhage frequently follow cardiac arrest caused by AFE, transfer to a trauma OR or hybrid OR with interventional radiology equipment will likely become necessary if the patient survives the initial insult.

If the patient survives the initial event, hemodynamic instability and pulmonary insufficiency frequently do not immediately resolve. Aggressively treat fever and consider therapeutic hypothermia, which may improve neurologic outcomes after cardiac arrest, but ongoing coagulopathy may be exacerbated by hypothermia. Avoid hyperglycemia. Nosocomial infections commonly develop. After return of spontaneous circulation, consideration for transfer to an interventional radiology suite for embolization of bleeding should be made, which may include stopping elective activities in that location.

A neonatal team should be immediately available and assume care of the infant postdelivery so the obstetric and anesthesia teams can continue to focus on the mother.

Further Reading

Society for Maternal-Fetal Medicine (SMFM) with the assistance of Pacheco LD, Saade G, et al. Amniotic fluid embolism: diagnosis and management. Am J Obstet Gynecol. 2016; 215:B16–24.

References

1. Pregnancy Mortality Surveillance System. Centers for Disease Control and Prevention. November 9, 2017. https://www.cdc.gov/reproductivehealth/maternalinfanthealth/pmss.html. Accessed on June 26, 2018.
2. Clark SL. Amniotic fluid embolism. Obstet Gynecol. 2014; 123(2):337–48.
3. Clark SL, Romero R, Dildy GA, Callaghan WM, Smiley RM, Bracey AW, Hankins GD, D'Alton ME, Pacheco LD, Vadhera RB, Herlihy P, Berkowitz RL, Belfort MA. Proposed diagnostic criteria for the case definition of amniotic fluid embolism in research studies. Am J Obstet Gyn. 2016; 215(4):408–12.
4. Royal College of Obstetricians and Gynecologists. UK Obstetric Surveillance System. March 31, 2015. https://www.npeu.ox.ac.uk/ukoss/current-surveillance/amf. Accessed on July 5, 2018.
5. The Australasian Maternity Outcomes Surveillance System. 2015. https://www.amoss.com.au/?q=content/amniotic-fluid-embolism-afe. Accessed on July 5, 2018.
6. Kobayashi H, Akasaka J, Naruse K, Sado T, Tsunemi T, Niiro E, Iwai K. Comparison of the different definition criteria for the diagnosis of amniotic fluid embolism. J Clin Diagnostic Res JCDR. 2017; 11(7):QC18–21. doi:10.7860/JCDR/2017/26746.10283.

7. Kramer MS, Rouleau J, Baskett TF, Joseph KS; Maternal Health Study Group of the Canadian Perinatal Surveillance System. Amniotic fluid embolism and medical induction of labour: a retrospective, population-based cohort study. Lancet 2006; 368:1444–48.

8. Knight M, UKOSS. Amniotic fluid embolism: active surveillance versus retrospective database review. Am J Obstet Gynecol. 2008; 199:e9.

9. Abenhaim HA, Azoulay L, Kramer MS, Leduc L. Incidence and risk factors of amniotic fluid embolisms: a population-based study on 3 million births in the United States. Am J Obstet Gynecol. 2008; 199:49.e1–8.

10. Kanayama N, Tamura N. Amniotic fluid embolism: pathophysiology and new strategies for management. J Obstet Gynaecol Res. 2014; 40(6):1507–17.

11. Kaur K, Bhardwaj M, Kumar P, Singhal S, Singh T, Hooda S. Amniotic fluid embolism. J Anaesthesiol Clin Pharm. 2016; 32(2):153–59. doi:10.4103/0970-9185.173356.

12. Births and Natality. National Center for Health Statistics. Centers for Disease Control and Prevention. March 31, 2017. https://www.cdc.gov/nchs/fastats/births.htm. Accessed on July 17, 2018.

13. Clark SL, Hankins GD, Dudley DA, Dildy GA, Porter TF. Amniotic fluid embolism: analysis of the national registry. Am J Obstet Gynecol. 1995; 172:1158–67.

14. Fitzpatrick KE, Tuffnell D, Kurinczuk JJ, Knight M. Incidence, risk factors, management and outcomes of amniotic-fluid embolism: a population-based cohort and nested case–control study. BJOG. 2016; 123:100–109.

15. Balinger KJ, Chu Lam MT, Hon HH, Stawicki SP, Anasti JN. Amniotic fluid embolism: despite progress, challenges remain. Curr Opin Obstet Gynecol. 2015, 27:398–405.

16. Clark SL, Pavlova Z, Horenstein J, Phelan JP. Squamous cells in the maternal pulmonary circulation. Am J Obstet Gynecol. 1986; 154:104–6.

17. Tamura N, Farhana M, Oda T, Itoh H, Kanayama N. Amniotic fluid embolism: pathophysiology from the perspective of pathology. J Obstet Gynaecol Res. 2017 Apr; 43(4):627–32.

18. Society for Maternal-Fetal Medicine (SMFM) with the assistance of Pacheco LD, Saade G, et al. Amniotic fluid embolism: diagnosis and management. Am J Obstet Gynecol. 2016; 215:B16–24.

19. Kleinman ME, Brennan EE, Goldberger ZD, Swor RA, Terry M, Bobrow BY, Gazmuri RJ, Travers AH, Rea T. Part 5: adult basic life support and cardiopulmonary resuscitation quality. Circulation. 2015; 132:S414–35.

20. Lavonas EJ, Drennan IR, Gabrielli A, Heffner AC, Hoyte CO, Orkin AM, Sawyer KN, Donnino MW. Part 10: special circumstances of resuscitation. Circulation. 2015; 132:S501–18.

21. Link MS, Berkow LC, Kudenchuk PJ, Halperin HR, Hess EP, Moitra VK, Neumar RW, O'Neil BJ, Paxton JH, Silvers SM, White RD, Yannopoulos D, Donnino MW. Part 7: adult advanced cardiovascular life support. Circulation. 2015;132:S444–64.

22. Stanten RD, Iverson LI, Daugharty TM, Lovett SM, Terry C, Blumenstock E. Amniotic fluid embolism causing catastrophic pulmonary vasoconstriction: diagnosis by transesophageal echocardiogram and treatment by cardiopulmonary bypass. Obstet Gynecol. 2003 Sep; 102(3):496–98.

23. Charbit B, Mandelbrot L, Samain E, Baron G, Haddaoui B, Keita H, Sibony O, Mahieu-Caputo D, Hurtaud-Roux MF, Huisse MG, Denninger MH, de Prost D. The decrease of fibrinogen is an early predictor of the severity of postpartum hemorrhage. J Thromb Haemost. 2007; 5(2):266–73.

24. Wikkelsø AJ, Edwards HM, Afshari A, Stensballe J, Langhoff-Roos J, Albrechtsen C, Ekelund K, Hanke G, Secher EL, Sharif HF, Pedersen LM, Troelstrup A, Lauenborg J, Mitchell AU, Fuhrmann L, Svare J, Madsen MG, Bødker B, Møller AM; FIB-PPH trial group. Preemptive treatment with fibrinogen concentrate for postpartum haemorrhage: randomized controlled trial. Br J Anaesth. 2015 Apr; 114(4):623–33.

25. Bell SF, Rayment R, Collins PW, Collis RE. The use of fibrinogen concentrate to correct hypofibrinogenaemia rapidly during obstetric haemorrhage. Int J of Ob Anesth. 2010 Apr; 19(2):218–23.

26. Wise EM, Harika R, Zahir F. Successful recovery after amniotic fluid embolism in a patient undergoing vacuum-assisted vaginal delivery. J Clin Anesth. 2016 Nov; 34:557–61.

27. Shen HP, Chang WC, Yeh LS, Ho M. Amniotic fluid embolism treated with emergency extracorporeal membrane oxygenation: a case report. J Reprod Med. 2009 Nov-Dec; 54(11–12):706–8.

28. Seong GM, Kim SW, Kang HS, Kang HW. Successful extracorporeal cardiopulmonary resuscitation in a postpartum patient with amniotic fluid embolism. J Thorac Dis. 2018 Mar; 10(3):E189–93.

29. Ho CH, Chen KB, Liu SK, Liu YF, Cheng HC, Wu RS. Early application of extracorporeal membrane oxygenation in a patient with amniotic fluid embolism. Acta Anaesthesiol Taiwan. 2009 Jun; 47(2):99–102.

30. Ogihara T, Morimoto K, Kaneko Y. Continuous hemodiafiltration for potential amniotic fluid embolism: dramatic responses observed during a 10-year period report of three cases. Ther Apher Dial. 2012; 16:195–97.

31. Weksler N, Ovadia L, Stav A, Ribac L, Iuchtman M. Continuous arteriovenous hemofiltration in the treatment of amniotic fluid embolism. Int J Obstet Anesth. 1994; 3:92–96.

32. Tamura N, Kimura S, Farhana M, Uchida T, Suzuki K, Sugihara K, Itoh H, Ikeda T, Kanayama N. C1 esterase inhibitor activity in amniotic fluid embolism. Crit Care Med. 2014; 42:1392–96.

33. Todo Y, Tamura N, Itoh H, Ikeda T, Kanayama N. Therapeutic application of C1 esterase inhibitor concentrate for clinical amniotic fluid embolism: a case report. Clin Case Rep. 2015; 3(7):673–75. doi:10.1002/ccr3.316.

34. Copper PL, Otto P, Leighton BL. Successful management of cardiac arrest from amniotic fluid embolism with ondansetron, metoclopramide, atropine and ketorolac: a case report. Society of Obstetric Anesthesiology and Perinatology Annual Meeting. 2013 Apr. San Juan, Puerto Rico.

35. Rezai S, Hughes AC, Larsen TB, Fuller PN, Henderson CE. Atypical amniotic fluid embolism managed with a novel therapeutic regimen. Case Rep Obstet Gynecol. 2017; 2017:8458375. doi:10.1155/2017/8458375.

36. Lynch W, McAllister RK, Lay JF Jr, Culp WC Jr. Lipid emulsion rescue of amniotic fluid embolism-induced cardiac arrest: a case report. A A Case Rep. 2017 Feb 1; 8(3):64–66.

Chapter 28

Anesthetic Management of Emergency Cesarean Delivery

M. Anthony Cometa and Adam L. Wendling

Summary Page
Symptoms:

Fetal:

- Fetal intolerance of labor
- Prolapsed umbilical cord
- Arrest of descent/shoulder dystocia unresolved

Maternal:

- Antepartum or intrapartum hemorrhage
- Uterine rupture
- Placental abruption with fetal distress

Differential Diagnosis:

- Malposition of fetal heart monitor
- Obstetrician apprehension

Introduction

Cesarean delivery has increased in the recent years. Lucas et al. described a classification system for urgency of cesarean delivery to assist with communication and clinical decision-making surrounding the time of delivery.[1] Their system rated urgency on a 1–4 scale:

1. Category 1—immediate threat to life of woman or fetus
2. Category 2—maternal or fetal compromise that is not immediately life-threatening
3. Category 3—needing early delivery but no maternal or fetal compromise
4. Category 4—elective

Such a system can assist the anesthesiologist in clinical decision-making surrounding allocating resources (prioritizing/delaying other surgical care, calling in more help from outside the hospital) and anesthetic options.

Emergent cesarean delivery is largely an unpredictable event. However, some accepted risk factors include induction of labor, trial of labor after previous cesarean, obesity, twin gestation, fetal macrosomia, maternal or gestational diabetes, and hypertensive disorders.

Emergency cesarean delivery is a stressful event on any labor and delivery unit. The anesthesiology, obstetrics, and nursing teams must all work in concert to provide the safest course of management to ensure a safe peripartum outcome for both the parturient and baby. The decision to proceed via general anesthesia versus neuraxial anesthesia requires careful thought. The risks and benefits of potential difficulties associated with airway management and aspiration risk in the parturient versus the neonatal sequelae that may be associated with potential delay of delivery to establish appropriate surgical anesthesia via neuraxial techniques (i.e., epidural or spinal anesthesia) need to be carefully considered. Communication between the anesthesiology provider and obstetrician is of key importance to ensure anesthetic management is appropriate according to the clinical presentation. At this time, the effects of maternal anesthetic management on neonatal outcomes require further study.

Management

Providing anesthesia to the parturient in an emergency setting is a multitasking, dynamic event. Regardless of the urgency, your priority is maternal safety, and communication with the obstetric and nursing team is critical to ensure your anesthetic plan is appropriate for the presenting maternal, fetal, and obstetric conditions.

Emergent cesarean deliveries typically occur on a labor and delivery ward, a "non–operating room (OR)-anesthesia" location. As labor and delivery occurs 24 hours a day regardless of weekends or holidays, many of these unexpected events will occur at a time and in a location where other anesthesia and surgical services are not located and are not familiar. Early activation of help if needed is essential. All elective activities on the labor and delivery floor should be held whenever possible. Labor inductions or augmentation should be temporarily withheld until the emergent delivery is stable.

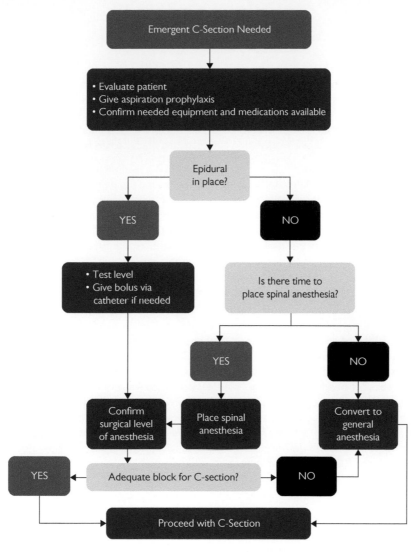

PS160336-9/14/21

Figure 28.1 Emergent cesarean section algorithm.

Step by Step

See Figure 28.1.

1. Evaluate the patient.

It is essential that the anesthesiology provider go to the bedside and evaluate the patient. Perform a history and physical and ensure a type and screen and labs have been sent. Evaluation of the patient's airway and whether or not the parturient has an established and appropriately functioning labor epidural will help determine next steps in clinical management. Communicate with the obstetrician to obtain any further critical information. Go to the OR to ensure your anesthesia workstation and team are ready to receive the patient.

2. Give aspiration prophylaxis.

The American Society for Anesthesiologists (ASA) Practice Guidelines for Obstetric Anesthesia recommend that aspiration prophylaxis be administered prior to surgical procedures. This can include nonparticulate antacids, H2-receptor blockers, and/or metoclopramide. In the setting of emergency cesarean delivery, administering 15–30 mL of sodium citrate PO to the parturient is appropriate. Administration of an H2-receptor blocker will begin to take effect at approximately 30 minutes, with maximal effect occurring at 60–90 minutes. This action may still be beneficial to mitigate any potential aspiration event that could occur during emergence.

Pearl: 255 mL of hydrochloric acid can be neutralized by 30 mL of sodium citrate.

3. Ensure availability of special equipment and medications.

Ensure you have difficult airway equipment available and ready to use including videolaryngoscopy and second-generation supraglottic airway devices. Additionally, consider the possible need for additional IV access and invasive monitoring (e.g., arterial line) if significant bleeding or severe hemodynamic instability is anticipated. If significant bleeding is anticipated during preoperative assessment, confirm blood product availability and the need to activate your institution's massive transfusion protocol. Hemorrhage during cesarean delivery can be significant. This is because uterine blood flow can range from 700 to 900 ml/min at term.

Ensure availability of additional uterotonics (e.g., methylergonovine or prostaglandin F2α) if needed.

4. Assess efficacy of existing epidural, if already in place.

If a labor epidural is already in place, it is essential to test the efficacy of the epidural to ensure surgical anesthesia coverage will be appropriate.

>> **Tip on Technique:** A bag full of ice applied onto the patient's abdomen is a quick and easy way to assess surgical anesthetic level.

If you think the existing epidural will be effective for surgery, aspirate the epidural catheter to assess if it is intravascular. If aspiration is negative, give preservative-free high-concentration local anesthetic through the catheter to establish surgical anesthesia. (See Table 28.1 for drugs and dosage options.) Neuraxial opioids such as fentanyl 50–100 mcg or sufentanil 5–20 mcg can work synergistically with high-concentration local anesthetics and can increase the likelihood of success of converting a previously sited epidural to a surgical anesthetic.

Overall, about 85–90% of labor epidurals should be able to be converted to a surgical anesthetic for cesarean section.[2] The goal is a T4–T6 level of anesthesia to cover the surgical area.

Table 28.1 Drugs Used for Epidural Surgical Anesthesia for Cesarean Delivery

Drug	Dose Range*	Duration (min)†
Local Anesthetics		
Lidocaine 2% with epinephrine 5 µg/ml	300–500 mg	75–100
2-Chloroprocaine 3%	450–750 mg	40–50
Bupivacaine 0.5%	75–125 mg	120–180
Ropivacaine 0.5%	75–125 mg	120–180
Opioids		
Fentanyl	50–100 µg	120–240
Sufentanil	10–20 µg	120–240
Morphine	3–4 mg	720–1440
Meperidine	50–75 mg	240–720

Source: Reprinted from Lawrence C. Tsen, *Chestnut's Obstetric Anesthesia: Principles and Practice*, 5th ed. Elsevier Saunders, Philadelphia, PA, Copyright 2014. With permission.

*Dose Range: dosage of medications below this range are not expected to have sufficient clinical effect and dosage above this range are expected to increase complications/side effects without clinical benefit.
†Duration: expected surgical anesthesia duration for each medication.

>> **Tip on Technique:** To help detect intravascular injection and reduce systemic absorption, use local anesthetic solutions with epinephrine. Epinephrine-containing solutions are acidic, which will reduce the unionized, lipid-soluble local anesthetic that must reach the intracellular sodium channel to generate a block. Alkalinization of the local anesthetic solution by addition of 1 mEq of bicarbonate for every 10 ml of stock solutions with epinephrine will speed the onset and increase the likelihood of a successful surgical anesthetic.

Caution! Unintentional intravascular injection of local anesthetic with epinephrine produces maternal tachycardia and hypertension. However, this may be difficult to distinguish in the setting of concurrent tachycardia.

>> **Tip on Technique:** For patients experiencing discomfort prior to surgery while utilizing the epidural catheter for cesarean delivery consider:

- Pull the catheter back 1–2 cm and give more local anesthetic.
- Give opioids through the epidural catheter.
- Give systemic sedation or convert to general anesthesia.

Caution! When providing high-concentration local anesthetic through a previously sited epidural catheter, be wary of systemic absorption/intravascular injection or unintended high neuraxial block.

‼ **Potential Complication:** High neuraxial block is the second most common serious complication of obstetric anesthetics.[3] It is manifested by respiratory insufficiency, upper extremity weakness, hypotension, and bradycardia. Typically, respiratory insufficiency predominates and ventilator support with positive pressure ventilation is often necessary.

5. **If no epidural is in place, discuss the possibility of spinal anesthesia with the surgeon.**

    The risks and benefits of proceeding with emergency cesarean delivery via general anesthesia versus neuraxial anesthesia must be carefully considered. It is important to discuss with the surgeons if the patient's presenting clinical conditions will allow placement of spinal anesthesia. IF THE ANSWER IS NO, PROCEED DIRECTLY TO STEP 7.

    If yes, proceed with a single-shot spinal technique. (See Table 28.2 for drug and dosage options.) The goal is a T4–T6 level of anesthesia to cover the surgical area. **Confirm that adequate spinal anesthesia is present before proceeding to step 6.**

Table 28.2 Drugs Used for Spinal Anesthesia for Cesarean Delivery

Drug	Dose Range*	Duration (min)[†]
Local Anesthetics		
Lidocaine	60–80 mg	45–75
Bupivacaine	7.5–15 mg	60–120
Levobupivacaine	7.5–15 mg	60–120
Ropivacaine	15–25 mg	60–120
Opioids		
Fentanyl	10–25 µg	180–240
Sufentanil	2.5–5 µg	180–240
Morphine	100–200 µg (0.1–0.2 mg)	720–1440
Meperidine[‡]	60–70 mg	60
Adjuvant Drugs		
Epinephrine[$]	100–200 µg (0.1–0.2 mg)	

*Dose Range: dosage of medications below this range are not expected to have sufficient clinical effect and dosage above this range are expected to increase complications/side effects without clinical benefit.

[†]Duration: expected surgical anesthesia duration for each medication.

[‡]Meperidine has both local anesthetic and opioid properties. The dose listed represents meperidine administered without additional local anesthetic.

[$]Epinephrine may augment local anesthetic duration of action.

NOTE: The meperidine dose for spinal administration is not to be combined with additional local anesthetic.

Source: Reprinted from Lawrence C. Tsen, *Chestnut's Obstetric Anesthesia: Principles and Practice*, 5th ed. Elsevier Saunders, Philadelphia, PA, Copyright 2014. With permission.

6. **Observe the patient and prepare for incision.**

    If the decision to proceed with emergency cesarean delivery was due to fetal indications, provide supplemental oxygen to maximize oxygen delivery to the fetus.

Make sure the patient is positioned supine with left uterine displacement (Figure 28.2). Supine hypotension syndrome is due to compression of the inferior vena cava by the gravid uterus. This decreased venous return can cause tachycardia, nausea and vomiting, and dizziness. Additionally, uteroplacental blood flow may be compromised, resulting in fetal distress.

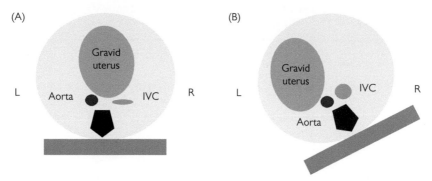

Figure 28.2 Left uterine displacement. A: Supine. Note compression of inferior vena cava (IVC) (light blue oval). B: Left uterine displacement and left tilt resulting in resolution of IVC compression.

>> **Tip on Technique:** Adverse effects of the supine position can be reduced by placing the mother in 15 degrees of lateral tilt.

While awaiting incision, ensure requested antibiotics have been administered. Make sure the surgeons test the efficacy of the neuraxial anesthetic technique prior to allowing them to make the first incision. If effective anesthesia has NOT been obtained, go directly to step 7.

If effective neuraxial anesthesia has been obtained, be prepared to treat hypotension with phenylephrine 50–100 mcg IV or ephedrine 5–10 mg IV. Phenylephrine results in less fetal acidemia compared to ephedrine.

Allow surgeons to proceed with incision and continue to watch the patient's reaction to incision. Treat vital signs according to clinical needs.

>> **Tip on Technique:** Occasionally, patients may begin to experience discomfort well after skin incision, during more stimulating surgical maneuvers such as uterine exteriorization and replacing the uterus in the pelvis or with strong surgical retraction.

For patients experiencing discomfort during surgery while utilizing the epidural catheter for surgical anesthesia, consider:
- Opioids delivered through the epidural catheter
- Systemic sedation:
- Inhaled nitrous oxide 30–70% in oxygen
- Ketamine 0.1–0.2 mg/kg IV in divided doses up to 0.5 mg/kg
- Midazolam 0.02–0.05 mg/kg IV
- Fentanyl 1–2 mg/kg IV
- Conversion to general anesthesia (step 7)

Which option depends on the degree to which the patient can tolerate the discomfort and the likely duration of discomfort (if significant discomfort occurs relatively early in the surgery, such as after delivery with uterine exteriorization, it may be better to induce general anesthesia than provide prolonged sedation).

Caution! When providing multiple sedatives and neuraxial anesthesia, respiratory depression can develop in the mother AND the neonate. If so, proceed to step 7.

Proceed on to delivery of infant and step 8.

7. **If no epidural is present or if the epidural is ineffective, proceed to general anesthesia.**

Preoxygenate the patient with 100% O_2. Ensure an assistant is present at the head of the bed to assist with rapid sequence induction.

Apply cricoid pressure and perform rapid sequence induction and intubation without ventilation.

Recommended induction drugs:

- Propofol 2–2.8 mg/kg IV (use with caution if hemodynamic instability is present)
- Ketamine 1–1.5 mg/kg IV (preferred if hemodynamic instability is present)
- Succinylcholine 1–1.5 mg/kg IV (preferred for rapid sequence induction)
- Rocuronium 1.2 mg/kg IV (if contraindication to succinylcholine)

Caution! The airway of the parturient may be particularly difficult.[4] Difficult airway equipment should be available. If intubation fails, place a second-generation supraglottic airway or perform mask ventilation until the baby is delivered to maximize oxygen delivery. After delivery, further attempts to secure the airway can be performed.

After general anesthesia has been induced and the airway has been secured, allow surgeons to proceed. If possible, delay giving any IV opioids until after delivery to minimize potential neonatal respiratory depression, but use your judgment if the clinical needs justify its use (e.g., maternal hemodynamic response to intubation/incision). Maintenance of anesthesia can be provided with isoflurane or sevoflurane in an oxygen/nitrous oxide mixture (assuming no contraindications to volatile agents).[5]

8. **After delivery of the infant, observe for delivery of the placenta and monitor for bleeding.**

If the placenta is unable to be delivered due to morbidly adherent pathology, be prepared for possible hysterectomy (see Chapter 29 for more details). If the decision has been made by the surgeons to proceed with hysterectomy due to concerns of morbidly adherent placenta, obtain additional IV access and place an arterial line. Confirm blood products are available and consider activating your hospital's massive transfusion protocol.

Give uterotonics after delivery of the placenta: Start an oxytocin infusion at a rate of <1 IU/min IV. Continue to observe the surgical field and ask the surgeon about uterine tone. Consider the use of additional uterotonics if uterine tone is insufficient:

- Methylergonovine: 0.2 mg IM (may be repeated once after 1 hour)
- Prostaglandin F2α: 0.25 mg IM (may be repeated every 15 minutes up to 2 mg)

> **WARNING!!** Methylergonovine is relatively contraindicated in patients with hypertension, peripheral vascular disease, ischemic heart disease, and preeclampsia. Methylergonovine administered too fast can cause cardiovascular complications such as coronary vasospasm, myocardial ischemia, and hypertension. Prostaglandin F2α is relatively contraindicated in patients with reactive airway disease and can cause bronchospasm and alter the ventilation-perfusion ratio in susceptible patients.

Despite delivery of the infant, it is important to maintain vigilance and communication with the surgical team to ensure uterine tone is sufficient to prevent postpartum hemorrhage. During this time, continue to ensure continued maternal comfort if the patient is under neuraxial anesthesia and give opioids if clinically required. Continue to maintain vigilance to observe for ongoing or unrecognized bleeding.

Other Management Considerations

Oftentimes, due to the emergent nature of surgery, cesarean delivery proceeds via general anesthesia. As such, neuraxial opioids may not have been given and postoperative pain may be significant, despite intraoperative use of IV opioids. A multimodal approach with different medications (e.g., acetaminophen, ketorolac) and techniques (e.g., transversus abdominis plane [TAP] block) should also be considered.

Emergency cesarean delivery has been associated with intraoperative awareness due to the avoidance of sedative premedications and the intentional use of low-concentration volatile agents, especially in hemodynamically unstable states. Although pregnancy reduces anesthetic requirements by 25–40%, delivery of volatile anesthetic at 0.5 MAC may not reliably provide an adequate depth of anesthesia to prevent intraoperative awareness. As such, balancing the needs of maternal safety and comfort with fetal outcome needs to be carefully considered.

Maternal anxiety during an emergency cesarean delivery is common and understandable. At times, the need to provide anxiolytic medication may be required. As previously mentioned, anxiolytic or hypnotic mediations may result in amnesia of the delivery event. Employing the assistance of available labor and delivery nurses to comfort the patient may be necessary to avoid administration of anxiolytics and the potential amnestic consequence; however, if maternal anxiety is causing a distraction and safety concern, anxiolytic administration may be clinically warranted.

On occasion, parturients will present with preexisting surgical hardware that may affect the ability to safely and efficiently perform a neuraxial anesthetic technique for cesarean delivery. It is important to try to identify these patients early and review any available imaging.

Obesity can have a significant effect on the ability to safely and efficiently perform a neuraxial technique in the setting of an emergency cesarean delivery. Additionally, the airway of the obese parturient may be quite challenging and of particular concern. As previously stated, it is essential that early communication and consultation with the obstetrician occurs to assess the urgency of the cesarean delivery to consider the risks/benefits of proceeding via a neuraxial versus general anesthetic technique.

References

1. Lucas DN, Yentis SM, Kinsella SM, et al. Urgency of caesarean section: a new classification. J R Soc Med 2000;93:346–50.

2. Bauer ME, Kountanis JA, Tsen LC, Greenfild ML, Mhyre JM. Risk factors for failed conversion of labor epidural analgesia to cesarean delivery anesthesia: a systematic review and meta-analysis of observational trials. Internat J Obstet Anesth 2012;21:294–309.

3. D'Angelo R, Smiley RM, Riley ET, Segal S. Serious complications related to obstetric anesthesia. Anesthesiology 2014;120:1505–12.

4. Hawkins JL, Chang J, Palmer SK, et al. Anesthesia-related maternal mortality in the United States: 1979–2002. Obstet Gynecol 2011 Jan;117(1):69–74.

5. Tsen LC. Anesthesia for cesarean delivery. In Chestnut's Obstetric Anesthesia: Principles and Practice (pp. 545–603). Philadelphia, PA: Elsevier Saunders; 2014.

Chapter 29

Anesthetic Management of Morbidly Adherent Placenta (Accreta/Increta/Percreta)

Brandon M. Lopez and M. Anthony Cometa

Summary Page

Symptoms:

- Often asymptomatic
- Painless vaginal bleeding

Differential Diagnosis

- Uterine atony
- Cervical lacerations
- Surgical injury
- Coagulopathies of pregnancy
- Trauma

Introduction

Morbidly adherent placenta (MAP) is a condition where the placenta attaches or invades into or through the uterus and does not normally detach from the uterus during childbirth. It is on the rise due to increased cesarean delivery rates and uterine instrumentation in the population. Abnormally adherent placentation rates as high as 1 in 500 pregnancies are now being quoted.[1] Placenta accreta can lead to an obstetric emergency, including massive hemorrhage and emergent hysterectomy, especially if undiagnosed prior to delivery.[2] Preparation and planning with a multidisciplinary team is key to success for these challenging deliveries.[2]

The risk of MAP (e.g., placenta accreta, placenta increta, placenta percreta) increases with the increased number of previous cesarean deliveries, especially if concurrent placenta previa is present.[3] Patient history that increases the chances of MAP include placenta previa, an anterior placenta, history of uterine instrumentation or scarring (dilation and curettage, fibroid surgery), and prior cesarean deliveries. Most patients have a lack of symptoms or painless vaginal bleeding as their only symptom. If the parturient has had one or more cesarean deliveries or prior uterine instrumentation, it is advised to investigate the location of the placenta. A previa or low-lying anterior placenta with a prior uterine scar is a sign that the suspicion for MAP should be heightened.[3] There are multiple patient comorbidities that can complicate a patient with MAP. Some of these include morbid obesity, history of prior abdominal surgeries, or a prior cardiac history.

Failure to anticipate a MAP can result in significant maternal hemorrhage with its associated morbidity and mortality. It is important to maintain vigilance in the preoperative assessment of parturients who have had multiple prior cesarean deliveries.[4] If risk of massive hemorrhage is high, consideration should be made to deliver the parturient in an operative suite with available help and away from potential distant birthing areas.[1]

Management

Ideally, the patient has had some prenatal care prior to delivery with an index of suspicion for MAP. Patients with a complete previa should have ultrasound imaging done to check for placental invasion. Magnetic resonance imaging (MRI) can also be used to further confirm the diagnosis.[5] Patients with a placenta previa and multiple cesarean deliveries have increasing odds of placenta accreta with each surgical delivery. This step-by-step guidance is for unplanned MAP, but it can be used during planned procedures as well.

Step by Step

1. **Call for help!**

    Activation of the institution-specific emergency response team is invaluable. The team should include anesthesiology, maternal-fetal medicine, gynecology-oncology, critical care medicine, and nursing support. Consider including general surgery or urology if placental invasion of periuterine structures is involved.

    Either the institution's massive transfusion protocol should be activated or the blood bank should be notified to prepare many units of packed red blood cells (PRBCs), fresh frozen plasma (FFP), and cryoprecipitate in anticipation of massive hemorrhage. Platelets should also be available.

    Unexpected MAP typically occurs on a labor and delivery location. As labor and delivery occurs 24 hours a day regardless of weekends or holidays, many of these unexpected events will occur at a time and in a location where other surgical services may not be located. Early calls for help are crucial to minimize morbidity and mortality. All other elective activities on the labor and delivery floor should be halted whenever possible. Labor inductions or augmentation should be temporarily withheld until the crisis is over.

2. **Convert to general anesthesia.**

Most cesarean deliveries occur under a regional anesthetic. When an unexpected MAP occurs, massive hemorrhage usually results. It is advised to convert to a general anesthetic in these situations, to better manage the patient's hemodynamics.[6]

> **WARNING!!** Emergent intubations in pregnant women, especially if in labor, can be difficult. Have appropriate airway equipment available including a videolaryngoscope, bougie, different direct laryngoscope blades, supraglottic airway devices, and flexible bronchoscopes.

>> **Tip on Technique:** Preoxygenate the patient with 100% O_2 via facemask. Ensure an assistant is present at the head of the bed to assist with rapid sequence induction (e.g., cricoid pressure).

Induction drugs: propofol 2–2.5 mg/kg IV and succinylcholine 1–2 mg/kg IV. Rocuronium 1.2 mg/kg IV can be used if a contraindication to succinylcholine exists.

Direct visualization with confirmation of end-tidal CO_2 is recommended.

> **Caution!** In the setting of hemorrhage and a regional anesthetic, caution should be taken regarding induction drug choice and dosing. In the setting of severe hypotension, the following induction drugs can be substituted: ketamine 0.5–2 mg/kg IV or etomidate 0.3–0.6 mg/kg IV.

3. **Place additional IV access and invasive monitors.**

Large-bore IV access is critical in unsuspected MAP due to the potential for large hemorrhage. Access should include 14- or 16-gauge IV catheters, an arterial line, and double-lumen or introducer central line (if peripheral access is unobtainable). Intraosseous (IO) access can also be used in an emergency; however, central venous access is preferred.

>> **Tip on Technique:** Placement of a radial arterial line is important for both continuous blood pressure monitoring and frequent blood sampling. An ultrasound is recommended for placement of central venous access due to patient position and surgical drapes.

4. **Prepare/give blood products.**

An RBC-to-FFP ratio of 2:1 or 1:1 is preferred in a massive transfusion situation. Early use of cryoprecipitate or fibrinogen concentrates may be preferred in obstetric hemorrhage as fibrinogen <200 mg/dL is associated with worse outcome.[7]

>> **Tip on Technique:** Transfusion should be guided by frequent arterial blood gases and patient hemodynamics. As a general rule, the patient should be transfused when the hemoglobin falls below 7 g/dL or continued bleeding and hypotension is present.

Caution! In the setting of a massive transfusion, caution should also be taken to not overtransfuse the patient after the bleeding has stopped. An endpoint for transfusion should be guided by arterial blood gases, patient hemodynamics, and viscoelastic testing, as described below.

On occasion, you may care for a patient whose religious beliefs may present a conflict for receiving blood products in the setting of MAP. It is important for the anesthesiology provider to have a discussion with the parturient detailing the significant risks of hemorrhage and the potential morbidity and mortality associated with the pathology of morbidly adherent placenta.

5. **Send off labs/use viscoelastic coagulation monitoring.**

Point-of-care laboratory testing using arterial or venous samples is key to evidence-based transfusion. Use the below labs to guide your transfusion and resuscitation. Send off the following labs: Complete blood count (CBC), prothrombin time/partial thromboplastin time/international normalized ratio (PT/PTT/INR), fibrinogen, arterial or venous blood gas, and thromboelastogram (TEG or rotational thromboelastography [ROTEM]).

TEG analysis can be very useful in assessing the cause and guiding management of hemorrhage (Figures 29.1 and 29.2). When interpreting a TEG from left to right, the straight line is the R value, or reaction time. This is dependent on clotting factors and best corrected with FFP. Next look at the alpha angle, which is the rate of clot formation. This is best corrected with fibrinogen. Then, look at the maximum amplitude (MA). This is the strength of the overall clot. This can be corrected with platelets. Last, look at the amplitude at 30 minutes. This shows the amount of lysis of the clot. If this is decreased, antifibrinolytics can be given, such as tranexamic acid.

>> **Tip on Technique:** If hyperfibrinolysis is suspected, use of lysine analogue tranexamic acid (1 gram IV) or epsilon aminocaproic acid (100 mg/kg IV) is recommended. Recombinant factor VIIa should be considered as a last resort.

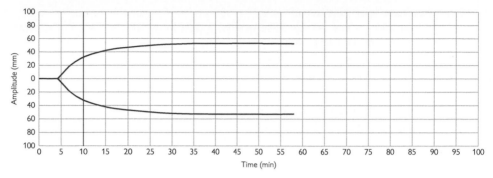

Figure 29.1 Normal thromboelastogram. Normal values include R: 4–8 min, alpha angle: 47–74 degrees, MA: 55–73 mm.

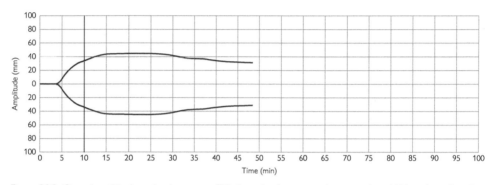

Figure 29.2 Coagulopathic thromboelastogram. This thromboelastogram shows a reduced MA and a reduced amplitude at 30 minutes. This patient would benefit from platelets and an antifibrinolytic in this setting.

7. Maintain hemodynamics.

Sometimes fluid and blood products are not enough to maintain appropriate hemodynamics. Target a goal mean arterial pressure of >65 mmHg. Use of the below drugs can be helpful:

- Norepinephrine 0.05 mcg/kg/min IV: this is the preferred vasopressor/inotrope
- Ephedrine 5–10 mg IV
- Phenylephrine 100–mcg IV
- Vasopressin 0.04 units/min IV

8. Alert interventional radiology (IR), if available.

IR can be valuable to help embolize areas of bleeding not amenable to surgical intervention. This is especially helpful for placenta percreta into surrounding structures or blood vessels.[7, 8-9]

9. Communicate with the team!

Communication is key during these events, especially when they are unexpected. Have frequent conversations with:

- Surgeons: regarding blood loss, coagulopathy, etc.
- Nursing: extra help, organization, crowd control
- Blood bank: availability of more products, etc.
- Anesthesia techs: need for more supplies

The response team should consist of the obstetrician and surgical assistant focusing on control of hemorrhage. The lead anesthesiologist should focus on coordination of extra IV access, arterial access, rapid transfusion setup, and blood product retrieval. The second assistant anesthesiologist or RN should coordinate transfusion of blood products at the direction of the lead anesthesiologist. The second assistant should also execute lab assessments such as TEG and blood gas analysis. The neonatal resuscitation team should evaluate and treat the neonate and then clear the location as soon as possible. The record keeper frequently is an anesthesia provider or RN. In addition to recording treatments, the record keeper should prompt the team for critical events. The runner should facilitate the delivery of lab tests and blood products and acquiring surgical equipment as needed.

10. Postoperative planning.

MAP is an obstetric emergency and usually manifests in massive hemorrhage. Discuss with the surgeon postoperative destination and planning. Most patients will need an intensive care unit (ICU) bed, preferably in a surgical ICU.[7] Due to large resuscitations, keeping the patient intubated is acceptable clinical practice. Contact needs to be made with the following:

- ICU charge nurse or bed board (acquiring bed space)
- Respiratory therapy regarding need for postoperative ventilation and transport
- ICU nursing to facilitate appropriate transfer of care

11. Debriefing and patient transport.

Debrief with surgeons and nursing staff regarding unfinished issues, concerns, and information to hand off to ICU staff.

>> **Tip on Technique:** Call for help if needed, including respiratory therapy, and transport the patient with appropriate monitoring to the ICU. Communicate issues and further needs to ICU staff for patient management. Comprehensive handoffs are extremely important in the critically ill patient.

Other Management Considerations

While some institutions recommend left uterine displacement to aid in caval decompression during routine cesarean delivery, many surgeons prefer the supine position for placenta accreta deliveries due to anatomy concerns. It has been shown in MRI studies that the amount of degrees needed to decompress the vena cava (30–45 degrees) is not optimal in this setting.[10] A discussion with your surgeon regarding preferred position is recommended, and manual left retraction of the uterus can be performed in the setting of severe hypotension during anesthetic induction or neuraxial sympathectomy.

Remember that MAP usually presents with no symptoms or painless vaginal bleeding. A hysterectomy for MAP is a major abdominal surgery, and postoperative pain considerations need to be addressed. Usually a midline incision is used due to need for exposure during these cases. If a neuraxial technique is employed, neuraxial opioids can be given. An epidural catheter can also be left in place for 24–48 hours to augment pain control. It is important to keep in mind that postoperative cesarean delivery pain has both somatic and visceral components and a multimodal approach with different medications (e.g., acetaminophen, ketorolac) and techniques (e.g., transversus abdominis plane block) should be considered, especially if general anesthesia is utilized.

> **Caution!** Before removal of an epidural catheter posthemorrhage, it is advised to check the international normalized ratio (INR) and platelet count. INR should be <1.5 and platelets >75,000 mm^3 if possible for safe removal of the catheter.

References

1. Grant TR, Ellinas EH, Kula AO, Muravyeva MY. Risk-stratification, resource availability, and choice of surgical location for the management of parturients with abnormal placentation: a survey of United States-based obstetric anesthesiologists. Int J Obstet Anesth. 2018 May;34:56–66. doi: 10.1016/j.ijoa.2018.01.008. Epub 2018 Feb 2. PMID: 29523485

2. Riveros-Perez E, Wood C. Retrospective analysis of obstetric and anesthetic management of patients with placenta accreta spectrum disorders. Int J Gynaecol Obstet. 2018 Mar;140(3):370–374. doi: 10.1002/ijgo.12366. Epub 2017 Nov 23. PMID: 29080306

3. Orbach-Zinger S, Weiniger CF, Aviram A, Balla A, Fein S, Eidelman LA, Ioscovich A. Anesthesia management of complete versus incomplete placenta previa: a retrospective cohort study. J Matern Fetal Neonatal Med. 2018 May;31(9):1171–1176. doi: 10.1080/14767058.2017.1311315. Epub 2017 Apr 16. PMID: 28335653

4. Sivasankar C. Perioperative management of undiagnosed placenta percreta: case report and management strategies. Int J Womens Health. 2012;4:451–454. doi: 10.2147/IJWH.S35104. Epub 2012 Sep 3. PMID: 23071415

5. Kuczkowski KM. Anesthesia for the repeat cesarean section in the parturient with abnormal placentation: what does an obstetrician need to know? Arch Gynecol Obstet. 2006 Mar;273(6):319–321. Epub 2005 Dec 9. Review. PMID: 16341867

6. Ioscovich A, Shatalin D, Butwick AJ, Ginosar Y, Orbach-Zinger S, Weiniger CF. Israeli survey of anesthesia practice related to placenta previa and accreta. Acta Anaesthesiol Scand. 2016 Apr;60(4):457–464. doi: 10.1111/aas.12656. Epub 2015 Nov 24. PMID: 26597396

7. Snegovskikh D, Clebone A, Norwitz E. Anesthetic management of patients with placenta accreta and resuscitation strategies for associated massive hemorrhage. Curr Opin Anaesthesiol. 2011 Jun;24(3):274–281. doi: 10.1097/ACO.0b013e328345d8b7. Review. PMID: 21494133

8. Peralta F, Wong CA. Interventional radiology in the pregnant patient for obstetric and nonobstetric indications: organizational, anesthetic, and procedural issues. Curr Opin Anaesthesiol. 2013 Aug;26(4):450–455. doi: 10.1097/ACO.0b013e3283625e89. Review. PMID: 23756912

9. Chu Q, Shen D, He L, Wang H, Zhao X, Chen Z, Wang Y, Zhang W. Anesthetic management of cesarean section in cases of placenta accreta, with versus without abdominal aortic balloon occlusion: study protocol for a randomized controlled trial. Trials. 2017 May 26;18(1):240. doi: 10.1186/s13063-017-1977-5. PMID: 28549439

10. Fujita N, Higuchi H, Sakuma S, Takagi S, Latif MAHM, Ozaki M. Effect of right-lateral versus left-lateral tilt position on compression of the inferior vena cava in pregnant women determined by magnetic resonance imaging. Anesth Analg. 2019 Jun;128(6):1217–1222. doi: 10.1213/ANE.0000000000004166. PMID: 31094791

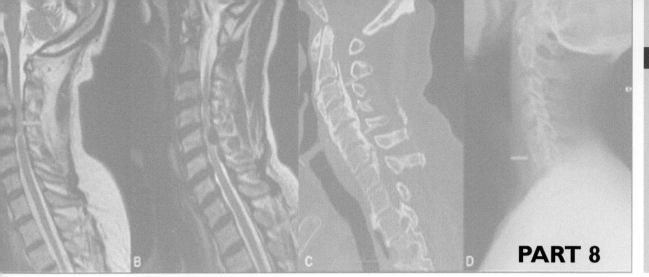
B   C   D

PART 8

EQUIPMENT, FACILITIES, CRM

Chapter 30

Anesthesia Machine Failures

Isaac Luria and Robert G. Loeb

Summary Page

Low Breathing Circuit Pressure:

Symptoms:

- Low circuit pressure alarm
- Bellows/reservoir bag collapse
- Inadequate patient tidal volumes
- Apnea alarm(s)—based on loss of pressure, flow, or carbon dioxide

Breathing Circuit Obstruction:

Symptoms:

- Low tidal volume or minute ventilation alarms
- Loss of capnography
- High airway pressure alarm
- Low airway pressure alarm
- High positive end-expiratory pressure
- Changes in flow-volume loops
- Changes in pressure-volume loops

Oxygen Pipeline Failure:

Symptoms:

- Low oxygen supply pressure alarm
- Low pressure on oxygen pipeline gauge
- Low pressure alarm on central pressure panel
- Oxygen flowmeter reading lower than previously set

- Nitrous oxide flowmeter reading lower than previously set
- Unable to drive bellows alarm
- Low circuit FiO_2 alarm
- Decreasing blood oxygen saturation

Hypoxic Oxygen Pipeline Mixture:

Symptoms:

- Low circuit FiO_2 alarm (from integrated oxygen analyzer or multigas analyzer)
- Circuit FiO_2 significantly lower than set
- Low patient oxygen saturation
- Condition worsens when increasing oxygen flow

Electrical Power Failure:

Symptoms:

- Electrical mains failure alarm on anesthesia machine
- Backup battery in use indicator light/message on anesthesia machine
- Loss of anesthesia machine electronic displays
- Ventilator failure
- Loss of power to other operating room equipment (including physiologic monitor)
- Loss of lighting

Differential Diagnosis:

- Medical causes of increased airway pressure (e.g., bronchospasm or surgical insufflation)
- Medical causes of patient hypoxia (i.e., atelectasis or bronchospasm)

Introduction

Anesthesia machine failures can be confusing for anesthesia providers.[1,2] It can be difficult in some cases to distinguish a patient's medical problems from a failure of equipment.[3] Under general anesthesia, the anesthesia machine functions as a life support system for the operative patient. While anesthesia machine or infrastructure failures are rare, they do happen.[4] Their rarity can make them difficult to diagnose, but the correct diagnosis cannot be made if it is not even on the list of considerations. The steps outlined in this chapter are important in their own right, but an important overarching lesson is to include equipment malfunction in the differential diagnosis of any intraoperative problem.

Caring for the safety of the patient first and foremost is vital when trying to diagnose what could be a machine problem. Resolving anesthesia machine failures should only be attempted after the safety of the patient has been otherwise secured. Such safety measures may include switching to a self-inflating rescue breathing device (SIRB), calling for help, or using a portable oxygen tank to completely remove the anesthesia machine variable from patient care.

A complete pre-use check will prevent many anesthesia machine problems, but the focus in this chapter is on failures that can appear during anesthesia despite a thorough pre-use check. This chapter provides an approach to the diagnosis and management of low breathing circuit pressure, breathing circuit obstruction, oxygen pipeline failure, hypoxic oxygen pipeline mixture, and anesthesia machine power failure.

Management

It is important to first ensure the safety of the patient before addressing any anesthesia equipment issues or failures. Ensure adequate oxygenation and ventilation, and hemodynamic stability. If the patient is unstable, disconnect the patient from the anesthesia machine and ventilate with a self-inflating rescue breathing device (SIRB)/bag-valve mask (BVM) and deliver oxygen from an oxygen tank. Once the patient is stable, the machine issues can be addressed.

Anesthesia machine and other equipment resources are stocked, maintained, repaired, and routinely checked by anesthesia technicians and clinical engineering support staff. Always be aware of these resources to call for help if needed or to execute safe judgment in situations where such help is likely to be slow or unavailable. Machine failures can be due to a variety of problems. Each type of problem will be addressed step by step separately.

A. Low Breathing Circuit Pressure

Step by Step

1. Diagnose and manage low breathing circuit pressure.

This will present as inadequate patient tidal volumes and the low circuit pressure or apnea alarms will go off.[5] If airway pressures are negative, immediately disconnect the patient from the anesthesia breathing circuit and ventilate via a SIRB/BVM (Figure 30.1).

> **WARNING!!** Sustained negative pressure within the breathing circuit can rapidly lead to negative pressure pulmonary edema!

>> **Tip on Technique:** A SIRB can be used to ventilate an unstable patient with room air until the anesthesia machine is repaired or replaced. Use a transport oxygen cylinder to provide supplemental oxygen as needed. Inhaled anesthetics cannot be administered if the anesthesia machine is not being used, so an alternate method of anesthesia will be required.

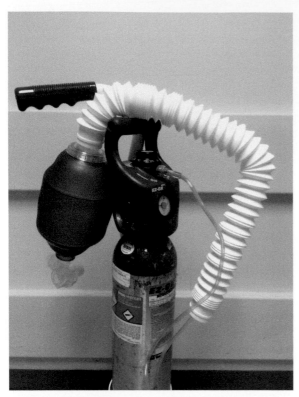

Figure 30.1 Self-inflating rescue breathing device (SIRB) and transport oxygen cylinder.

2. Increase anesthesia machine fresh gas flow.

Increase the anesthesia machine fresh gas flow to 10 L/min of 100% oxygen.

>> **Tip on Technique:** This will overcome most leaks and allow a search for the problem. Quantifying an anesthesia machine leak rate can help determine where the leak may be located and whether or not it is clinically significant. Most anesthesia machines have a visual indicator of breathing circuit volume at end exhalation: during manual ventilation it is the size of the breathing bag at end exhalation; in a bellows ventilator it is the size of the bellows at end exhalation; with a piston or impeller-driven ventilator (where the breathing bag remains in the circuit during mechanical ventilation) it is the size of the breathing bag at end exhalation.

To quantify the leak, set the fresh gas flow to 10 L/min and slowly turn down the fresh gas flow until the indicator of circuit volume at end exhalation just begins to decrease with each breath. The minimum flow at which it does not decrease is the leak rate. A significant leak that causes total loss of circuit volume at high fresh gas flow will certainly need to be addressed quickly; however, a small leak that can be masked by 500 mL/min of fresh gas flow may not need to be addressed urgently based on clinical judgment.

3. Look for common sources of low circuit pressure.

Easily visible sources of leak include:
- Endotracheal tube (ETT) or supraglottic airway (SGA) disconnected from breathing circuit
- Circuit tubing disconnected from anesthesia machine

- Accidental total or partial extubation, or SGA displacement
- Lack of fresh gas flow
- Low tidal volume or inspiratory pressure ventilator settings
Hidden sources of leak include:
- Open carbon dioxide absorber canister
- Leak around the ETT cuff or SGA
- Nasogastric/orogastric suction tube misplaced in trachea
- Opened vaporizer filling port

4. Rule out a ventilator problem.

Switch to manual ventilation and close the adjustable pressure-limiting (APL) valve.

If the breathing bag does not fill at 10 L/min of fresh gas flow, then look for large leaks in the breathing circuit or suction being applied to the breathing circuit (e.g., from a malpositioned gastric tube). All other causes of such a large leak are likely to be internal to the machine or scavenging system, the diagnosis of which is beyond the scope of this chapter. Request further assistance in resolving the machine problem or replacing the machine while utilizing backup ventilation equipment (e.g., SIRB) to support the patient.

5. Perform a circuit leak check.

Disconnect the patient from the breathing circuit and perform a circuit leak check as one would during a pre-use check: occlude the Y-piece, close the APL valve, turn off fresh gas flow, and pressurize the circuit to between 30 and 40 cm H_2O. If there is a leak in the breathing circuit, squeezing the breathing bag while listening for the leak can help locate it. A stable circuit pressure suggests no circuit leak.

If there is not a leak, the problem is probably within the patient, for example, an ETT cuff leak or unplanned extubation, a misplaced gastric tube, or a bronchial or tracheal fistula. The problem could also be a malfunctioning scavenger system. Check for this by fully opening the APL valve while occluding the Y-piece. If the circuit pressure becomes negative, disconnect the malfunctioning scavenger system.

>> **Tip on Technique**: Titrating fresh gas flow to assess leak rate in mL/min can provide additional information in deciding if a leak is clinically significant or urgent. A small leak can likely wait for a safe time to evaluate, while a large leak will likely need to be addressed sooner rather than later.

B. Breathing Circuit Obstruction

Step by Step

1. Diagnose and manage breathing circuit obstruction.

Circuit obstruction can present as low tidal volumes, loss of capnography, or high peak end-expiratory pressure (PEEP) and will trigger airway pressure alarms. Immediately disconnect the patient from the breathing circuit if sustained airway pressure is present.

> **WARNING!!** If peak and nadir airway pressures are high, sustained positive pressure within the breathing circuit can rapidly lead to barotrauma and cardiovascular collapse!

2. Locate the site of circuit obstruction.

Obstructions within the patient or ETT tend to cause high peak airway pressure but normal nadir airway pressure (PEEP). Go to step 3 for management.

Obstructions on the inspiratory side of the breathing circuit tend to cause low peak airway pressure. Go to step 4 for management.

Obstructions on the expiratory side of the breathing circuit or scavenger system tend to cause high peak and nadir airway pressures. Go to steps 4 and 5 for management.

3. Look for and correct obstruction within the lungs of the patient or the ETT.

Consider bronchospasm, pneumothorax, mainstem intubation, abdominal insufflation or ascites, a kinked ETT, heavy secretion burden, or mucous plugging as a source of obstruction.

>> **Tip on Technique:** Passing a suction catheter down the ETT can aid in such a diagnosis and fix a problem caused by secretion plugging.

4. Look for and correct obstruction within the breathing system.

Consider as a cause wrong breathing tubing connections; improperly placed humidifiers or unidirectional PEEP valves; external crimping of the circuit; internal obstruction, such as by mucous plug or water; plastic wrapping or caps left on the CO_2 absorbent; a rubber stopper between the anesthesia machine and breathing circuit (such stoppers are part of an automated check for some machines); or a stuck inspiratory or expiratory valve. Remove/fix any of these problems if detected.

>> **Tip on Technique:** Pay special attention to any component that may have been changed or adjusted since the anesthesia machine pre-use check.

5. Look for and correct obstruction of the scavenger system.

Consider and correct if detected:

- Scavenger system is disconnected from waste anesthesia gas outlet
- External crimping of hose between breathing circuit and scavenger system
- Internal obstruction of hose between breathing circuit and scavenger system
- Failure of APL valve that leads to scavenger system
- Failure of ventilator relief valve that leads to scavenger system

A failed underpressurization valve will cause the scavenging system to suck gas out of the breathing circuit instead of drawing in room air like it should. This will cause loss of breathing circuit volume and low breathing circuit pressure, and even negative breathing circuit pressure. A failed overpressurization valve will cause a closed scavenging system to back up when flow from the breathing circuit exceeds the vacuum flow rate, rather than venting to the room as it should. This will produce high peak and nadir circuit pressures, which worsen with increased fresh gas flow.

C. Oxygen Pipeline Failure

Step by Step

1. Diagnose and manage pipeline pressure failure.

Check pipeline pressure to verify that it is below 30 PSIG (200 kPa). Notify others that you are concerned about possible O_2 pipeline failure.

> **WARNING!!** Such a failure could affect other rooms or even the entire hospital.

>> **Tip on Technique:** On a machine that does not have mechanical gauges, you may need to configure the display to see compressed gas supply pressures (Figure 30.2).

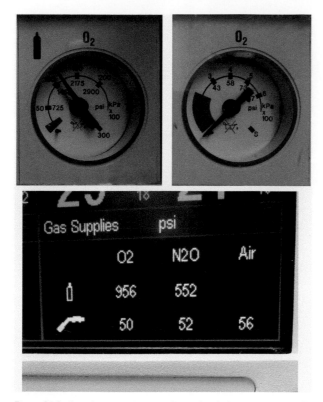

Figure 30.2 Anesthesia machine mechanical and electronic gauges. Older anesthesia machines may have mechanical cylinder (top left) and pipeline (top right) pressure gauges. Mechanical gauges are in a constant location and typically display pressures in units of PSIG and kPa. Newer anesthesia machines may have electronic displays of pipeline and cylinder pressures (bottom). Electronic displays may require user action, which varies by anesthesia machine model, to be displayed and alter the units.

2. Open the backup oxygen cylinder.

Opening the backup oxygen cylinder should "fix" the problem. See Figure 30.3 on how to open the cylinder. Verify the pressure on the anesthesia machine cylinder pressure gauge and that the cylinder is delivering flowed oxygen to the patient.

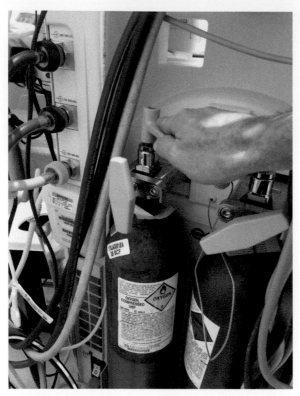

Figure 30.3 How to open the O$_2$ cylinder. The backup oxygen cylinder is opened by using a tank wrench to turn the valve counterclockwise. The cylinder is often located on the back of the anesthesia machine. It should be left closed when not in use.

3. Conserve the limited oxygen supply.

Take the following actions:

- Switch to manual ventilation and ventilate by hand or have the patient breathe spontaneously.
- Reduce total fresh gas flow and oxygen concentration as the patient tolerates.
- Confirm the auxiliary oxygen flowmeter (as used with nasal cannulas) is off.
- Request additional oxygen cylinders.

>> **Tip on Technique:** Switching to manual ventilation is an important step in conserving a limited oxygen supply in a bellows ventilator that uses oxygen as a drive gas. This step is not needed in piston- or impeller-type ventilators, or in bellows ventilators that use air as a drive gas. If unsure of ventilator type, it is safest to switch to manual ventilation.

4. Calculate running time on current backup cylinder.

Figure 30.4 shows how to calculate the time remaining in the cylinder using current cylinder pressure and oxygen consumption. If a pipeline oxygen problem is affecting the entire operating room (OR) suite, knowing the current runtime is an important factor in triaging who needs extra cylinders first.

$$\text{Time Remaining} = \frac{\text{Content of Tank}}{\text{Anesthesia Machine Oxygen Consumption}}$$

where Content of Tank = (Pressure in Tank/Pressure of Full Tank) × Content of Full Tank

and Anesthesia Machine Oxygen Consumption = Fresh Gas + Ventilator Drive Gas + Auxiliary
= Fresh Gas + (Tidal Volume ×
Respiratory Rate) + Auxiliary

In this Example:

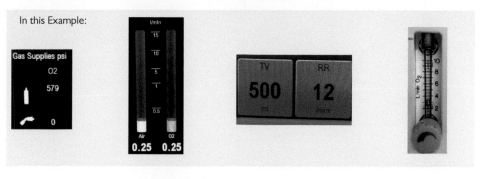

$$\text{Time Remaining} = \frac{(579\text{psi}/2200\text{psi}) \times 660\text{L}}{0.25\text{L/min} + (0.5\text{L} \times 12\text{breaths/min}) + 3\text{L/min}}$$

$$= \frac{174\text{L}}{0.25\text{L/min} + 6\text{L/min} + 3\text{L/min}}$$

$$= 19 \text{ min}$$

Figure 30.4 How to calculate time remaining. Calculating the time remaining when using an oxygen e-cylinder. As can be seen in the example, more gas is typically used to power a bellows ventilator than for the fresh gas flow. The importance of turning off the auxiliary oxygen is also shown. The time remaining would go from 19 minutes to over 11 hours if the ventilator and auxiliary oxygen were turned off. Note that electrically powered ventilators (e.g., piston and turbine) do not consume oxygen.

> **Caution!** DO NOT assume that every E size cylinder is a potential source of backup oxygen for the anesthesia machine. Many patient transport oxygen cylinders are E size but do not have the proper fitting to attach to an anesthesia machine yoke (Figure 30.5). If unsure, ask for help from someone with experience in changing anesthesia machine backup cylinders.

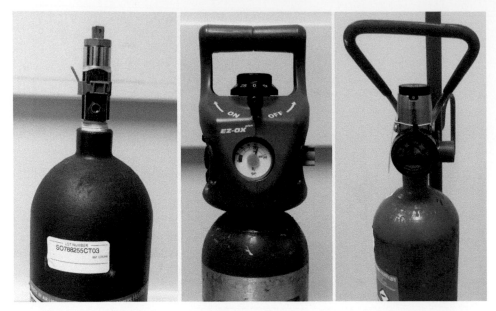

Figure 30.5 Oxygen cylinders with and without regulators. Transport oxygen cylinders often incorporate an integrated regulator/flowmeter. The two cylinders on the right are examples of such cylinders. Only the cylinder on the left can be mounted to an anesthesia machine yoke to provide backup oxygen. Note that the middle cylinder does have a DISS fitting (left side, not shown) that can be attached to the pipeline inlet of an anesthesia machine using a compatible hose.

D. Hypoxic Oxygen Pipeline Mixture

Step by Step

1. Diagnose and manage a hypoxic oxygen pipeline mixture.

> **WARNING!!** Such a failure could affect other rooms or even the entire hospital. Notify others that you are concerned about contamination of the central O_2 supply.

A hypoxic oxygen pipeline mixture will result in inadequate oxygen delivery to the patient, causing oxygen desaturation due to the delivery of an FiO_2 much lower than what is set on the machine. This should trigger the low circuit FiO_2 alarm from the oxygen analyzer.

Another potential cause for inadequate oxygen delivery to the patient is low-flow anesthesia, where the circuit oxygen concentration is predictably less than the dialed concentration. Malignant hyperthermia or other hypermetabolic conditions, which further decrease circuit oxygen concentration compared with dialed concentration, can also result in inadequate oxygen delivery.

2. Turn off all gases other than oxygen at high flow.

>> **Tip on Technique:** If the circuit oxygen concentration increases to 100%, then the problem was insufficient flow of oxygen into the breathing circuit. Consider a leak in the oxygen flowmeter (very rare event) if circuit oxygen concentration was lower than predicted based on fresh gas flows. If the concentration does NOT increase to 100%, consider and manage a hypoxic oxygen pipeline mixture via the steps below.

3. Open the backup oxygen cylinder and disconnect the oxygen pipeline from the anesthesia machine.

> **WARNING!!** Disconnecting the oxygen pipeline source is vital! Otherwise, gas will continue to flow from the oxygen pipeline source. Verify the pressure on the anesthesia machine cylinder pressure gauge.

Anesthesia machines regulate internal gas pressures to preferentially draw compressed gas from the pipeline over the backup cylinder so as not to drain the cylinder when it isn't needed. If there is concern that the pressurized gas in the pipeline is NOT oxygen, the pipeline MUST be disconnected before the cylinder oxygen will flow.

Possible causes of a hypoxic gas supply include:

- Contaminated central supply
- Crossed central supply pipelines, especially during or after construction/renovation
- Wrong cylinder attached to device (wrong cylinder problems almost always involve equipment that has been tampered with and important safety features removed)
- Oxygen hose attached to the wrong outlet (wrong attachment problems almost always involve equipment that has been tampered with and important safety features removed)
- Crossed lines within an anesthesia machine, especially after maintenance
- Unfamiliar equipment in line (e.g. an air/gas mixer at the oxygen pipeline outlet)

4. Conserve the limited oxygen supply.

Take the following actions:

- Switch to manual ventilation and ventilate by hand or have the patient breathe spontaneously.
- Reduce total fresh gas flow and oxygen concentration as the patient tolerates.
- Confirm the auxiliary oxygen flowmeter (as used with nasal cannulas) is off.
- Request additional oxygen cylinders.

> **>> Tip on Technique:** Switching to manual ventilation is an important step in conserving a limited oxygen supply in a bellows ventilator that uses oxygen as a drive gas. This step is not needed in piston- or impeller-type ventilators, or in bellows ventilators that use air as a drive gas. If unsure of ventilator type, it is safest to switch to manual ventilation.

5. Calculate running time on current backup cylinder.

Figure 30.4 shows how to calculate the time remaining in the cylinder using current cylinder pressure and oxygen consumption. If a pipeline oxygen problem is affecting the entire OR suite, knowing the current runtime is an important factor in triaging who needs extra cylinders first.

> **Caution!** DO NOT assume that every E size cylinder is a potential source of backup oxygen for the anesthesia machine. Many patient transport oxygen cylinders are E size but do not have the proper fitting to attach to an anesthesia machine yoke (see Figure 30.5). If unsure, ask for help from someone with experience in changing anesthesia machine backup cylinders.

E. Electrical Power Failure

Step by Step

1. Assess the degree of electrical power failure.

Is just the anesthesia machine affected? This is loss of power to only the anesthesia machine. Assess its connection to the main power outlet, and reconnect if disconnected. Ensure that the power switch (often located on the back of the machine, where the power cord is connected) is turned on.

Are some but not all pieces of electrical equipment in the OR affected? This is a tripped circuit breaker or ground fault interrupt circuit (GFIC) causing loss of power to one or a few outlets.

Unplug the last piece of equipment that was plugged in. Plug the anesthesia machine (and other crucial equipment) into other "live" outlets until the circuit breaker or GFIC is reset. A tripped circuit breaker or GFIC results when too much equipment is plugged into a single circuit breaker or when a short-circuited piece of equipment is plugged into a GFIC. The last piece of equipment plugged in or powered on either overloaded the circuit or contained a short circuit; it should be checked.

Are most or all pieces of equipment affected with loss of lighting? This is power failure to the entire OR, and perhaps the facility or region. Pieces of equipment with backup battery will continue uninterrupted, but lighting and other equipment will not function until facility backup power starts. Backup power will not supply all outlets. During a power failure of the entire OR, facility, or region, ensure that the anesthesia machine and other crucial equipment are connected to a red outlet that provides power from a backup generator.

>> **Tip on Technique:** New anesthesia machines have battery backup that powers all functions. Older anesthesia machines may not power the ventilator while on battery, and manual ventilation may be needed until power is restored.

2. If main power is not restored, ensure that the ventilator functions on battery, and conserve battery power.

Consider switching to manual or spontaneous ventilation to conserve battery life (especially with a piston or impeller ventilator). The machine will continue to function with limited capabilities if the battery fails. Manual ventilation with oxygen will still be possible, but the ventilator will stop working.

Depending on the anesthesia machine, fresh gas may be controlled with a different knob and gas flows other than oxygen may be lost. Flow may be measured on a separate flowmeter (of total flow) and administration of volatile anesthetics may stop. Reference the anesthesia machine user manual for specific capabilities and instructions.

Caution! Systemwide considerations to address if electrical power is lost in multiple locations:
- Elective cases should be canceled or delayed during a generalized failure unless the facility has backup generators that are expected to power the facility indefinitely.
- Backup generators are powered by liquid fuels, which need to be replenished.
- Backup generators are often located at ground level and are susceptible to failure during flooding.

Other Management Considerations

It is important to be able to distinguish an oxygen pipeline pressure failure from a hypoxic oxygen pipeline. While both of these scenarios will require similar (but not identical) interventions, the presentation may be different enough to warrant explanation. Oxygen pipeline failure is specifically a loss of pressure in the central oxygen pipeline. The anesthesia machine will no longer have oxygen pressure to supply fresh gas flow and ventilator bellows drive gas; the oxygen pipeline pressure gauge will read low pressure; the fail-safe valves will terminate the flow of nitrous oxide and other non-oxygen-containing gases; and alarms will report low oxygen supply pressure. In the case of a hypoxic oxygen pipeline mixture, pressurized gas is available to the anesthesia machine, but this gas is not pure oxygen. There will be no low-pressure alarms, and pipeline pressure gauges will read normal. This scenario is more confusing to providers because the first indication may not be an anesthesia machine alarm but rather a patient alarm such as low SpO_2. This can lead to tunnel vision in searching for an abnormal patient condition when the true problem is in the equipment. The anesthesia machine may also sound an alarm that circuit oxygen is low (frequently set to an inspired oxygen concentration of 18–21%). Assuming adequate fresh gas flow and a properly calibrated oxygen analyzer, such an alarm always indicates a hypoxic gas in the breathing circuit, either from a hypoxic oxygen supply or a leak at the oxygen flowmeter. The response to a hypoxic oxygen pipeline mixture is the same as for an oxygen pipeline failure except that in the former, disconnecting the pipeline oxygen supply is vital.

Further Reading

Loeb RG. Anesthesia machines: prevention, diagnosis, and management of malfunctions. In: UpToDate, Nussmeier, NA (Ed), UpToDate, Waltham, MA. (2017): https://www.uptodate.com/contents/anesthesia-machines-prevention-diagnosis-and-management-of-malfunctions

References

1. Buffington CW, Ramanathan S, Turndorf H. Detection of anesthesia machine faults. Anesth Analg 1984; 63:79.
2. Larson ER, Nuttall GA, Ogren BD, et al. A prospective study on anesthesia machine fault identification. Anesth Analg 2007; 104:154.
3. Webb RK, Russell WJ, Klepper I, Runciman WB. The Australian Incident Monitoring Study. Equipment failure: an analysis of 2000 incident reports. Anaesth Intensive Care 1993; 21:673.
4. Cassidy CJ, Smith A, Arnot-Smith J. Critical incident reports concerning anaesthetic equipment: analysis of the UK National Reporting and Learning System (NRLS) data from 2006–2008. Anaesthesia 2011; 66:879.
5. Raphael DT, Weller RS, Doran DJ. A response algorithm for the low-pressure alarm condition. Anesth Analg 1988; 67:876.

Chapter 31

Operating Room Fires

Jennifer R. Matos and David Gutman

Summary Page
Symptoms:

- Popping/crackling sound heard
- Smell of smoke
- Seeing flames/smoke in the operating room, or near or on the patient

Differential Diagnosis:

Fire within the patient's airway (see Chapter 1 on Airway Fires)

Introduction

Operating room (OR) fires that occur in the OR theater can be divided into those that occur within the airway versus on or around the patient or drapes. The Emergency Care Research Institute (ECRI) estimates that 90–100 surgical fires occur every year.[1] As such, an OR fire is a very rare but potentially devastating event that can lead to significant morbidity or mortality. For a fire to occur, there must be three elements present: an oxidizer, an ignition source, and a fuel. This is known as the "fire triad," and if any one of these is not present, a fire cannot happen (Figure 31.1).

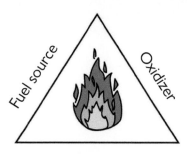

Ignition source

Oxidizers	Fuel
Oxygen	Patient
Nitrous Oxide	Drapes
	Gauzes
Ignition Sources	Dressings
Electrocautery	Gowns
Heating Probes	Endotracheal Tubes
Defibrillators	02 Masks
Fiberoptic Scopes	Intestinal Gases
Electrosurgical Devices	Blankets
Static Electricity	Sponges
Lasers	Gloves
	Prep-Solutions
	Ventilator Circuits

Figure 31.1 Fire triad.

An analysis of malpractice claims involving an OR fire from the American Society of Anesthesiologists Closed Claims Database found that 90% of claims involved electrocautery as the primary ignition source, with 95% having supplemental oxygen as the oxidizer source.[2] Of the electrocautery-induced OR fires, 85% of these events occurred during head, neck, and upper chest surgery. The analysis also revealed that 83% of the fires occurred during monitored anesthesia care (MAC) and sedation cases where oxygen was delivered via an open delivery system (nasal cannula or facemask).

High-risk procedures are those where an ignition source contacts an oxidizer-rich environment and may include:

- Any case involving the airway (i.e., tonsillectomy, tracheostomy, removal of laryngeal papillomas) is at increased risk since electrocautery or lasers can potentially be used in an oxygen-rich area, causing combustion.
- MAC (cataract excisions, etc.) cases are at higher risk since they employ an open system for supplemental oxygen delivery, leading to an oxygen-rich environment.

- Removal of lesions on the head, neck, and face is also higher risk given the proximity to the airway and supplemental oxygen.
- Procedures employing ignition sources (lasers, electrocautery, fiberoptic scopes) all increase the risks of OR fire given that they can ignite a fuel source such as the drapes or wet prep.

Note: The treatment of airway fires is covered in Chapter 1.

Treatment

The first step of OR fire management should be fire prevention.

Prevention strategies for fire include:

- During the surgical timeout, if there is a higher risk of surgical fires (head/neck, upper chest, etc.) this should be identified and discussed, and it should be ensured that appropriate equipment (extra saline, etc.) is available, and potential personnel assignments in the event of a fire should be assigned.
- Since open oxygen delivery systems (nasal cannula, facemask) were involved in most of the OR fires, use of a closed oxygen delivery system (endotracheal tube [ETT], supraglottic airway [SGA]) should be considered for head and neck surgeries.
- Cuffed endotracheal tubes should be used for all surgeries involving the airway.
- The lowest oxygen concentration possible should be used for patients with the goal of <30% FiO_2 for MAC cases involving the head and neck. For patients with pulmonary comorbidities (i.e., chronic obstructive pulmonary disease, prior lung resection) who cannot tolerate an FiO_2 of 30% or less, an SGA or ETT should be considered.
- The surgeon should give advanced warning before electrocautery is used in the airway to allow reduction in the FiO_2.
- Laser-resistant ETTs should be used for laser surgery.
- For high-risk cases, electrocautery should be limited to short bursts and preferentially bipolar electrocautery used.
- Nitrous oxide should be avoided in cases at high risk for fire.
- Prep solutions may act as a fuel source for fires. Patients with more body hair and those with excess or lax skin tissue that forms multiple folds may allow pooling of the prep solution, leading to inadequate drying. This increases the risk of a surgical fire. Consider the use of a timer to ensure adequate drying of surgical prep solutions. At least 3 minutes is recommended.[3]
- Improper draping can lead to oxygen trapping under the occlusive drapes, leading to an oxygen-rich environment; suctioning of gases under the drapes for head and neck procedures can be done to reduce oxygen concentrations.
- Moisten sponges and gauze when an ignition source is used in close proximity.

Step by Step

Note: This sequence should follow the recommended RACE acronym:

- **R**escue (assist anyone in immediate danger to a safe area)
- **A**lert/**A**larm (others to presence of fire)
- **C**ontain (confine fire by closing doors behind you during evacuation)
- **E**xtinguish (attempt to put out the fire)/evacuate if needed

1. **Recognize that a fire is present.**

    A fire should be suspected if a popping/crackling sound is heard, there is the smell of smoke, or flames or smoke is seen in the OR, near the patient, or on the patient. Failure to act promptly or a delay in treatment must be avoided. While the smell of charred body tissue is not uncommon in the OR, extra vigilance and speed of reaction must be increased for high-risk cases in which fire is considered.

WARNING!!   Fires under the drapes may present as smoke only.

---

2. **Rescue or relocate anyone in immediate danger.**

    If personnel are standing next to the fire, tell them to move. If they are unable to move themselves, direct other personnel to remove them from the flames while you ensure patient safety.

3. **Immediately alert all personnel to the presence of a fire.**

    Clearly announce that there is a fire. Ensure that ALL members of the OR team are alerted.

    Call for additional help. The moment a fire is either suspected or detected and this is vocalized, it must be promptly verbalized and the entire team must respond in accordance with fire algorithms expediently to best take care of the patient.

4. **Stop the procedure.**

    Immediately halt the operation. Turn off any ignition sources: electrocautery, laser, fiberoptic scopes, etc.

5. **Remove all burning and flammable material from patient.**

    Remove all drapes or equipment that is burning or smoking. Remove all hot or burning debris from the patient.

6. **Contain the fire and extinguish any burning material.**

    Use saline to extinguish flames and any burning material, **EXCEPT** for electrical fires.

    >> **Tip on Technique:** If unable to extinguish burning material with saline, a CO_2 fire extinguisher can be used on the patient.

    How to use a fire extinguisher to extinguish flames (PASS):
    - **P**ull the locking pin from its place.
    - **A**im nozzle at the base of the flames.
    - **S**queeze the handles together.
    - **S**weep the spray from side to side at the base of the fire.

    Stop the flow of all airway gases or other contributors to the fire. Stop ALL ignition (laser, electrocautery, flexible bronchoscopes, etc.) and oxidizer sources (oxygen, nitrous oxide) (see Figure 31.1) of the fire triad.

    If the fire is in close proximity to the patient's face or chest and an open source of oxygen is being used (nasal cannula or facemask), turn off the oxygen source. If a laser is being used, confirm it is turned off. If electrocautery is being used, tell the surgeon to turn it off.

    Ensure the OR doors are closed. Attempt to disconnect appliances as able. With anesthesiology approval, the oxygen shutoff valve can be used to discontinue oxygen flow to the OR if necessary.

7. **Activate the fire alarm system, if appropriate.**

Pull the fire alarm switch. Call the hospital operator or institution fire services line and provide vital information. Call 911 and provide vital information.

8. **Evacuate the area, if appropriate.**

If the fire is not controlled, consider relocating the patient to another OR if stable. If under general or neuraxial anesthesia, the patient can be rolled out of the OR on the OR table or lowered to the floor on a sheet and dragged to safety. The anesthesia team should stay with the patient to continue to provide care.

If the situation allows and the patient is stable, the surgeon can close the incision prior to moving the patient. If the patient or situation is not stable enough for timely suturing, the surgeon can pack the wound with wet laps and assist with moving the patient out of harm's way. If the patient only received local anesthesia and is stable, they can be assisted out of the room.

Evacuate all nonessential personnel not providing care to the patient.

9. **Assess the patient for injury.**

Assess the patient for burns. Remove all coverings from the patient to facilitate a thorough exam.

Assess the depth (degree of burn), location, and extent of any burns sustained by the patient:

- First-degree burns: superficial, only affecting the epidermis, appears red and painful, without blisters (i.e., mild sunburn)
- Second-degree burns: involve epidermis and dermis, appear red and blistered
- Third-degree burns: epidermis and dermis are destroyed, may appear white or blackened and charred
- Fourth-degree burns: damage all layers of skin and deeper tissues, may involve muscle and bone

Patients undergoing MAC or sedation with supplemental oxygen via nasal cannula may have experienced an inhalational burn injury. If there is melted plastic or debris on their face/neck or charring of the hair in the nares, or if they endorse any respiratory compromise, immediately intubate them as they can experience profound airway edema quickly (see Chapter 1 on airway fires).

For major burns, the patient should be transferred to a burn center for definitive care.

Burn center referral criteria include:

- Second degree (partial thickness) >10% total body
- Burns involving face, hands, feet, genitalia, perineum, or major joints
- Third-degree burns
- Electrical or chemical burns
- Inhalation injury
- Patients with preexisting medical disease that could complicate management, prolong recovery, or affect mortality
- Patients with trauma where burns are the greatest risk of morbidity and mortality
- Burns in children in hospitals without qualified personnel or equipment to care for children
- Burns in patients who will require special social, emotional, or rehabilitative intervention

10. Provide burn care if indicated.

All patients with significant risk for inhalation injury should have a thorough airway examination, and intubation should be performed early when the airway is compromised. Preemptive intubation of patients with inhalation injury can be lifesaving but should be performed for clear indications. Succinylcholine may be used for the initial intubation but should be avoided 48 hours onward from burn injury due to concern for exaggerated hyperkalemic response.

For patients with inhalational injury, bronchodilators (i.e., albuterol) may be used for bronchospasm, but corticosteroids should be avoided secondary to an increased risk of infection.

Initially, saline-soaked gauze can be applied to small and moderate-sized burn areas to cool the area to minimize the injury zone. Core temperature should be monitored to ensure the patient does not develop systemic hypothermia.

For more severe burns (nonsuperficial), topical antibiotics should be applied. A burn center should be called and consulted for the appropriate topical antibiotic prior to transfer.

For moderate to severe burns, fluid resuscitation with crystalloid solutions using the Parkland or Brooke fluid resuscitation formula can be used. The Parkland formula for fluid resuscitation is 4 ml/kg/% body surface area with the first half given in first 8 hours and the second half over next 16 hours. Ensure proper warming as these patients may be prone to excess heat loss.

11. Hold a postevent debriefing.

Involve intraoperative staff and OR coordinators. Review and document all steps that were taken and outcomes. Notify senior management of the event. Hold a family meeting including the patient and provide full disclosure of intraoperative events. Provide reassurance and counseling, including short- and long-term posttraumatic stress disorder counseling as needed. Coordinate care with patient representatives, if applicable.

Report the fire to the local fire department. Report the sentinel event to the state health department. Contact risk management and advise them of the event, and follow any additional institutional protocols.

Other Management Considerations

Fire prevention is a team approach and is difficult to predict or prepare for. All hospital employees and especially OR staff should have mandatory yearly or even more frequent reeducation and updates on fire protocols and procedures.

Steps that can be taken to reduce fire risk in the OR include:

- Working areas should be kept free of debris.
- Unsafe equipment and conditions must be addressed.
- Flammable material should be properly stored.
- Doors should not be wedged, propped open, or in any way secured in an open position.

Employees should be aware of the location of fire alarm stations, fire extinguishers, exit routes, and means of reporting and securing assistance in their immediate work areas. Everyone should be aware of the institutional acronyms for dealing with fires both in the OR and in the medical center as a whole (i.e., PASS, RACE, REACT).

PASS (fire extinguisher use):

- **P**ull the locking pin.
- **A**im the nozzle at the base of the flames.
- **S**queeze the handles together.
- **S**weep the spray.

RACE:

- **R**escue (assist anyone in immediate danger to a safe area).
- **A**lert/**A**larm (others to presence of fire).
- **C**ontain (confine fire by closing doors behind you during evacuation).
- **E**xtinguish (attempt to put out the fire)/evacuate if needed.

REACT:

- **R**emove those in immediate danger.
- **E**nsure all doors are closed.
- **A**ctivate the fire alarm.
- **C**all the fire department.
- **T**ry to extinguish the fire.

Further Reading

Gaba DM, Fish KJ Howard SK, Burden AR. Chapter 5: Operating Room Fire. In DM Gaba, KJ Fish, SK Howard, AR Burden, editors. *Crisis Management in Anesthesiology*. Philadelphia: Elsevier/Saunders; 2015:122–124.

Day AT, Rivera E, Farlow JL, Gourn CG, Nussenbaum B. Surgical fires in otolaryngology: a systematic and narrative review. *Otolaryngol Head Neck Surg*. 2018 Apr;158(4):598–616.

Rinder CS. Fire safety in the operating room. *Curr Opin Anaesthesiol*. 2008 Dec;21(6):790–795.

References

1. ECRI Institute. Surgical Fire Prevention. https://www.ecri.org/solutions/accident-investigation-services/surgical-fire-prevention/ Accessed August 23, 2022.

2. Mehta S, Bhananker S, Posner K, et al. Operating room fires: a closed claims analysis. *Anesthesiology*. 2013;118(5):1133–1139. doi:10.1097/ALN.0b013e31828afa7b.

3. Apfelbaum J, Caplan R, Barker S, et al. Practice Advisory for the Prevention and Management of Operating Room Fires. *Anesthesiology*. 2013;118(2):271–290. doi:10.1097/aln.0b013e31827773d2.

Chapter 32
Crisis Resource Management

Lauren C. Berkow and Keith Ruskin

Introduction

Anesthesia was the first medical specialty to recognize the role of human factors and crisis resource management (CRM) in improving patient safety. This chapter will review the basics of CRM, including teamwork, communication, shared mental models, and situation awareness. Lack of good communication is one of the most common causes of adverse events and medical errors. Good communication fosters clear team roles and collective decision-making. Strategies that improve communication, foster teamwork, and anticipate and plan for emergencies can have a significant impact on outcome. The use of checklists and cognitive aids can help standardize patient care as well as ensure that vital steps are not skipped in the emergent setting. The use of simulation and team training can improve communication in the operating room.

Management

Step by Step

1. Know your environment.

Being familiar with the environment you work in is vital when emergencies occur. This includes:

- Knowing the physical environment:
    - Be familiar with the equipment used in routine and emergency situations.
    - Perform all required machine and safety checks.
    - Confirm that you have all necessary equipment and medications available for use.
- Knowing the personnel in the environment:
    - What procedures are usually performed by a surgeon or other physician?
    - Are the nurses or other support staff familiar with the planned procedure?
    - Are there personnel who can help during a critical event?
- Knowing what equipment is available and where to find it

Pearl: Operating room briefings or "timeouts" provide an opportunity for all the members of the team to introduce themselves. Making this routine practice will breed familiarity in the team.

!! **Potential Complication**: Lack of familiarity with colleagues can affect communication during an emergency. Lack of available equipment can result in the lack of ability to carry out an intended plan or action during an emergency.

WARNING!!   Nurses and proceduralists may not be familiar with terminology commonly used by anesthesiologists. If you need a piece of equipment or help with a technical procedure, use simple language whenever possible. For example, instead of asking for "cricoid pressure," show the assistant what you need.

---

2. Anticipate and plan for emergencies.

Effective response and treatment of an anesthetic emergency starts before the emergency even occurs. Anticipate what emergency could happen for any case, both elective and emergent, and plan for the response to that emergent event.

Advance planning for possible complications and emergencies also makes the anesthesia provider more aware and vigilant to watch for these events.

Know where the emergency equipment, such as the crash cart, defibrillator, or difficult airway cart, is located. If the possibility of needing this equipment is high, have it in the room just in case before the procedure begins.

>> **Tip on Technique**: Review potential complications with the entire team at the briefing or "timeout" at the beginning of the day to allow the entire team to anticipate problems and plan for an emergency response. Use the Risk Assessment Matrix tool as an aid to planning (Figure 32.1).[1]

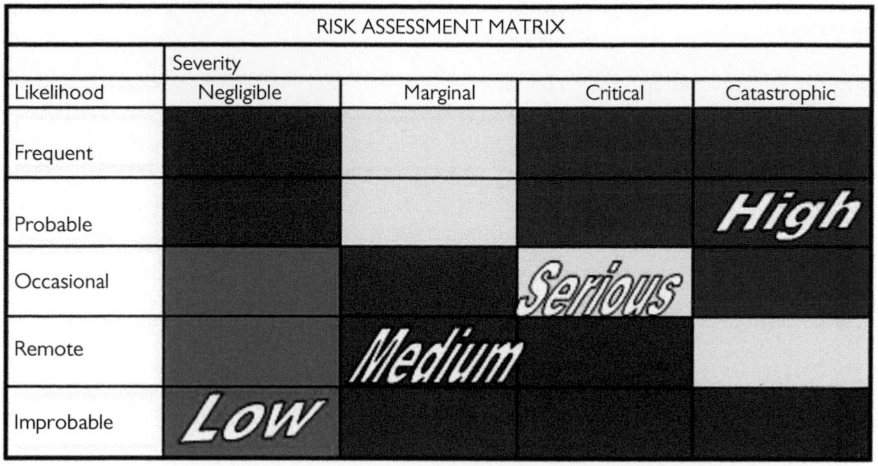

RISK ASSESSMENT MATRIX				
	Severity			
Likelihood	Negligible	Marginal	Critical	Catastrophic
Frequent				
Probable				*High*
Occasional			*Serious*	
Remote		*Medium*		
Improbable	*Low*			

Figure 32.1 Risk Assessment Matrix Tool, developed by the US Federal Aviation Administration. Source: https://www.faa.gov/regulations_policies/handbooks_manuals/aviation/media/risk_management_hb_change_1.pdf

‼ **Potential Complication**: Lack of preparation and planning for emergencies may delay recognition and response to an emergency should it occur.

Caution! Ensure that equipment and/or cognitive aids that will be required during the initial management of a high-risk critical event are present before starting the procedure.

3. Call for help early and mobilize all available resources.

This simple but important step is often delayed in the initial chaotic moments of an anesthesia emergency.

Have a mechanism in place to rapidly call for help in the operating room environment and ensure that all team members are familiar with that mechanism. This will decrease the time required for help to arrive. Help should include additional personnel to help as well as needed medications and equipment.

>> **Tip on Technique**: Examples of mechanisms that can allow for rapid response to a call for help include a button to push or a clear message paged overhead such as "anesthesia stat" or "code blue."

WARNING!! If a procedure is taking place outside of the main operating room, help may take longer than usual to arrive. This delay should be anticipated and included in the decision to call for help.

‼ **Potential Complication**: A lack of additional/available resources can prohibit effective and timely response to an emergency. Simulation of an emergency can identify gaps in needed resources and also educate providers on how to mobilize resources effectively.[2]

>>**Tip on Technique**: In an emergency, use all available personnel. For example, a medical student or nurse can help to move equipment or retrieve a piece of equipment that is urgently needed.

>> **Tip on Technique**: Having certain specialized emergency equipment already compiled together into a cart, tackle box, or other receptacle can simplify the emergency response by not having to travel to different locations to obtain equipment or medications.

4. **Set priorities and use cognitive aids.**

Cognitive aids can be very useful to set priorities and may include checklists, briefing or debriefing tools, and published algorithms. See Figure 32.2 for an example of a cognitive aid for airway management. See Figure 32.3 for a checklist for management of delayed emergence.

>> **Tip on Technique**: Cognitive aids may be used to confirm a diagnosis, verify drug dosages, and ensure that all critical steps are taken to resolve an event.[3] Use of a cognitive aid may increase the probability of a successful outcome.

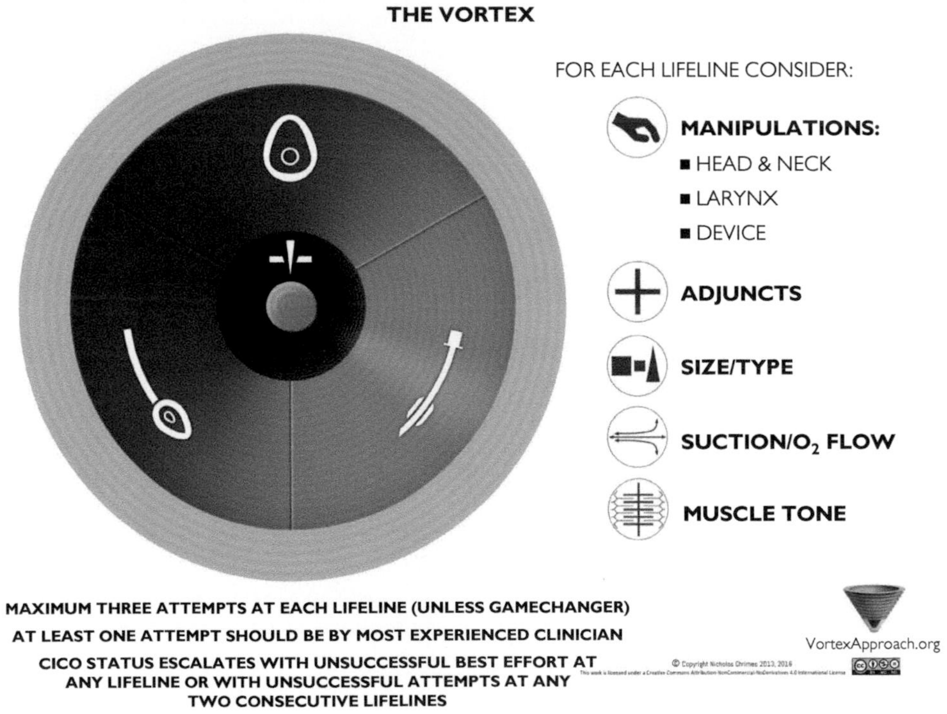

THE VORTEX

FOR EACH LIFELINE CONSIDER:

MANIPULATIONS:
- HEAD & NECK
- LARYNX
- DEVICE

ADJUNCTS

SIZE/TYPE

SUCTION/O$_2$ FLOW

MUSCLE TONE

MAXIMUM THREE ATTEMPTS AT EACH LIFELINE (UNLESS GAMECHANGER)
AT LEAST ONE ATTEMPT SHOULD BE BY MOST EXPERIENCED CLINICIAN
CICO STATUS ESCALATES WITH UNSUCCESSFUL BEST EFFORT AT
ANY LIFELINE OR WITH UNSUCCESSFUL ATTEMPTS AT ANY
TWO CONSECUTIVE LIFELINES

VortexApproach.org

© Copyright Nicholas Chrimes 2013, 2016
This work is licensed under a Creative Commons Attribution-NonCommercial-NoDerivatives 4.0 International License

Figure 32.2 The Vortex Cognitive Aid is an example of a cognitive aid to assist with emergency airway management. With permission from Dr. Nicholas Chrimes.

DELAYED EMERGENCE

By Stanford Anesthesia Cognitive Aid Group

CHECK

1. Confirm that all anesthetic agents (inhalation/IV) are **OFF**.

2. Check for residual muscular paralysis (if patient is asleep, use twitch monitor), and reverse accordingly.

CONSIDER

Consider:

1. Opioid reversal: start with **naloxone** 40 μg IV; repeat every 2 minutes, increasing up to 400 μg.

2. Benzodiazepine reversal: start with **flumazenil** 0.2 mg IV every 1 minute; max dose = 1 mg.

3. Scopolomine reversal (e.g. Patch): **Physostigmine** 1 mg IV (Potential cholinergic crisis, including severe bradycardia, so have atropine ready).

CHECK

1. Monitors: Check **Hypoxemia**? **Hypercarbia**? **Hypothermia**?

2. Complete **Neuro exam**, as able, for focal neurologic deficits (if intubated look for: pupils, asymmetric movement, gagging, etc.)

   If abnormal exam or **suspect stroke**, obtain **stat Head CT scan** and consult neurology/neurosurgery.

3. **Hypoglycemia**: check glucose (glucometer).

4. Labs: **ABG plus electrolytes**. Rule out CO_2 narcosis from Hypercarbia, Hypo- or Hypernatremia.

5. Check for **medication swap** or dosing error.

TREATMENT

1. Correct any abnormalities in oxygenation, ventilation, laboratory values, or temperature.

2. If residual mental status abnormalities, monitor the patient in the ICU with **neurological follow up**, including serial exams. Repeat Head CT or MRI as needed.

END

10 DELAYED EMERGENCE

Figure 32.3 The delayed emergence checklist from the Stanford Anesthesia Emergency Anesthesia Manual. Source: http://emergencymanual.stanford.edu https://creativecommons.org/licenses/by-nc-nd/3.0/deed.en_US

!! **Potential Complication**: Cognitive aids that are outdated may have inaccurate information. Ensure that all cognitive aids used for critical events are continuously updated to reflect the state of the art.

> **WARNING!!** Cognitive aids may contain generalized information that is applicable to a broad range of emergencies. Each patient is different. Use clinical judgment to ensure that the correct diagnosis and treatment are used. Electronic checklists that are integrated with a specific patient record may reduce this risk.

> **Caution!** Memory and judgment can be impaired during periods of high workload. Using a cognitive aid may help to ensure that the correct steps are taken to resolve the problem.

In the chaos of an emergency, it is important to set priorities and tackle the most important and lifesaving maneuvers first.

>> **Tip on Technique**: The team leader is ultimately responsible for setting priorities, but team members must speak up if they believe that a different course of action is in the best interest of the patient.

!! **Potential Complication:** If priorities are not identified and set, less urgent steps may be taken before more important ones, resulting in complications or patient harm. Checklists can be useful to set and identify priorities in an emergency.

> **WARNING!!** The only thing worse than no plan is two different plans.

5. Distribute the workload.

Distributing the workload allows several tasks to be performed simultaneously or in quick succession. It also allows all team members to have a role and reduces risk of cognitive overload.[4] Having a clear definition of a team leader whose primary role is to distribute the workload and assign tasks is essential. The team leader should make decisions, prioritize tasks, and ensure that essential tasks are completed.

> **WARNING!!** Lack of a clear team leader can cause team members to become confused about their roles, producing an unbalanced distribution of the workload. This can prevent or delay resolution of the emergency.

> **Caution!** The team leader should avoid performing specific tasks or should designate another leader if he or she is the only person that can accomplish a task.

>> **Tip on Technique:** Assigning team members different roles permits each team member to have a different perspective during an emergency, reducing the risk of fixation errors.

6. Communicate effectively and use all available information.

Lack of good communication is one of the most common causes of adverse events and medical errors. Good communication fosters clear team roles and collective decision-making. Close the loop:

- Confirm that the provider received the communication and is performing the requested task.
- The person receiving the instruction should repeat the communication back to confirm it was received.
- Cross and double check: correlate and confirm data and results.
- All team members should be empowered to speak up.

>> **Tip on Technique**: A noisy environment will make communication more difficult. Do not raise your voice unless absolutely necessary. Ask all other personnel to keep conversation to a minimum.

>> **Tip on Technique**: Unnecessary alarms can contribute to noise pollution and will also make it difficult to detect new problems.[5] Acknowledge and silence alarms while the problem is being addressed.

!! **Potential Complication:** Vague statements may not convey the appropriate sense of urgency. As an example, "The patient is in ventricular fibrillation with no pulse. Start CPR now!" is clearer and conveys a higher state of urgency than "That rhythm looks abnormal and I have no pulse. We should probably start CPR now."

>> **Tip on Technique**: Use the SBAR technique for effective communication:[6]

- State the **S**ituation: Example: "Mr. X is having trouble breathing."
- Present the **B**ackground: Example: "He was extubated 2 hours ago and his oxygen saturation is now 82%."
- State the **A**ssessment: Example: "I think we should reintubate him."
- Provide a **R**ecommendation: Example: "I agree. Let's get the equipment and medications ready for intubation."

>> **Tip on Technique**: Another communication technique is CUS[7]:

- I am **C**oncerned.
- I am **U**ncomfortable.
- This is a **S**afety issue!

Each statement indicates an increasing level of attention that the situation requires. For example:

- I am concerned. The blood pressure is low.
- I am uncomfortable. Sustained hypotension in a patient with cerebrovascular disease may cause a stroke.
- This is a safety issue! The patient is now having electrocardiogram (ECG) changes.

7. Reevaluate and reassess the situation.

> As an emergency unfolds and actions are taken, priorities and patient conditions may rapidly change. It is important to regularly reevaluate the patient and the situation.

> >> **Tip on Technique:** Elicit input from all members of the team to obtain different perspectives and avoid fixation errors or situational bias.

> >> **Tip on Technique:** Consider using the "Rule of Three."[8] When treating any problem, consider at least three possible diagnoses. After treating the problem twice and before treating the problem a third time, reconsider the alternative diagnoses.

Other Management Considerations

Simulation and team training exercises can be very useful to increase familiarity with one's environment, including getting to know all the personnel in the working environment. Regular checks to ensure that equipment needed for emergencies is stocked in the correct amounts and in the correct locations can reduce the risk of missing equipment in the emergent setting.

Many published algorithms, cognitive aids, and checklists have been published for use in the operating room. Examples include:

- World Health Organization Surgical Safety Checklist[9]
- American Society for Anesthesiology Difficult Airway Algorithm[10]
- Stanford Cognitive Aid[11]

References

1. https://www.faa.gov/regulations_policies/handbooks_manuals/aviation/media/risk_management_hb_change_1.pdf
2. Gaba D. Crisis resource management and teamwork training in anaesthesia. Brit J Anaesth. 2010;105(1):3–6.
3. Burian BK, Clebone A, Dismukes K, Ruskin KJ. More than a tick box: medical checklist development, design, and use. Anesth Analg. 2018 Jan;126(1):223–232.
4. Hall M, Dieckmann, P. Crisis resource management to improve patient safety. Euroanethesia. 2005. https://www.guysandstthomas.nhs.uk/resources/education-training/sail/reading/crisis-mgt-pt-safety.pdf
5. Ruskin KJ, Hueske-Kraus D. Alarm fatigue: impacts on patient safety. Curr Opin Anaesthesiol. 2015 Dec;28(6):685–690.
6. Bracco D, Videlier E, Ramadori F. Anesthesia crisis resource management. Anesthesiol Rounds. 2009;8(4).
7. Improving Communication and Teamwork in the Surgical Environment Module. Content last reviewed May 2017. Agency for Healthcare Research and Quality, Rockville, MD. https://www.ahrq.gov/professionals/quality-patient-safety/hais/tools/ambulatory-surgery/sections/implementation/training-tools/cus-tool.html
8. Stiegler MP, Ruskin KJ. Decision-making and safety in anesthesiology. Curr Opin Anaesthesiol. 2012 Dec;25(6):724–729.
9. https://www.who.int/patientsafety/safesurgery/checklist/en/
10. Apfelbaum JL, Hagberg CA, Connis RT, Abdelmalak BB, Agarkar M, Dutton RP, Fiadjoe JE, Greif R, Klock Jr PA, Mercier D, Myatra SN. American Society of Anesthesiologists practice guidelines for management of the difficult airway. Anesthesiology. 2022 Jan; 136(1):31–81.
11. http://emergencymanual.stanford.edu/

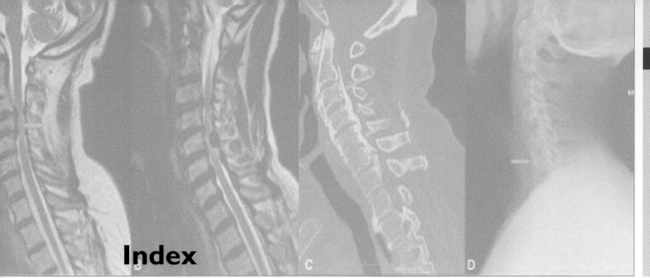

Index

For the benefit of digital users, indexed terms that span two pages (e.g., 52–53) may, on occasion, appear on only one of those pages

Tables, figures, and boxes are indicated by *t*, *f*, and *b* following the page number

accreta/increta/perceta. *See* morbidly adherent placenta
ACE inhibitor, angioedema associated with, 236, 237*f*, 240
acetaminophen
  fever/transfusion reaction-associated, 190
  tonsillar hemorrhage, pediatric patients, 182
  ventilation/intubation weaning, 92
acid-base disorders, arrhythmia-associated, 72
acute coronary syndrome algorithm, 100*f*
acute hemolytic reaction, 164
adenosine
  stable VT/VF, 122
  supraventricular tachycardia, 78
adult cardiac arrest algorithm, 110*f*
Airtraq, 198*f*
airway block, 51*f*, 51
airway fires
  burned material aspiration, 6
  characterization, 4
  complications, 7
  documentation/reporting, 7
  fire triad, 4*f*, 4
  fuel control, 8
  higher risk procedures, 4*b*, 5
  patient desaturation, 6
  postoperative care, 7
  prevention/risk reduction, 4, 6, 8
  procedure, 5*f*, 5–7
  tonsillar hemorrhage, 181
  tracheostomy, 57
airway foreign body
  blind finger sweep, 18

characterization, 16*f*, 16, 23
emergence/extubation, 22
esophageal perforation, 22
glottic opening, 19
history/physical/imaging, 18*f*, 18
inhaled inductions, 20
IV access, 19
lithium disc battery, 22
postoperative care, 23
procedure, 17–23
respiratory failure/hypoxia, 17
ventilation/intubation, 17, 18, 19
ventilation/intubation regimens, 20–21, 22
albuterol
  anaphylactic reactions, 232
  bronchospasm, 13, 38
Amicar (ε-aminocaproic acid), 161
aminophylline, for angioedema-associated bronchospasm, 239
amiodarone
  atrial fibrillation, 81
  long-term oral use complications, 82
  stable VT/VF, 122
  unstable VT/VF, 118
  ventricular premature beats, 82
amniotic fluid embolism
  characterization, 264*f*, 264
  CPR, 266
  diagnosis, 265
  medical agent regimens, 267, 268–69
  perimortem cesarean delivery, 269
  procedure, 265–69
  thromboelastography, 267, 268*f*
  treatment, 265, 268–69

anaphylaxis
    anaphylactoid reactions vs., 233
    bronchospasm, 13
    characterization, 228f, 228
    diagnosis, 229–30, 233
    epinephrine, 231, 232, 232t
    histamine levels collection, 233
    medical agent regimens, 231, 232–33
    procedure, 229–33
    serum tryptase collection, 233
    severity grades, 230, 230t
    signs/symptoms, 229t
    supraglottic airway, 231
anesthesia machine failures
    backup oxygen cylinders, 301, 302f
    breathing circuit obstruction, 297–98
    characterization, 295
    circuit leak check, 297
    electrical power failure, 304
    hypoxic oxygen pipeline mixture, 302–3,
        305
    low breathing circuit pressure, 295–97, 296f
    management, 295
    mechanical/electronic gauges, 299f
    oxygen cylinder, opening, 300f
    oxygen pipeline failure, 299f, 299–301, 300f,
        301f, 302f, 305
    time remaining calculation, 300–1, 301f
    ventilator problem exclusion, 297
angiocatheters complications, 127
angioedema
    ACE inhibitor-induced, 236, 237f, 240
    anaphylaxis-associated, 228, 229t, 230t, 231,
        238
    bronchospasm, 239
    characterization, 236
    diagnosis, 236–38, 237f
    hereditary, 236, 238, 239–40
    histamine-mediated, 236
    medical agent regimens, 239–40
    nasotracheal intubation contraindicated, 239
    patient comorbidities, 240
    procedure, 236–40
    transfusion reactions, 188
    treatment, 236
antibiotics, for transfusion reaction, 190
arrhythmias
    atrial fibrillation, 76t, 80–81
    atrial flutter, 76t, 79f, 79–80
    bradyarrhythmias, 72–76
    bronchospasm-associated, 12
    characterization, 72
    emergency craniotomy, 214

    myocardial ischemia/infarction, 98–99
    pacemakers/defibrillators, 82–83
    tachyarrhythmias, 76–82
    ventricular premature beats, 76t, 81–82
aspirin, for myocardial ischemia/infarction, 99
asystole. See PEA/asystole
atrial fibrillation, 76t, 80–81
atrial flutter, 76t, 79f, 79–80
atropine
    airway foreign body/RSI, 20
    amniotic fluid embolism, 268
    arrhythmias, 99
    bradycardia, 73
    high/total spinal anesthesia, 219
    high/total spinal anesthesia bradycardia, 220
    laryngospasm, 30
    spinal cord injury, 197
AV blocks
    first degree, 73t, 74f, 74
    myocardial ischemia/infarction, 99
    permanent pacing of, 83
    procainamide contraindications, 82
    second degree, 73t, 74f, 74–75, 75f, 83
    third degree, 73t, 75f, 75–76, 83
AV fistula, IV placement and, 134

barcode sign, 125
Beck's triad, 86, 88
Berinert, hereditary angioedema, 239
beta agonists, hyperkalemia, 164
beta blockers
    contraindications, 98
    myocardial ischemia/infarction, 98, 99
    sinus tachycardia, 77
    ventricular premature beats, 81
bleeding/intraoperative
    acidosis, 170
    blood product dosages/expected impacts, 175t
    characterization, 168
    coagulation factor deficits, 173f, 174
    hypocalcemia, 170
    hypofibrinogenemia, 173f, 174
    hypovolemia, 170, 174
    maximum allowable blood loss, 169t
    procedure, 168–74, 172f, 173f, 174f
    thrombocytopenia, 173f, 174
    transfusion trigger values, 171–72
    treatment, 168
bleeding/post-tonsillectomy. See tonsillar
        hemorrhage
Bougie, 198f
bradyarrhythmias
    AV block, first degree, 73t, 74f, 74

AV block, second degree, 73t, 74f, 74–75, 75f, 83
AV block, third degree, 73t, 75f, 75–76, 83
sinus bradycardia, 73f, 73–74, 73t
treatment, 72–76
types of, 73t
bradycardia
  bronchospasm, 12
  characterization, 104
  high/total spinal anesthesia, 220
  laryngospasm, 28, 31
  laryngospasm notch pressure application, 30f,
    30
  myocardial ischemia/infarction, 99
  neuraxial anesthesia, 220
  spinal cord injury, 197
breathing circuit obstruction, 297–98
bronchoscope, flexible, 198f
bronchoscopy
  airway fires, 5, 7
  airway foreign body, 19
  tracheostomy and, 61
bronchospasm
  albuterol, 13
  angioedema, 239
  characterization, 10
  IgE mediated, 14
  inability to oxygenate/ventilate regimens, 38
  ipratropium, 13
  patient positioning, 12f, 12
  procedure, 10–13, 11f
  response algorithm, 11f, 27f
  risk reduction, 13
  suctioning, 13
bupivacaine, for cesarean delivery, 277t, 278t
burn assessment, 311
burn center referral criteria, 311

calcium channel blockers, for ventricular premature
    beats, 81
calcium chloride/calcium gluconate
  hyperkalemia, 164
  hypocalcemia, 161, 164
  transfusion reactions, 191
cardiac arrest algorithm, 110f
cardiac tamponade
  causes of, 86, 87t
  characterization, 86
  electrical alternans, 88, 89f
  emergence/extubation, 92
  general anesthesia induction, 91
  hemodynamic compromise, 89f, 89
  hemodynamic stability, fluid bolus regimens, 90
  one-lung ventilation, 91

pericardial effusion causing, 89f, 92f, 92–93, 93f
  pericardiocentesis, 90, 92–93, 93f
  procedure, 87–92, 88f, 89f
  sedation regimens, 91
  signs/symptoms, 88f, 88–89
  subxiphoid drainage, 90
carotid sinus massage, supraventricular
    tachycardia, 78
central line associated bloodstream infections
    (CLABSIs), 141
central venous catheter, multiorifice, 150f, 150–51
central venous line (CVL), 134, 140–44, 141f, 143f,
    197
cesarean delivery/emergency. See also morbidly
    adherent placenta
  algorithm, 275f
  aspiration prophylaxis, 276
  characterization, 274
  epidural agents/discomfort, 279
  epidural assessment, 276–78, 277t
  hydrochloric acid neutralization, 276
  hypotension agent regimens, 279
  induction agents, 280
  intraoperative awareness, 281
  maternal anxiety, 281
  medical agent regimens, 276, 277t, 278t, 279
  neuraxial anesthesia, 278, 278t, 279
  obesity and, 281
  patient positioning, 279f, 279
  procedure, 276–81
  uterine tone agents, 280–81
chloroprocaine, cesarean delivery, 277t
chylothorax, 142
clopidogrel, hemorrhage and, 165
cognitive aids, 318f, 318–20
COPD, tension pneumothorax and, 124
coronary artery disease, sinus tachycardia and, 77
corticosteroids
  amniotic fluid embolism, 268
  anaphylactic reactions, 233
  angioedema, 239
  transfusion reactions, 189
  transfusion reactions/delayed, 190–91
CPR
  amniotic fluid embolism, 266
  PEA/asystole, 106
  unstable VT/VF, 114, 116
  venous air embolism, 151–52
cricothyroid membrane identification, 50f, 50
cricothyrotomy, 56
crisis resource management procedure, 316–22,
    317f, 318f, 319f
CRM procedure, 316–22, 317f, 318f, 319f

cryofibrinogen regimen, 164
CUS technique, 321

Dantrium, 256f, 256–57
DAPT, for myocardial ischemia/infarction, 99
delayed emergence checklist, 319f
desflurane, bronchospasm, 13
dexamethasone
    airway edema, 52
    airway foreign body, 22
    angioedema, 239
    brain relaxation, emergency craniotomy, 213
    bronchospasm, 13
    tonsillar hemorrhage, 181
    transfusion reactions, 189
dexmedetomidine
    airway foreign body, 20, 21
    CMRO$_2$ reducing, emergency craniotomy, 213
    spinal cord injury, 201
diazepam
    emergency craniotomy, 212
    seizures, LAST-associated, 247
difficult airway
    airway foreign body, 20
    awake intubation, 50–51, 51f
    awakening patient, 48
    cart, example, 45f, 46f
    characterization, 44f, 44–45
    complications, 46, 48, 49
    extubation assessment, 52
    inability to oxygenate/ventilate, 37–39
    PEA/asystole, 107
    postoperative care, 52
    procedure, 45f, 45–52
    reattempted intubation, 48–49
    supraglottic airway devices, 44, 45, 47,
        48, 49
    supraglottic airway placement, 47–48
    surgical airway, 46, 47, 48, 49–50, 50f
    tracheostomy, 59, 67–68
    two-person mask ventilation technique, 46–47,
        47f
    ventilation/intubation, 13
diltiazem
    atrial fibrillation, 81
    atrial flutter, 80
    supraventricular tachycardia, 78
diphenhydramine
    anaphylactic reactions, 232
    angioedema, 239
    transfusion reactions, 189
disseminated intravascular coagulation (DIC), 186,
    189, 265, 269

dobutamine
    amniotic fluid embolism, 267
    venous air embolism, 152
dopamine
    transfusion reactions, 189
    unstable VT/VF, 121
double-lumen tubes, 34f, 35–36, 36f
Durant maneuver, 151

Ecallantide, hereditary angioedema, 239
electrical power failure, 304
electrocautery, 57
electrolyte disorders, arrhythmia-associated, 72
emergency cesarean delivery. See cesarean
        delivery/emergency
emergency craniotomy
    arterial line placement indications, 209
    blood pressure/ICP guidelines, 212
    brain relaxation agents, 213
    characterization, 208f, 208
    CMRO$_2$ reducing medications, 213
    complications, 214
    critical medications, 212
    glucose levels, 214
    induction medications, 210
    intranasal probes/nasotracheal tubes
        contraindicated, 214
    patient positioning, 210–11, 211f
    procedure, 209–14
endocrine surgery, arrhythmia and, 72
end-tidal capnography (EtCO$_2$), 150
ephedrine
    bleeding/intraoperative, 171
    cardiac tamponade, 90, 91
    cesarean delivery/hypotension, 279
    high/total spinal anesthesia, 219
    high/total spinal anesthesia hypotension, 220
    morbidly adherent placenta, 287
    spinal cord injury, 197
    unstable VT/VF, 118
epidural hematoma anesthesia procedure, 221–23,
    222f
epinephrine
    ACLS protocol, PEA/asystole, 107
    anaphylactic reactions, 231, 232, 232t
    angioedema, 239
    bleeding/intraoperative, 171
    blood pressure maintenance, 160
    bronchospasm, 38
    cesarean delivery/emergency, 278t
    LAST, 248
    spinal cord injury, 197
    tension pneumothorax, 127

transfusion reactions, 188
   unstable VT/VF, 121
esmolol
   atrial fibrillation, 81
   emergency craniotomy, 210
esophageal perforation, IV access, 19
esophagoscopy, airway foreign body, 19
etomidate
   cardiac tamponade, 91
   CMRO$_2$ reducing, emergency craniotomy, 213
   emergency craniotomy, 210
   spinal cord injury, 201

famotidine, for transfusion reactions, 189
fentanyl
   cardiac tamponade, 91
   cesarean delivery/emergency, 276, 277t, 278t
   cesarean delivery/epidural agents, 279
   CMRO$_2$ reducing, emergency craniotomy, 213
   emergency craniotomy, 210
   spinal cord injury, 201
   tonsillar hemorrhage, pediatric patients, 182
fire extinguisher operation, 310, 313
fire triad, 4f, 4, 308f
flumazenil, to reverse benzodiazepines, 48
foreign bodies. See airway foreign body
furosemide, emergency craniotomy, 213

gastroesophageal reflux disease (GERD), 26
glossopharyngeal nerve block, for SCI, 202f, 202
glucose/dextrose, hyperkalemia, 164
glycopyrrolate
   airway foreign body, 21
   airway foreign body/RSI, 20
   arrhythmias, 99
   bradycardia, 73
   spinal cord injury, 197, 200
Goldenhar syndrome, 182–83
granuloma, foreign bodies and, 16

H2 blockers, transfusion reactions, 189
heart attack. See myocardial ischemia/infarction
Heimlich flutter valve, 128–29, 129f
HELLP syndrome, 223
hemophilia A/B, 165
hemopneumothorax, 129
hemorrhage
   characterization, 158
   conditions predisposing to, 165
   ethical issues in, 165
   fibrinogen levels, 161
   hyperkalemia, 164f, 164
   hypocalcemia, 161, 164

   massive transfusion protocol, 160–61
   postoperative care, 164–65
   procedure, 158–65, 159f, 162f, 163f
   transfusion reactions, 164
hemothorax, 127, 129, 130, 142
heparin, for myocardial ischemia/infarction, 99
hiatal hernia, tension capnothorax and, 127
high/total spinal anesthesia procedure, 218–20
histamine antagonists, for anaphylactic reactions, 232
Horner's syndrome, 130
human fibrinogen concentrate (RiaSTAP) regimen, 164
hydrocortisone
   amniotic fluid embolism, 268
   anaphylactic reactions, 233
   spinal cord injury, 201
hypertonic saline, emergency craniotomy, 212
hypoxic oxygen pipeline mixture, 302–3, 305

ibutilide
   atrial fibrillation, 81
   atrial flutter, 80
Icatibant, hereditary angioedema, 239
IgA deficiency, 188
implantable cardioverter-defibrillator (ICD), 82–83
increta/perceta/accreta. See morbidly adherent placenta
insulin, hyperkalemia, 164
intercostal nerve injury, tube thoracostomy and, 127, 128
intraoperative bleeding. See bleeding/intraoperative
intraosseous (IO) access, 134, 137–40, 138f, 139f
ipratropium, bronchospasm, 13
isoflurane
   airway foreign body, 21
   bronchospasm, 13
   CMRO$_2$ reducing, emergency craniotomy, 213

Jehovah's Witness patients, 165, 286
Johans connector, 150f, 150–51

ketamine
   airway foreign body, 20, 21
   bronchospasm, 38
   cardiac tamponade, 91
   cesarean delivery/epidural agents, 279
   cesarean delivery/induction agents, 280
   spinal cord injury, 201
   tonsillar hemorrhage, 180
ketorolac, amniotic fluid embolism, 268

labetalol, myocardial ischemia/infarction, 98
laryngeal surgery, airway fires and, 5
laryngectomy stoma, tracheostomy *vs.*, 64*f*, 64–66,
    65*f*
laryngoscopy
    contraindications, 65
    tracheostomy, 67
laryngospasm
    airway foreign body, 21
    characterization, 26
    diagnosis, 26
    laryngospasm notch pressure application, 30*f*,
        30
    medical agent regimen, 30–31
    partial/glottic spasm, 26
    patient positioning, 26, 28*f*
    positive pressure ventilation, 26–28
    procedure, 26–31, 28*f*, 29*f*, 30*f*
    recurrence risk management, 31
    response algorithm, 27*f*
laser airway surgery, airway fires and, 8
LAST
    absorption rate, 249
    ASRA checklist, 245*f*
    ASRA Rescue Kit, 246*f*, 249
    characterization, 244
    development of, 249
    lipid emulsion therapy, 246, 248–49
    medical agent regimens, 247, 248
    prevalence by block type, 221
    prevention, 249
    procedure, 221, 244–49
    seizures, 221
    stages of, 221
    treatment, 244–49
latex products, 230, 240
left ventricular assist device (LVAD), 115
levetiracetam, emergency craniotomy, 212
levobupivacaine, for cesarean delivery, 278*t*
lidocaine
    airway foreign body/RSI, 21
    awake intubation, 51
    bronchospasm, 38
    cesarean delivery/emergency, 277*t*, 278*t*
    glossopharyngeal nerve block, 202
    maximum dose without epinephrine, 203
    recurrent laryngeal nerve block, 203
    spinal cord injury, 201
    superior laryngeal nerve block, 203
    toxicity, indications, 82
    ventricular premature beats, 82
lipid emulsion therapy
    amniotic fluid embolism, 268
    LAST, 246, 248–49

local anesthetic systemic toxicity. *See* LAST
lorazepam
    emergency craniotomy, 212
    seizures, LAST-associated, 247
low breathing circuit pressure, 295–97, 296*f*
lung point sign, 125
lymph node dissection, IV placement and, 134

magnesium
    angioedema-associated bronchospasm, 239
    bronchospasm, 38
    unstable VT/VF, 119
malignant hyperthermia
    activated charcoal filters, 258*f*, 258
    characterization, 254
    dantrolene regimen, 256*f*, 256–57, 257*f*
    hyperkalemia, 259
    hypoxic oxygen pipeline mixture, 302–3
    management, 254–55
    MH Hotline, 259
    procedure, 255–59, 258*f*
    team composition, 255
mannitol
    emergency craniotomy, 212
    transfusion reactions, 189
Marfan's syndrome, 124
massive transfusion protocol (MTP), 160–61
mastectomy, IV placement and, 134
maximum allowable blood loss, 169*t*
Medic Alert Registry, 52
meperidine, cesarean delivery, 277*t*, 278*t*
methylene blue, anaphylactic reactions, 231
methylergonovine, uterine tone, 280–81
methylprednisolone
    anaphylactic reactions, 233
    angioedema, 239
    transfusion reactions, 189
metoprolol
    atrial fibrillation, 81
    sinus tachycardia, 77
midazolam
    airway foreign body, 20, 21
    cardiac tamponade, 91
    cesarean delivery/epidural agents, 279
    emergency craniotomy, 212
    high/total spinal anesthesia seizures, 220
    LAST, 221
    seizures, LAST-associated, 247
    spinal cord injury, 202
    tension pneumothorax, 127
morbidly adherent placenta. *See also* cesarean
        delivery/emergency
    characterization, 284
    ethical issues in, 286

hemorrhage/TEG analysis, 286, 287f
medical agent regimens, 285, 287
patient positioning, 288
postoperative pain, 288–89
procedure, 284–88
response team members/roles, 288
morphine, cesarean delivery, 277t, 278t
myasthenia gravis, procainamide contraindications, 82
myocardial ischemia/infarction
acute coronary syndrome algorithm, 100f
arrhythmias, 98–99
characterization, 96
diagnosis, 96–97, 97f
drug regimens, 98, 99
NSTEMI, 96, 97f, 99
patient in preoperative phase, 101
postoperative in recovery room, 101
procedure, 96–101
risk factors, 96
sinus tachycardia-associated, 77
STEMI, 96, 97, 99

naloxone, to reverse opioids, 48
needle thoracostomy, 62
neuraxial anesthesia
bradycardia, 220
cesarean delivery/emergency, 278, 278t, 279
complications, 218
epidural hematoma procedure, 221–23, 222f
hemodynamics support agents, 220
high/total spinal procedure, 218–20
seizure agents, 220
systemic toxicity procedure, 221
neuromuscular-blocking agents, anaphylaxis and, 230
nitric oxide, amniotic fluid embolism, 267
nitroglycerin
contraindications, 98
myocardial ischemia/infarction, 98
nitrous oxide
cesarean delivery/epidural agents, 279
contraindications, 6
venous air embolism, 152
norepinephrine
amniotic fluid embolism, 267
bleeding/intraoperative, 171
blood pressure maintenance, 160
morbidly adherent placenta, 287
spinal cord injury, 197
unstable VT/VF, 121
North American Malignant Hyperthermia Registry, 259

NSAIDs, angioedema associated with, 240

obesity
bronchospasm, 12
cesarean delivery and, 281
difficult airway, 47
laryngospasm and, 26
tonsillar hemorrhage complications, 182–83
tracheostomy and, 56
obstructive sleep apnea (OSA), 26, 47, 182–83
ondansetron
amniotic fluid embolism, 268
high/total spinal anesthesia nausea/vomiting, 220
tonsillar hemorrhage, 181–82
one-lung ventilation
bronchial blockers, 35–36, 36f
cardiac tamponade, 91
characterization, 34
converting, 37
difficult intubation, 36–37
double-lumen tubes, 34f, 34, 35–36, 36f
extubation management, 40–41
hemodynamic instability during, 39
inability to oxygenate/ventilate, 37–39
inadequate isolation, 35–36, 36f
single-lumen tubes, 35–36, 37
surgical field/operative lung deflation, 39–40
tube placement difficulties, 35–36, 36f
opioids
cesarean delivery/epidural agents, 276, 277t, 278t, 279
tonsillar hemorrhage, pediatric patients, 182
OR fires
burn assessment, 311
burn center referral criteria, 311
characterization, 308–9
fire extinguisher operation, 310, 313
ignition sources, 308f, 308–9
inhalational burn injury, 311–12
prevention strategies, 309, 312
procedure, 309–12
osteomyelitis, 137
osteopenia, 137
overdrive pacing, stable VT/VF, 122
oxygen contraindications, 6
oxygen pipeline failure, 299f, 299–301, 300f, 301f, 302f, 305

paradoxical air embolism, 148
Parkland fluid resuscitation formula, 312
PASS mnemonic, 310, 313
patent foramen ovale (PFO), 148, 149f

patient positioning
  bronchospasm, 12f, 12
  central venous access, 140
  cesarean delivery/emergency, 279f, 279
  CPR, 106, 114, 151
  emergency craniotomy, 210–11, 211f
  epidural hematoma procedure, 223
  infants/children, 12
  laryngospasm, 26, 28f
  left lateral decubitus, 151
  morbidly adherent placenta, 288
  sitting position craniotomy, 152, 153f
  spinal cord injury, 197
  tonsillar hemorrhage, 179, 182
  tube thoracostomy, 128f, 128
PEA/asystole
  ACLS protocol agents, 107
  adult cardiac arrest algorithm, 110f
  causes of, 104, 109
  characterization, 104, 105f
  chest compression rate, 106
  compression-to-ventilation ratio, 106
  differential diagnosis, 108–9, 108t
  difficult airway, 107
  $EtCO_2$ values, 106, 108
  management, 104–5
  medication patches, 106
  pacemakers/defibrillators, 106
  pregnancy, 109
  procedure, 105–9
pediatrics
  airway foreign body, 16f, 16
  inhaled inductions, 20
  IV access, 19
  laryngoscopy blade sizing, 180t
  laryngospasm, 31
  laryngospasm/patient positioning, 28f
  respiratory failure/hypoxia, 17
  tonsillar hemorrhage, 179, 180t, 181
  tonsillar hemorrhage complications, 182–83
  tonsillar hemorrhage medical agents, 182
  transfusion ethics, 165
  transfusion reactions, 191
  ventilation/intubation, 18
pentobarbital
  $CMRO_2$ reduction, craniotomy, 213
  craniotomy, 212
perceta/accreta/increta. See morbidly adherent placenta
pericardiocentesis, 90, 92–93, 93f
pericarditis, cardiac tamponade-associated, 86, 88f
peripheral IV access, 134–37, 136f

phenylephrine
  bleeding/intraoperative, 171
  blood pressure maintenance, 160
  cardiac tamponade, 90, 91
  cesarean delivery/hypotension, 279
  contraindications, 98
  high/total spinal anesthesia, 219
  high/total spinal anesthesia hypotension, 220
  inability to oxygenate/ventilate, 38
  morbidly adherent placenta, 287
  myocardial ischemia/infarction, 98
  spinal cord injury, 197
  tension pneumothorax, 127
  venous air embolism, 152
phenytoin, emergency craniotomy, 212
Pierre-Robin sequence, 182–83
placenta accreta/increta/perceta. See morbidly adherent placenta
pneumonia/postobstructive, foreign bodies and, 16
pneumopericardium, cardiac tamponade-associated, 86
pneumothorax. See tension pneumothorax
postdecompression syndrome, 92
prednisolone, transfusion reactions/delayed, 190–91
pregnancy
  amniotic fluid embolism (see amniotic fluid embolism)
  cesarean delivery/emergency (see cesarean delivery/emergency)
  difficult airway, 47
  HELLP syndrome, 223
  PEA/asystole, 109
  placenta accreta/increta/perceta (see morbidly adherent placenta)
  ventilation/intubation in, 285
procainamide
  atrial flutter, 80
  contraindications, 82
  stable VT/VF, 122
  ventricular premature beats, 82
propofol
  airway foreign body, 20, 21
  airway foreign body/RSI, 20
  cesarean delivery/induction agents, 280
  $CMRO_2$ reducing, emergency craniotomy, 213
  emergency craniotomy, 210
  high/total spinal anesthesia seizures, 220
  laryngospasm, 28
  LAST, 221
  malignant hyperthermia, 255
  morbidly adherent placenta, 285
  seizures, LAST-associated, 247
  spinal cord injury, 201

prostacyclin (epoprostenol), amniotic fluid embolism, 267
prostaglandin F2α, uterine tone, 280
prothrombin complex concentrates (PCCs), 163–64
pulseless electrical activity. See PEA/asystole

Queckenstedt maneuver, 151

RACE mnemonic, 309, 313
ranitidine, transfusion reactions, 189
rapid sequence intubation
    airway foreign body, 19, 20–21
    post-tonsillectomy hemorrhage, 178f
    spinal cord injury, 200–1
REACT mnemonic, 313
recombinant factor VIIa (rFVIIa), 163–64
recurrent laryngeal nerve block, for SCI, 203
remifentanil
    airway foreign body, 21
    CMRO$_2$ reducing, emergency craniotomy, 213
    emergency craniotomy, 213
    spinal cord injury, 202
resuscitative endovascular ballooning of the aorta (REBOA), 159f, 159
Revonto, 256f, 256–57
Risk Assessment Matrix Tool, 317f
rocuronium
    cardiac tamponade, 91
    cesarean delivery/induction agents, 280
    difficult airway, 48
    emergency craniotomy, 210
    laryngospasm, 31
    morbidly adherent placenta, 285
    tonsillar hemorrhage, 180
ropivacaine, cesarean delivery, 277t, 278t
rotational thromboelastogram (ROTEM), 161, 162f, 163f, 172f, 172–73, 172t, 173f, 174f
RSI. See rapid sequence intubation
Ruconest, hereditary angioedema, 239
Ryanodex, 257f, 257

salbutamol, bronchospasm, angioedema-associated, 239
SBAR technique, 321
seashore sign, 125f, 125
self-inflating rescue breathing device (SIRB), 295, 296f
sevoflurane
    airway foreign body, 21
    bronchospasm, 13
    CMRO$_2$ reducing, emergency craniotomy, 213
    inhaled inductions, 20

sinus bradycardia, 73f, 73–74, 73t
sinus tachycardia, 76–77, 77f
sitting position craniotomy, 152, 153f
sniffing position, 28f
sodium bicarbonate
    hyperkalemia, 164
    transfusion reactions, 189
sotalol, stable VT/VF, 122
spinal cord injury
    airway equipment, 198f, 198–200
    bradycardia, 197
    characterization, 196
    extubation criteria/ICU, 203–4
    induction medications, 201–2
    manual in-line stabilization, 200f, 200, 204
    medical agents, 197
    nerve blocks, 202f, 202–3
    neurogenic shock, 198
    patient positioning, 197
    procedure, 196–204, 200f
    treatment, 196
Still disease, 86
stylet, lighted, 198f
subcutaneous emphysema, tracheostomy and, 59
succinylcholine
    airway foreign body/RSI, 20
    cardiac tamponade, 91
    cesarean delivery/induction agents, 280
    emergency craniotomy, 210
    high/total spinal anesthesia, 220
    high/total spinal anesthesia seizures, 220
    laryngospasm, 30
    LAST, 221
    morbidly adherent placenta, 285
    spinal cord injury, 201
sufentanil
    cesarean delivery, 276, 277t, 278t
    CMRO$_2$ reducing, craniotomy, 213
sugammadex
    anaphylaxis risk, 231
    difficult airway, 48
    laryngospasm, 31
superior laryngeal nerve block, 51f, 51, 203
supraglottic airway (SGA)
    anaphylactic reactions, 231
    characterization, 198f
    difficult airway, 44, 45, 47, 48, 49
    PEA/asystole, 107
    tracheostomy, 59, 67
supraventricular tachycardia, 76t, 78f, 78–79
SVT. See supraventricular tachycardia

synchronized cardioversion
    atrial fibrillation, 81
    atrial flutter, 80
    contraindications, 80, 81
    myocardial ischemia/infarction, 98
    supraventricular tachycardia, 78
    unstable VT/VF, 119–21
systemic toxicity anesthesia procedure, 221

tachyarrhythmias
    atrial fibrillation, 76t, 80–81
    atrial flutter, 76t, 79f, 79–80
    sinus tachycardia, 76–77, 77f
    supraventricular tachycardia, 76t, 78f, 78–79
    treatment, 76–82
    types of, 76t
    ventricular premature beats, 76t, 81–82
TACO, 164, 189–90, 190t
Takotsubo cardiomyopathy, 214
tension capnothorax, 127
tension pneumothorax
    airway foreign body IV access, 19
    barcode/seashore signs, 125f, 125
    central venous access, 142
    characterization, 124
    complications, 127, 130
    diagnosis, 124
    nitrous oxide and, 124
    procedure, 124–30, 125f, 126f, 128f, 129f
    tracheostomy and, 59, 61, 62
    tracheostomy tube in false track, 60f, 66
terbutaline, for anaphylactic reactions, 232
thrombocytopenia, cancer and, 165
thrombocytopenia, procainamide
        contraindications, 82
thromboelastogram (TEG), 161, 172f, 172–73,
        172t, 173f, 174f
tonsillar hemorrhage
    airway fires, 181
    cricoid pressure issues, 181
    lab testing, 179
    laryngoscopy blade sizing, 180t
    medical agents, 180, 181–82
    patient positioning, 179, 182
    pediatric patients, 179, 180t, 181, 182
    pediatric patients complications, 182–83
    prevalence, 182
    procedure, 178–82
    response algorithm, 178f
tonsillectomy, airway fires and, 5
torsades de pointes, ibutilide-associated, 81
tracheostomy
    accidental decannulation/preexisting
        tracheostomy, 67

airway fires, 57
airway pressure increase/cardiovascular
        collapse, 62–63
    bleeding during dissection, 62–63, 63f, 68
    characterization, 56–57
    contraindications, 56t
    cuff damage management, 58–59
    cuff damage prevention, 57–58, 58f
    cuff pressure/tidal volume loss, 58–59
    difficult airway, 59, 67–68
    in ICU setting, 67–68
    inability to ventilate post-insertion, 59–61,
        60f, 61f
    inability to ventilate via existing tracheostomy,
        66
    laryngectomy stoma vs., 64f, 64–66, 65f
    malposition, 59, 60f, 61f, 61, 62
    positive pressure breaths contraindicated, 59
    preexisting, complications of, 64–67
    stenosis, 68
    tube in false track, 60f, 66
    upper airway patency, 64f, 66
tracheotomy, airway fires and, 5
trach-innominate fistula, 68
TRALI, 164, 189–90, 190t
tranexamic acid
    amniotic fluid embolism, 267
    bleeding/intraoperative, 169
    hyperfibrinolysis prevention, 161
transcutaneous pacing, bradycardia, 74
transfusion reactions
    characterization, 186
    complications, treatment, 191
    delayed, treatment, 190–91
    etiologies, 186t
    hemorrhage, 164
    medical agents, 188, 189
    normal/abnormal responses signs/symptoms,
        187f
    pediatrics, 191
    procedure, 187–91
    transfusion-associated graft-versus-host disease
        (TA-GVHD), 191
    transfusion-transmitted infection (TTI), 191
transient jugular venous compression, 151
transport oxygen cylinder, 295, 296f
trauma
    tonsillar hemorrhage complications, 182–83
    transfusion ethics, 165
traumatic brain injury (TBI), 196, 197, 208,
        210, 214
trisomy 21, 182–83
troponin, 96
two-person mask ventilation technique, 46–47, 47f

upper respiratory tract infection (URI), 26

VAE. *See* venous air embolism
valproate, emergency craniotomy, 212
Valsalva maneuver, supraventricular tachycardia, 78
vascular access
    central venous line (CVL), 134, 140–44, 141*f*,
        143*f*, 197
    complications, 144
    intraosseous (IO), 134, 137–40, 138*f*, 139*f*
    peripheral IV, 134–37, 136*f*
vasopressin
    ACLS protocol, PEA/asystole, 107
    anaphylactic reactions, 231
    bleeding/intraoperative, 171
    blood pressure maintenance, 160
    inability to oxygenate/ventilate, 38
    LAST, 248
    morbidly adherent placenta, 287
    spinal cord injury, 197
    transfusion reactions, 189
    unstable VT/VF, 118
    venous air embolism, 152
vecuronium CMRO$_2$ reduction, 213
venous air embolism
    characterization, 148
    clinical presentation, 151, 152
    diagnostic monitors, 149–51, 150*f*
    gas lethal volume, 152
    nitrous oxide contraindicated, 152
    patient positioning, 151, 152
    procedure, 151–52
    risk by procedure type, 148*t*

    risk factors, 153
    sitting position craniotomy, 152, 153*f*
ventilation/intubation
    airway fires, 6
    airway foreign body, 17, 19
    airway foreign body regimens, 20–21, 22
    bronchospasm, 12, 13
    difficult airway, 13
    one-lung (*see* one-lung ventilation)
    in pregnant women, 285
    suctioning, 13
    tracheostomy (*see* tracheostomy)
    two-person mask ventilation technique, 46–47,
        47*f*
    unstable VT/VF, 116
    weaning, medical regimen, 92
ventricular premature beats, 76*t*, 81–82
ventricular tachycardia/fibrillation
    characterization, 114, 122
    defibrillation sequence, 116, 117*f*
    ECG tracing/pulseless, 115*f*, 119*f*
    PEA *vs.*, 104
    stable, procedure, 121*f*, 121–22
    ultrasound examination, 115
    unstable, procedure, 114–21, 115*f*, 117*f*, 119*f*
    unstable, treatment algorithm, 118*f*
    VADs and, 115
verapamil, supraventricular tachycardia, 78
video laryngoscope, 198*f*
von Willebrand disease, 165
Vortex Cognitive Aid, 44*f*, 318*f*

warfarin, hemorrhage and, 165